3D-Printed Dental Materials

3D-Printed Dental Materials

Guest Editor

Ji-Man Park

MDPI

Basel • Beijing • Wuhan • Barcelona • Belgrade • Novi Sad • Cluj • Manchester

Guest Editor
Ji-Man Park
Department of Prosthodontics
Yonsei University
Seoul
Korea

Editorial Office
MDPI AG
Grosspeteranlage 5
4052 Basel, Switzerland

This is a reprint of the Special Issue, published open access by the journal *Materials* (ISSN 1996-1944), freely accessible at: https://www.mdpi.com/journal/materials/special_issues/3D_printed_dental.

For citation purposes, cite each article independently as indicated on the article page online and as indicated below:

Lastname, A.A.; Lastname, B.B. Article Title. *Journal Name* **Year**, *Volume Number*, Page Range.

ISBN 978-3-7258-7843-7 (Hbk)
ISBN 978-3-7258-7844-4 (PDF)
https://doi.org/10.3390/books978-3-7258-7844-4

Contents

About the Editor vii

Preface ix

Filiberto Mastrangelo, Rossella Battaglia, Dario Natale and Raimondo Quaresima
Three-Dimensional (3D) Stereolithographic Tooth Replicas Accuracy Evaluation: In Vitro Pilot Study for Dental Auto-Transplant Surgical Procedures
Reprinted from: *Materials* **2022**, *15*, 2378, https://doi.org/10.3390/ma15072378 1

Nawal Alharbi, Amal Alharbi and Reham Osman
Stain Susceptibility of 3D-Printed Nanohybrid Composite Restorative Material and the Efficacy of Different Stain Removal Techniques: An In Vitro Study
Reprinted from: *Materials* **2021**, *14*, 5621, https://doi.org/10.3390/ma14195621 12

Soo-Yeon Yoo, Seong-Kyun Kim, Seong-Joo Heo, Jai-Young Koak and Joung-Gyu Kim
Dimensional Accuracy of Dental Models for Three-Unit Prostheses Fabricated by Various 3D Printing Technologies
Reprinted from: *Materials* **2021**, *14*, 1550, https://doi.org/10.3390/ma14061550 23

Wonjoon Moon, Seihwan Kim, Bum-Soon Lim, Young-Seok Park, Ryan Jin-Young Kim and Shin Hye Chung
Dimensional Accuracy Evaluation of Temporary Dental Restorations with Different 3D Printing Systems
Reprinted from: *Materials* **2021**, *14*, 1487, https://doi.org/10.3390/ma14061487 36

Malte Hartmann, Markus Pfaffinger and Jürgen Stampfl
The Role of Solvents in Lithography-Based Ceramic Manufacturing of Lithium Disilicate
Reprinted from: *Materials* **2021**, *14*, 1045, https://doi.org/10.3390/ma14041045 45

Kyung Chul Oh, June-Sung Shim and Ji-Man Park
In Vitro Comparison between Metal Sleeve-Free and Metal Sleeve-Incorporated 3D-Printed Computer-Assisted Implant Surgical Guides
Reprinted from: *Materials* **2021**, *14*, 615, https://doi.org/10.3390/ma14030615 63

Seung-Ho Shin, Jung-Hwa Lim, You-Jung Kang, Jee-Hwan Kim, June-Sung Shim and Jong-Eun Kim
Evaluation of the 3D Printing Accuracy of a Dental Model According to Its Internal Structure and Cross-Arch Plate Design: An In Vitro Study
Reprinted from: *Materials* **2020**, *13*, 5433, https://doi.org/10.3390/ma13235433 73

André Edelmann, Lisa Riedel and Ralf Hellmann
Realization of a Dental Framework by 3D Printing in Material Cobalt-Chromium with Superior Precision and Fitting Accuracy
Reprinted from: *Materials* **2020**, *13*, 5390, https://doi.org/10.3390/ma13235390 85

Ui-Lyong Lee, Jun-Young Lim, Sung-Nam Park, Byoung-Hun Choi, Hyun Kang and Won-Cheul Choi
A Clinical Trial to Evaluate the Efficacy and Safety of 3D Printed Bioceramic Implants for the Reconstruction of Zygomatic Bone Defects
Reprinted from: *Materials* **2020**, *13*, 4515, https://doi.org/10.3390/ma13204515 96

Tamaki Hada, Manabu Kanazawa, Maiko Iwaki, Toshio Arakida, Yumika Soeda, Awutsadaporn Katheng, et al.
Effect of Printing Direction on the Accuracy of 3D-Printed Dentures Using Stereolithography Technology
Reprinted from: *Materials* **2020**, *13*, 3405, https://doi.org/10.3390/ma13153405 . . . . **109**

Shuaishuai Cao, Jonghyeuk Han, Neha Sharma, Bilal Msallem, Wonwoo Jeong, Jeonghyun Son, et al.
In Vitro Mechanical and Biological Properties of 3D Printed Polymer Composite and β-Tricalcium Phosphate Scaffold on Human Dental Pulp Stem Cells
Reprinted from: *Materials* **2020**, *13*, 3057, https://doi.org/10.3390/ma13143057 . . . . **121**

Seong Ryoung Kim, Sam Jang, Kang-Min Ahn and Jee-Ho Lee
Evaluation of Effective Condyle Positioning Assisted by 3D Surgical Guide in Mandibular Reconstruction Using Osteocutaneous Free Flap
Reprinted from: *Materials* **2020**, *13*, 2333, https://doi.org/10.3390/ma13102333 . . . . **135**

Soohyun Bae, Min-Ho Hong, Hyunwoo Lee, Cheong-Hee Lee, Mihee Hong, Jaesik Lee and Du-Hyeong Lee
Reliability of Metal 3D Printing with Respect to the Marginal Fit of Fixed Dental Prostheses: A Systematic Review and Meta-Analysis
Reprinted from: *Materials* **2020**, *13*, 4781, https://doi.org/10.3390/ma13214781 . . . . **146**

Bartłomiej Konieczny, Agata Szczesio-Wlodarczyk, Jerzy Sokolowski and Kinga Bociong
Challenges of Co–Cr Alloy Additive Manufacturing Methods in Dentistry—The Current State of Knowledge (Systematic Review)
Reprinted from: *Materials* **2020**, *13*, 3524, https://doi.org/10.3390/ma13163524 . . . . **160**

About the Editor

Ji-Man Park

Ji-Man Park is a professor in the Department of Prosthodontics at Seoul National University School of Dentistry, Seoul, Republic of Korea. His research focuses on digital dentistry, including the accuracy of intraoral scanners, additive manufacturing of dental materials, digital denture workflows, AI-assisted CAD software, robotic implant surgery, and the standardization of dental CAD/CAM technologies. He has contributed to national and international research collaborations in the field of digital dental medicine and has been actively involved in academic, editorial, and standardization activities related to dental materials, digital workflows, and prosthodontic rehabilitation.

Preface

Additive manufacturing has become an important area of digital dentistry, providing new possibilities for the fabrication of dental models, surgical guides, provisional restorations, dentures, metal frameworks, ceramic restorations, patient-specific implants, and regenerative scaffolds. This Reprint was prepared to gather the contributions published in the Special Issue "3D-Printed Dental Materials" and to present them as a focused collection for readers interested in the scientific and clinical development of dental 3D printing. The included articles reflect the diversity of this field, ranging from material processing and dimensional accuracy to biological response and clinical application. I hope that this Reprint will serve as a useful resource for researchers, clinicians, dental technicians, and manufacturers who are working to translate additive manufacturing technologies into reliable and evidence-based dental care.

Ji-Man Park
Guest Editor

materials

MDPI

Article

Three-Dimensional (3D) Stereolithographic Tooth Replicas Accuracy Evaluation: In Vitro Pilot Study for Dental Auto-Transplant Surgical Procedures

Filiberto Mastrangelo [1,*], Rossella Battaglia [2], Dario Natale [3] and Raimondo Quaresima [4,*]

1 Department of Clinical and Experimental Medicine, University of Foggia, 71100 Foggia, Italy
2 Independent Researcher, 71100 Foggia, Italy; rossellabattaglia1994@gmail.com
3 Independent Researcher, 76125 Trani, Italy; darionatale87@gmail.com
4 Department of Civil Engineering, Architecture and Environment, University of L'Aquila, 67100 L'Aquila, Italy
* Correspondence: filiberto.mastrangelo@unifg.it (F.M.); raimondo.quaresima@univaq.it (R.Q.)

Abstract: After immediate tooth extraction or after alveolar socket healing, tooth transplants are increasingly used for functional restoration of edentulous maxillary areas. Recent studies have shown the periodontal ligament (PDL) viability and the tooth housing time in the adapted neo-alveolus as key factors for transplantation success. During surgical time, 3D stereolithographic replicas are used for fitting test procedures. In this paper, the accuracy of 3D dental replicas, compared with the corresponding natural teeth, is assessed in surgical transplantation. Lamb skulls were selected and submitted to Cone Beam Computer Tomography (CBCT). Scanning information, converted into Standard Digital Imaging and Communications in Medicine (DICOM) and Standard Triangulation Language (STL), was sent to the Volux X-ray Centre for 3D replica printing. After the tooth extractions, all lambs' incisors were measured with a digital caliber and compared with the 3D replicas. Volume and dimensional error values were evaluated. All replicas showed macroscopically smaller volume (45.54%). Root replicas showed higher variations compared with the crown areas, with several unreplicated apical root areas. The cement–enamel junction tooth area was replicated quite faithfully, and the base area relative error showed 9.8% mean value. Even further studies with a larger number of replicas are needed. Data obtained confirmed high volumes of macroscopic discrepancies with several unreproduced apical root sites. The achieved accuracy (90.2%) confirmed that the 3D replicas cannot be used to reduce the surgical time during transplantation predictable procedures.

Keywords: 3D-printed replica; cone beam computer tomography; tooth transplantation; DICOM-STL; accuracy

1. Introduction

The full digital revolution is inducing rapid developments throughout the world of modern dentistry. Integration of digital technologies in surgical treatment has allowed a transition from a two-dimensional to a three-dimensional (3D) clinical approach, and recently, dental clinicians have increased the utilization of digital scanners, cone beam computed tomography, and 3D printers. Digital technology promotes several advantages for practitioners and patients in all common treatments. However, the lack of accuracy and strictness in the stereolithographic model or replicas could lead to the failure of the surgical procedures [1–3].

Oral surgery is also developing techniques and procedures to reduce surgical times, reduce invasiveness and complications, and increase patient compliance and treatment success rates. Currently, dental auto-transplantation can be considered a predictable procedure to replace a missing tooth, and as a valid alternative to modern osseointegrated dental implantology. During the last 15 years, several studies evaluated the viability of the periodontal ligament (PDL) fibers as a key factor in increasing the dental transplant success rate [4,5]. In 2012 Andersson et al., explained how periodontal ligament vitality can prevent failure or ankyloses in the tooth transplant procedures [6]. Therefore, during the fitting procedures, the elapsed time from the tooth extraction and its re-placement into the neo-alveolus prepared site plays a crucial role in preserving the PDL integrity and viability. Another crucial factor is the tooth's anatomical root conformation. Obviously, similar anatomical conformation of the donor element with the extracted tooth reduces the surgical procedure time. However, in the oral cavity, there are no teeth completely equal and several surgical procedures are needed to adapt the maxillary neo-alveolus to the donor root morphology [7]. Conventional dental transplant procedures used the extracted donor tooth as a template to prepare the receiving neo-alveolus site and to verify the dental adaptation, increasing both the extra-alveolar time tooth permanence and risk of failure of the dental transplant procedure [8–10]. In recent years, several authors have promoted the use of 3D stereolithographic tooth replicas as a "fit test", in order to drastically reduce the tooth extra-alveolar time permanence and minimize the graft manipulation [11,12]. Several autotransplantation studies have reported a short extraoral time of the donor tooth resulted in high success and survival rates of 80.0–91.1%, compared with control cases with increased extra-oral time and lower percentages [13]. Nevertheless, several cases revealed limitations of the teeth replicas due to their linear and volume dimensions, if compared with the donor tooth [14].

Therefore, the surgical procedures became more complex and ineffective due to the necessary adaptations without obtaining the expected results [15–18]. A full digital pre-surgical procedure endorses the cone beam computed tomography (CBCT) of the donor tooth to evaluate the dental volumes, the anatomical characteristics and the root configuration. In this way, after data processing, a printed 3D stereolithographic replica can be used to organize the surgical neo-alveolus site preparation and reduce the surgical variables and risks [12,18]. However, several 3D replica cases revealed more linear discrepancies and smaller size dimensions compared with the donor tooth [19,20].

The aim of the present study was to assess, in a lamb animal model, the 3D dental replica's accuracy and the mean error value compared with the corresponding natural mono-radicular extracted tooth.

2. Materials and Methods

In 2019, at the Clinical and Experimental Medicine Department School of Dentistry of Foggia University, five lamb skulls were selected, and cone beam computer tomography (CBCT) was performed. After radiological scanning, eight mono-radicular incisors were used to record linear and volume data. Data scans were then converted in Standard Digital Imaging and Communications in Medicine (DICOM) and Standard Triangulation Language (STL) and sent to the Volux X-ray Centre for 3D replica printing. After radiological procedures, all incisor teeth were gently, surgically extracted. All specimens were analyzed with a precision caliber and compared with the 3D replicas. Volume and dimensional error values were detected.

2.1. Radiological Acquisition and 3D Printing

Cone beam computer tomography (CBCT) technology (NewTom GiANO®, Cefla, Imola, Italy) with a Field of View (FOV) of 11 × 8 cm was used and the scan was displayed using NNT-Viewer software. The files obtained were converted in Digital Imaging and Communications in Medicine (DICOM) and Standard Triangulation Language (STL) format and sent to the Volux X-ray Centre (Santarcangelo di Romagna, Rimini, Italy) for 3D tooth stereolithographic replica printing. After the DICOM file was recorded, a pool of three engineers extrapolated each dental element using special Amira-Fei® Software (Thermo Fisher Scientific—Waltham, MA, USA) and converted it to an STL file (Figure 1).

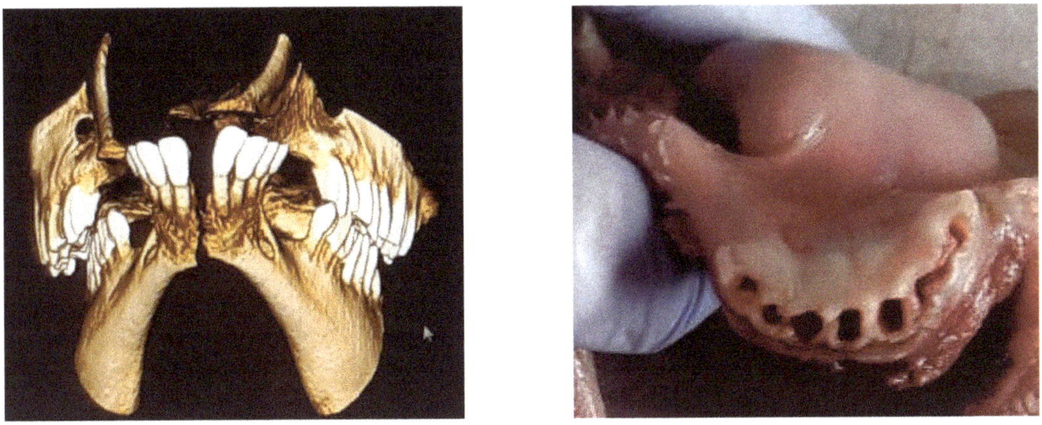

(a) (b)

Figure 1. The tridimensional reconstruction of lamb before: (**a**) teeth extraction in DICOM format and (**b**) clinical view of lamb skull after teeth extraction.

In the digital file reconstruction, the overlapping and the dental anomalous inclination were analyzed, and a single block of teeth connected by the crowns was evaluated. Single crowns and roots were then separated and the portion of the cement–enamel junction was detected. All crowns were digitally cut in a sagittal way at the interproximal level preserving the teeth landmarks. The digital files obtained for all incisors were sent to a stereolithographic printing machine, DWS DIGITALWAX 020D® (professional resin 3D printer from DWS Additive Manufacturing—DWS-020D Aniwaa Pte Ltd., Singapore) and 3D tooth replica models were produced using polymerized fluid resin (Polyamide 6).

Mesio-distal measurements on the midpoint of the mesial face, and buccal-lingual measurements on the midpoint of the distal face, of each tooth replica were carried out with a digital caliber (TACKLIFE DC02— Plainview, NY, USA) and all diameters were evaluated. All distances between the midpoints of the mesial, distal, buccal, and lingual faces and the apex were also measured in triplicate and the arithmetic means was obtained for each replica.

2.2. *Tooth Extraction and Samples Measurement*

Eight dental elements were selected for each lamb skull. After the radiological procedures were carried out, the lamb mono-radicular incisors were gently extracted (Figure 1b) and immersed in 0.5% sodium hypochlorite solution for 1 h. All samples were then gently cleaned and the fibrous periodontal ligament and bone residues were removed. All incisors were stored in a 0.9% weight/volume NaCl physiological solution. Mesio-distal measurements on the midpoint of the mesial face, and buccal-lingual measurements on the midpoint of the distal face, of each tooth were carried out with a digital caliber (TACKLIFE DC02, Plainview, NY, USA) and all diameters were evaluated (Figure 2).

For each tooth all distances between the midpoints of the mesial, distal, buccal and lingual faces and the apex were measured in triplicate and the arithmetic means were calculated. In order to obtain an assimilated geometric model of the natural tooth and replicas, a rhombic-based pyramid model for the root was adopted (Figure 3).

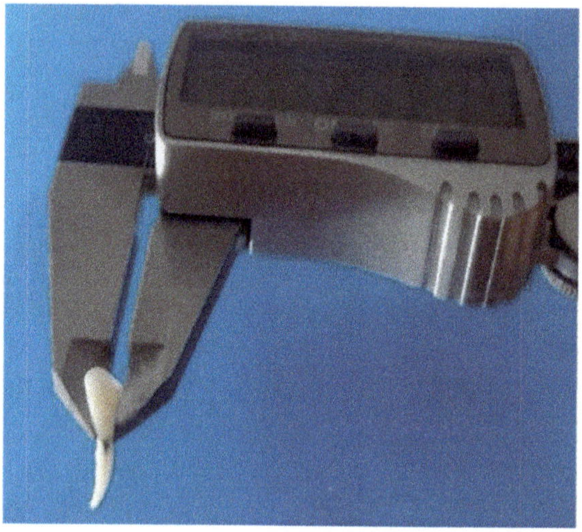

Figure 2. Digital caliber measurements of the mesio-distal and buccal-lingual diameters (hundredths millimeter precision). In the first case the locating branches of the caliber were placed on the midpoint of the mesial face and midpoint of the distal face of the tooth, likewise it was carried out for the measurement of the buccal-lingual diameter.

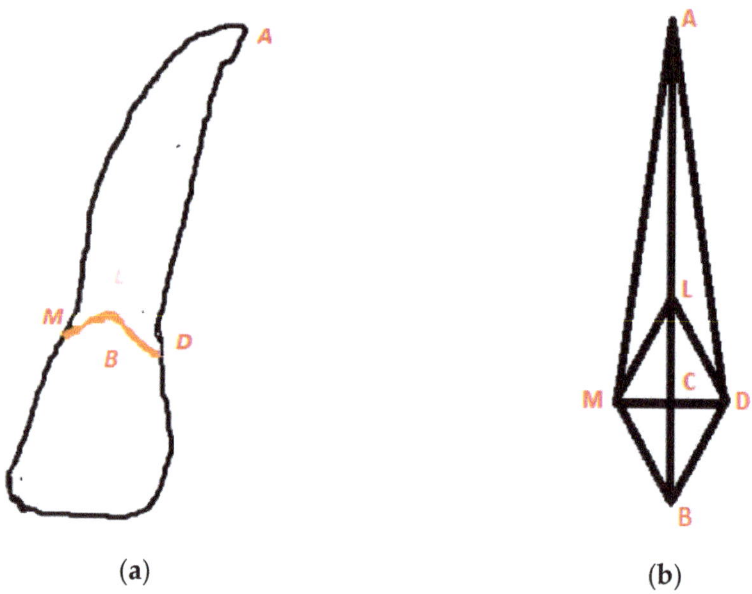

Figure 3. Dental root representation and geometric measurements: (**a**) assimilation to a polyhedric figure with a pyramidal shape as a base (i.e., the crown, delimited by the cement–enamel junction) and (**b**) a rhombus and a vertex that stands for dental apex. Legend: Natural tooth root midpoints: (A) Apex; (M) Mesial; (D) Distal; (B) Buccal. Tooth root replica geometric model: (A) Apex: (MD) Mesial-distal diagonal; (BL) Buccal-lingual diagonal; (C) Intersection point between mesial-distal and buccal-lingual diagonals.

The root volume was calculated as a product of the mesio-distal (MD) and buccal-lingual (BL) diagonals (base area of the rhombus) by the height of the pyramid (*h* coincides with the longitudinal axis of the tooth/replica) as:

$$\mathrm{V} = \frac{1}{3}\,[(MD)(BL)\,h] \tag{1}$$

Distances between four points to the cement–enamel junction (CEJ) and the apex (A), AM (mesial point apex), AD (distal point apex), BA (buccal point apex) and LA (lingual point apex) were evaluated with a digital caliber.

To calculate the height of the pyramid on the buccal-lingual plane, the triangular sections (ACM and ACD triangles) were considered. The height was calculated, according to Pythagoras' theorem, as segment AC, where C is the intersection point of MD and BL diagonals (Figure 3b), as:

$$AC = \sqrt{AM^2 - \frac{1}{2}MD^2} \tag{2}$$

In the same way on the mesio-distal plane the height of the pyramid, taking into account the triangles ACV and ACL (Figure 3b), was calculated as:

$$AC = \sqrt{AV^2 - \frac{1}{2}VL^2} \tag{3}$$

The two heights obtained were mathematically averaged and the value replaced in the formula Equation (1) to calculate the volume.

Linear and volume measurement percentage errors were analyzed between the natural tooth and the replicas using the equation:

$$\text{Linear Er\%} = \frac{\textit{Measurements on natural tooth} - \textit{Measurements on 3D model}}{\textit{Measurements on natural tooth}}\,100 \tag{4}$$

$$\text{Volume Er\%} = \frac{\text{Natural tooth volume} - \text{3D model volume}}{\text{Natural tooth volume}}\,100 \tag{5}$$

3. Results

All 3D replicas appeared smaller than the natural teeth (Figure 4) and showed linear and volume error percentages (Table 1).

The CEJ Mesio/distal and buccal/lingual mean value error were 0.04 and 0.06 with a 4.17 (SD ± 0.0025) and 6.19 (SD ± 0.09) percentage, respectively. The root mean value linear error was higher in all specimens with 0.39 in M/A and D/A, 0.43 in B/A, and 0.40 in L/A measurements. The relative percentage root error was 39.42 (SD ± 0.11) in M/A, 39.22 (SD ± 0.099) in D/A, 43.11 (SD ± 0.09) in B/A, and 39.92 (SD ± 0.087) in L/A. (Table 1) In the CEJ portion, all replicas showed macroscopically good features and a low discrepancy value compared with the natural tooth with 9.8% (SD ± 0.083) error mean value. (Table 2) Relatively shorter root volume was macroscopically evaluated in all replicas compared with the natural tooth, and several apex zones showed high discrepancies and low accuracy grades, with the lack of several features. The replica's volume showed 0.46 mean value error with a 45.54% (SD ± 0.082) (Table 3).

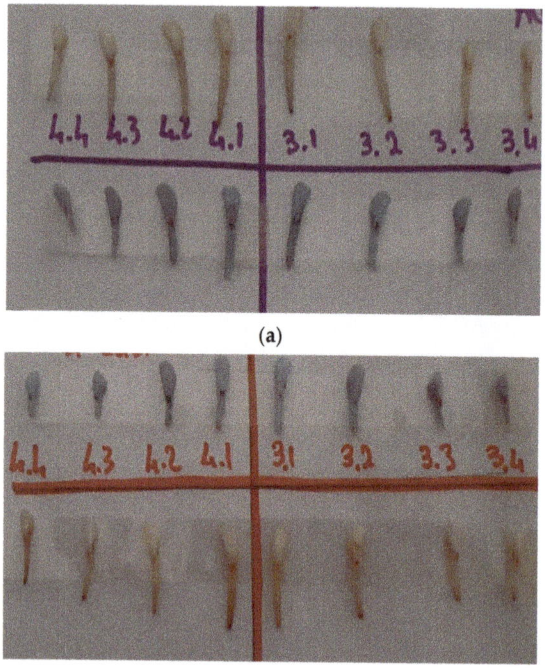

(**a**)

(**b**)

Figure 4. Comparison of natural teeth once extracted and their 3D replicas: (**a**) first lamb skull; (**b**) second lamb skull.

Table 1. Cement–Enamel Junction (CEJ) and Root percentage error evaluation at mesial, distal, buccal, and lingual points in all natural tooth and replica specimens. All measurements were calculated using the aforementioned formula. Legend: a1 = lamb skull 1; a2 = lamb skull 2; M/A = mesial point and apex; D/A = distal point and apex; B/A = buccal point and apex; L/A = lingual point and apex.

Error Percentage (%)						
	CEJ		Root			
Tooth	**Mesio/Distal**	**Vestib/Lingual**	**M/A**	**D/A**	**B/A**	**L/A**
3.1 a1	0.01	0.04	0.29	0.33	0.37	0.35
3.2 a1	0.04	0.02	0.33	0.37	0.53	0.54
3.3 a1	0.04	0.02	0.39	0.39	0.42	0.40
3.3 a1	0.04	0.07	0.42	0.43	0.53	0.42
4.1 a1	0.05	0.09	0.26	0.27	0.23	0.24
4.2 a1	0.03	0.00	0.39	0.35	0.41	0.33
4.3 a1	0.07	0.01	0.59	0.59	0.41	0.39
4.4 a1	0.01	0.02	0.51	0.53	0.53	0.45
3.1 a2	0.06	0.03	0.26	0.26	0.35	0.30
3.2 a2	0.02	0.36	0.29	0.31	0.40	0.37
3.3 a2	0.05	0.07	0.32	0.39	0.39	0.41
3.3 a2	0.06	0.03	0.32	0.30	0.36	0.35
4.1 a2	0.07	0.03	0.29	0.30	0.34	0.31
4.2 a2	0.02	0.00	0.45	0.37	0.50	0.42
4.3 a2	0.01	0.15	0.56	0.51	0.55	0.55
4.4 a2	0.07	0.00	0.53	0.51	0.52	0.52
Average	0.04	0.06	0.39	0.39	0.43	0.40
Error (%)	4.17	6.13	39.42	39.22	43.11	39.92
Stand Dev	0.02	0.09	0.11	0.09	0.09	0.08

Table 2. Percentage error calculated through the ratio between the base area of the natural tooth and the prototype.

Error Percentage (%)	
Tooth Number	**Basic Area**
3.1 a1	0.05
3.2 a1	0.06
3.3 a1	0.05
3.3 a1	0.11
4.1 a1	0.14
4.2 a1	0.04
4.3 a1	0.08
4.4 a1	0.03
3.1 a2	0.09
3.2 a2	0.38
3.3 a2	0.12
3.3 a2	0.09
4.1 a2	0.10
4.2 a2	0.02
4.3 a2	0.14
4.4 a2	0.07
Average	0.098
Error (%)	9.80
Stand Dev	0.083

Table 3. Assessment of the percentage error calculated by evaluating the difference between the volume of the natural tooth and the prototyped tooth. For problems of a technical nature, the top third of the models was reduced and this justified its high error percentage. (see Figure 4).

Error Percentage (%)	
Tooth Number	**Volume**
3.1 a1	0.37
3.2 a1	0.48
3.3 a1	0.44
3.3 a1	0.52
4.1 a1	0.38
4.2 a1	0.40
4.3 a1	0.55
4.4 a1	0.53
3.1 a2	0.36
3.2 a2	0.36
3.3 a2	0.46
3.3 a2	0.39
4.1 a2	0.38
4.2 a2	0.42
4.3 a2	0.62
4.4 a2	0.57
Average	0.46
Error (%)	45.54
Stand Dev	0.082

4. Discussion

In 1956, Hale et al., described autogenous molar transplantation clinical technique [21]. Several manuscripts with descriptions of surgical techniques and clinical case reports of mono-radicular vs. pluri-radicular transplanted teeth have been reported [22]. Compared with dental implants, the tooth transplantations showed important advantages to periodontal ligament and proprioception preservation cheapness, and finally it could be performed in young patients in which an implant could not be performed [23]. The risks described were ankylosis, root resorption, and transplantation failure [22–25]. In literature, two different tooth transplantation surgical techniques were described: In the first, the tooth atraumatic placement was immediately realized into a fresh alveolar socket after the tooth extraction. In the second technique, the surgeon used a surgical burs action to create a new alveolar socket site into the maxillary bone before tooth atraumatical placement [22,23]. In literature, biomaterials and membrane were described, to close the 2/3 mm gap between the transplanted tooth and the receiving bone site [26]. In 2001, Czochrowska et al., after 35 years of surgical procedures, showed a 90–92% success rate in transplanted procedures [27], whereas in 2008, Reich et al., and Jonsson described heterogeneous results during follow-up time observation [22,28]. In 2020, Boschini, L et al., observed an 89.69% success rate in open apex tooth transplants compared with complete formed apex transplants (80%) [29]. The authors hypothesized these differences since, in open apex transplants, pulp stem cells may maintain a higher differentiation rate, whereas after complete apex formation, the transplants could have an endodontic treatment two weeks later in order to reduce pulp and periodontal complications [23]. In 2018, Jakobsen et al., confirmed root formation and the reduction in traumaticity were the crucial factors to obtaining a high tooth transplanted success rate [25], whereas Kafourou et al., in 2017 described the higher diameter of the apex (1–2 mm) with the potential of revascularization and the rate of the tooth eruption in the maxilla as important key points for the success of the procedure [30]. In 2017, Tang et al., in 23 Chinese patients, showed a high success rate related to the shape of the root, which appeared to be preferable when conical and smooth [31]. In 2017, Strabac et al., in a five-year human cohort study, showed better results in the upper arch compared with the lower arch, perhaps due to the reduced thickness of bone [32]. In 2013, Denys et al., and in 2015, Ronchetti et al., showed a higher negative effect rate in multiple-root teeth (81.6%) compared with mono-radicular teeth (33.8%) [33]—perhaps related to the root anatomy—with more trauma induced by extraction procedures [34]. In order to reduce the intra-and extra-oral surgical time of tooth transplantation, maintain the periodontal tissue vitality, reduce the complications, and increase the procedure success rate, several authors have proposed transplanted tooth 3D replicas from CBCT using a surgical template [23,35,36]. In 2016, Verweij et al., and in 2019, Ezeldeen et al., established that this technique could improve the survival rate up to 92% [1,35]. In 1990, Andreasen et al., recommended keeping tooth extra-oral time to less than 18 min during dental surgical transplantation procedures to achieve periodontal healing [24]. However, in 2019, Wu Y affirmed that 3D replica errors may be related to surgical procedures having a longer duration of up to 3.5–4 min [26]. In 2020, Vinci et al., found similar kinds of inaccuracies between DICOM data and stereolithographic models in an implant guided surgery study [37]. Several factors may be responsible for the lack of the replica's accuracy, such as areas of shrinkage, thinness of layers, or even angulation of 3D printing [38,39], as well as the voxel CBCT data conversion in STL and DICOM format [40]. Concerning shrinkage, it must be considered that every crystalline and/or amorphous, fluid or melting material could be used for 3D printing. The results of the present pilot study have shown a significant linear and volume lack of accuracy in all 3D replicas compared with the natural tooth; all 3D replicas have reported high discrepancy and low accuracy grade of the apex zone with lack of details and features. The root mean value of the linear errors was 0.39 in M/A and D/A, 0.43 in B/A, and 0.40 in L/A measurements, whereas the relative percentage root error was 39.42 (SD $\pm$ 0.11) in M/A, 39.22 (SD $\pm$ 0.099) in D/A, 43.11 (SD $\pm$ 0.09) in B/A, and 39.92 (SD $\pm$ 0.087) in L/A. The replica's volume showed 0.46 mean value error with a 45.54% (SD $\pm$ 0.082) overall error. This overall linear and volumetric error, in addition to the complete lack of multiple details and characteristics of the tooth apex area, plays a crucial role during the autotransplant surgical procedures. It is not possible to prepare an adequate area of bone in which to place the donor tooth and maintain the vitality of the cells of the periodontal ligament, which for the clinician is the crucial objective of the surgical procedure.

The factors that contribute to the low accuracy (distortion and shrinkage) of the 3D replica include the resin used [41], the processing parameters [41–43], and object shape [44,45]. The high critical defects macroscopically observed on all the replicas in the root apex zone, as well as the low accuracy grade, seem to be correlated to the resin used and to the digital file reconstruction. Considering that the shrinkage rate of the polyamide polymer used (PA6-Poly(azepan-2-one); poly(hexano-6-lactam)) ranges within 0.5–1.6% [46,47] the main remaining error percentage seem to be ascribed to the accuracy of the complex radiological acquisition (CBCT combined with NNT-Viewer software) and STL conversion procedures.

5. Conclusions

Further studies with a greater number of specimens and a comparison of different software and polymeric materials will be needed to confirm the present pilot study. However, the results confirmed that the 3D replicas from CBCT scans of the jaws were not accurate in linear and volume measurements. Currently, the 3D replicas' high lack of volume accuracy (around 45%) does not indicate their use would contribute to the reduction in surgical times needed to improve the success rate during dental transplant procedures. Indeed, the 3D tooth replicas' high error rates regarding the apical areas are crucial during the tooth placement procedures into the neo-alveolus site. Further information will have to be evaluated for multi-rooted elements in order to verify whether the margin of error of the 3D replicas recorded in this study will remain constant or will be different in the presence of a further variable given by the complex anatomy of the transplanted multi-rooted tooth.

Author Contributions: Conceptualization, F.M., R.B., D.N.; Data curation, R.B., R.Q., F.M.; Investigation, F.M., R.B., R.Q.; Methodology, F.M., R.Q., R.B.; Project administration, F.M., R.Q.; Resources, R.Q., F.M.; Writing—original draft, F.M., R.B., D.N.; Writing—review and editing, F.M., R.Q. All authors have read and agreed to the published version of the manuscript.

Funding: This research received no external funding.

Institutional Review Board Statement: Not applicable.

Informed Consent Statement: Not applicable.

Data Availability Statement: Data presented in this study are available on request from the corresponding author.

Conflicts of Interest: The authors declare no conflict of interest.

Abbreviations

A	Apex
AD	Distal point apex
AM	Mesial point apex
CBCT	Cone Beam Computer Tomography
CEJ	Cement–enamel junction
DICOM	Digital Imaging and Communications in Medicine
FOV	Field of View
LA	Lingual point apex
MD	Mesio-distal
PDL	Periodontal ligament
SD	Standard Deviation
STL	Standard Triangulation Language
BA	Buccal point apex
BL	Buccal lingual

References

1. Verweij, J.P.; Jongkees, F.A.; Moin, D.A.; Wismeijer, D.; Van Merkesteyn, J.P.R. Autotransplantation of teeth using computer-aided rapid prototyping of a three-dimensional replica of the donor tooth: A systematic literature review. *Int. J. Oral Maxillofac. Surg.* **2017**, *46*, 1466–1474. [CrossRef] [PubMed]
2. Tian, Y.; Chen, C.; Xu, X.; Wang, J.; Hou, X.; Li, K.; Lu, X.; Shi, H.; Lee, E.-S.; Jiang, H.B. A Review of 3D Printing in Dentistry: Technologies, Affecting Factors, and Applications. *Scanning* **2021**, *2021*, 9950131. [CrossRef] [PubMed]
3. Park, J.M.; Hong, Y.S.; Park, E.J.; Heo, S.J.; Oh, N. Clinical evaluations of cast gold alloy, machinable zirconia, and semiprecious alloy crowns: A multicenter study. *J. Prosthet. Dent.* **2016**, *115*, 684–691. [CrossRef] [PubMed]
4. Andreasen, J.O.; Paulsen, H.U.; Yu, Z.; Schwartz, O. A long-term study of 370 auto transplanted premolars. Part III. Periodontal healing subsequent to transplantation. *Eur. J. Orthod.* **1990**, *12*, 25–37. [CrossRef] [PubMed]
5. Ahlberg, K.; Bystedt, H.; Eliasson, S.; Odenrick, L. Long-Term Evaluation of Autotransplanted Maxillary Canines with Completed Root Formation. *Acta Odontol. Scand.* **1983**, *41*, 23–31. [CrossRef]
6. Andersson, L.; Andreasen, J.O.; Day, P.; Heithersay, G.; Trope, M.; Di Angelis, A.J.; Kenny, D.J.; Sigurdsson, A.; Bourguignon, C.; Flores, M.T.; et al. International Association of Dental Traumatology guidelines for the management of traumatic dental injuries: 2. Avulsion of permanent teeth. *Dent. Traumatol.* **2020**, *28*, 370–375. [CrossRef]
7. Armstrong, L.; O'Reilly, C.; Ahmed, B. Autotransplantation of third molars: A literature review and preliminary protocols. *Br. Dent. J.* **2020**, *228*, 247–251. [CrossRef]
8. Anssari Moin, D.; Verweij, J.P.; Waars, H.; van Merkesteyn, R.; Wismeijer, D. Accuracy of Computer-Assisted Template-Guided Autotransplantation of Teeth with Custom Three-Dimensional Designed/Printed Surgical Tooling: A Cadaveric Study. *J. Oral Maxillofac. Surg.* **2017**, *75*, 925.e1–925.e7. [CrossRef]
9. Tsukiboshi, M. Autotransplantation of teeth: Requirements for predictable success. *Dent. Traumatol.* **2002**, *18*, 157–180. [CrossRef]
10. Verweij, J.P.; Moin, D.A.; Mensink, G.; Nijkamp, P.; Wismeijer, D.; van Merkesteyn, J.P.R. Autotransplantation of Premolars With a 3-Dimensional Printed Titanium Replica of the Donor Tooth Functioning as a Surgical Guide: Proof of Concept. *J. Oral Maxillofac. Surg.* **2016**, *74*, 1114–1119. [CrossRef]
11. Berry, E.; Brown, J.M.; Connell, M.; Craven, C.M.; Efford, N.D.; Radjenovic, A.; Smith, M.A. Preliminary experience with medical applications of rapid prototyping by selective laser sintering. *Med. Eng. Phys.* **1997**, *19*, 90–96. [CrossRef]
12. Sokolowski, A.A.; Sokolowski, A.A.; Kammerhofer, J.; Madreiter-Sokolowski, C.T.; Payer, M.; Koller, M.; Jakse, N.; Wegscheider, W.A. Accuracy assessment of 3D-printed tooth replicas. *Int. J. Comput. Dent.* **2019**, *22*, 321–329. [CrossRef] [PubMed]
13. Rebong, R.E.; Stewart, K.T.; Utreja, A.; Ghoneima, A.A. Accuracy of three-dimensional dental resin models created by fused deposition modeling, stereolithography, and Polyjet prototype technologies: A comparative study. *Angle Orthod.* **2018**, *88*, 363–369. [CrossRef] [PubMed]
14. Park, J.M.; Jeon, J.; Koak, J.Y.; Kim, S.K.; Heo, S.J. Dimensional accuracy and surface characteristics of 3D-printed dental casts. *J. Prosthet. Dent.* **2020**, *126*, 427–437. [CrossRef]
15. Teixeira, C.S.; Pasternak, B., Jr.; Vansan, L.P.; Sousa-Neto, M.D. Autogenous transplantation of teeth with complete root formation: Two case reports. *J. Endod.* **2006**, *39*, 977–985. [CrossRef]
16. Jang, J.H.; Lee, S.J.; Kim, E. Autotransplantation of Immature Third Molars Using a Computer-aided Rapid Prototyping Model: A Report of 4 Cases. *J. Endod.* **2013**, *39*, 1461–1466. [CrossRef]
17. Lee, S.J.; Kim, E. Minimizing the extra-oral time in autogeneous tooth transplantation: Use of computer-aided rapid prototyping (CARP) as a duplicate model tooth. *Restor. Dent. Endod.* **2012**, *37*, 136–141. [CrossRef]
18. Van der Meer, W.J.; Jansma, J.; Delli, K.; Livas, C. Computer-aided planning and surgical guiding system fabrication in premolar autotransplantation: A 12-month follow up. *Dent. Traumatol.* **2015**, *32*, 336–340. [CrossRef]
19. Chang, P.S.; Parker, T.H.; Patrick, C.W., Jr.; Miller, M.J. The Accuracy of Stereolithography in Planning Craniofacial Bone Replacement. *J. Craniofac. Surg.* **2003**, *14*, 164–170. [CrossRef]
20. Lill, W.; Solar, P.; Ulm, C.; Watzek, G.; Blahout, R.; Matejka, M. Reproducibility of three-dimensional CT-assisted model production in the maxillofacial area. *Br. J. Oral Maxillofac. Surg.* **1992**, *30*, 233–236. [CrossRef]
21. Hale, M.L. Autogenous transplants. *Oral Surg.* **1956**, *9*, 76. [CrossRef]
22. Reich, P.P. Autogenous Transplantation of Maxillary and Mandibular Molars. *J. Oral Maxillofac. Surg.* **2008**, *66*, 2314–2317. [CrossRef] [PubMed]
23. Pecci Lloret, M.P.; Martínez, E.P.; Rodríguez Lozano, F.J.; Pecci Lloret, M.R.; Guerrero Gironés, J.; Riccitiello, F.; Spagnuolo, G. Influencing Factors in Autotransplantation of Teeth with Open Apex: A Review of the Literature. *Appl. Sci.* **2021**, *11*, 4037. [CrossRef]
24. Andreasen, J.O.; Paulsen, H.U.; Yu, Z.; Bayer, T.; Schwartz, O. A long-term study of 370 autotransplanted premolars. Part II. Tooth survival and pulp healing subsequent to transplantation. *Eur. J. Orthod.* **1990**, *12*, 14–24. [CrossRef]
25. Jakobsen, C.; Stokbro, K.; Kier-Swiatecka, E.; Ingerslev, J.; Thorn, J.J. Autotransplantation of premolars: Does surgeon experience matter? *Int. J. Oral Maxillofac. Surg.* **2018**, *47*, 1604–1608. [CrossRef] [PubMed]
26. Wu, Y.; Chen, J.; Xie, F.; Liu, H.; Niu, G.; Zhou, L. Autotransplantation of mature impacted tooth to a fresh molar socket using a 3D replica and guided bone regeneration: Two years retrospective case series. *BMC Oral Health* **2019**, *19*, 248. [CrossRef]
27. Czochrowska, E.M.; Stenvik, A.; Bjercke, B.; Zachrisson, B.U. Outcome of tooth transplantation: Survival and success rates 17–41 years posttreatment. *Am. J. Orthod. Dentofac. Orthop.* **2002**, *121*, 110–119. [CrossRef]

28. Jonsson, T.; Sigurdsson, T.J. Autotransplantation of premolars to premolar sites. A long-term follow-up study of 40 consecutive patients. *Am. J. Orthod. Dentofac. Orthop.* **2004**, *125*, 668–675. [CrossRef]
29. Boschini, L.; Melillo, M.; Berton, F. Long term survival of mature autotransplanted teeth: A retrospective single center analysis. *J. Dent.* **2020**, *98*, 103371. [CrossRef]
30. Kafourou, V.; Tong, H.J.; Day, P.; Houghton, N.; Spencer, R.J.; Duggal, M. Outcomes and prognostic factors that influence the success of tooth autotransplantation in children and adolescents. *Dent. Traumatol.* **2017**, *33*, 393–399. [CrossRef]
31. Tang, H.; Shen, Z.; Hou, M.; Wu, L. Autotransplantation of mature and immature third molars in 23 Chinese patients: A clinical and radiological follow-up study. *BMC Oral Health* **2017**, *17*, 163. [CrossRef]
32. Strbac, G.D.; Giannis, K.; Mittlböck, M.; Fuerst, G.; Zechner, W.; Stavropoulos, A.; Ulm, C. Survival rate of autotransplanted teeth after 5 years—A retrospective cohort study. *J. Cranio Maxillofac. Surg.* **2017**, *45*, 1143–1149. [CrossRef] [PubMed]
33. Denys, D.; Shahbazian, M.; Jacobs, R.; Laenen, A.; Wyatt, J.; Vinckier, F.; Willems, G. Importance of root development in autotransplantations: A retrospective study of 137 teeth with a follow-up period varying from 1 week to 14 years. *Eur. J. Orthod.* **2013**, *35*, 680–688. [CrossRef] [PubMed]
34. Ronchetti, M.F.; Valdec, S.; Pandis, N.; Locher, M.; van Waes, H. A retrospective analysis of factors influencing the success of autotransplanted posterior teeth. *Prog. Orthod.* **2015**, *16*, 42. [CrossRef] [PubMed]
35. Ezeldeen, M.; Wyatt, J.; Al-Rimawi, A.; Coucke, W.; Shaheen, E.; Lambrichts, I.; Willems, G.; Politis, C.; Jacobs, R. Use of CBCT Guidance for Tooth Autotransplantation in Children. *J. Dent. Res.* **2019**, *98*, 406–413. [CrossRef] [PubMed]
36. Kim, E.; Jung, J.Y.; Cha, I.H.; Kum, K.Y.; Lee, S.J. Evaluation of the prognosis and causes of failure in 182 cases of autogenous tooth transplantation. *Oral Surg. Oral Med. Oral Pathol. Oral Radiol. Endodontol.* **2005**, *100*, 112–119. [CrossRef]
37. Vinci, R.; Manacorda, M.; Abundo, R.; Lucchina, A.G.; Scarano, A.; Crocetta, C.; Lo Muzio, L.; Gherlone, E.F.; Mastrangelo, F. Accuracy of Edentulous Computer-Aided Implant Surgery as Compared to Virtual Planning: A Retrospective Multicenter Study. *J. Clin. Med.* **2020**, *9*, 774. [CrossRef]
38. Barker, T.M.; Earwaker, W.J.S.; Lisle, D.A. Accuracy of stereolithographic models of human anatomy. *Australas. Radiol.* **1994**, *38*, 106–111. [CrossRef]
39. Hada, T.; Kanazawa, M.; Iwaki, M.; Arakida, T.; Soeda, Y.; Katheng, A.; Otake, R.; Minakuchi, S. Effect of Printing Direction on the Accuracy of 3D-Printed Dentures Using Stereolithography Technology. *Materials* **2020**, *13*, 3405. [CrossRef]
40. Kim, Y.H.; Jung, B.Y.; Han, S.S.; Woo, C.W. Accuracy evaluation of 3D printed interim prosthesis fabrication using a CBCT scanning based digital model. *PLoS ONE* **2020**, *15*, e0240508. [CrossRef]
41. Ligon, S.C.; Liska, R.; Stampfl, J.; Gurr, M.; Mülhaupt, R. Polymers for 3D Printing and Customized Additive Manufacturing. *Chem. Rev.* **2017**, *117*, 10212–10290. [CrossRef] [PubMed]
42. Gundrati, N.B.; Chakraborty, P.; Zhou, C.; Chung, D.D.L. Effects of printing conditions on the molecular alignment of three-dimensionally printed polymer. *Compos. Part B Eng.* **2018**, *134*, 164–168. [CrossRef]
43. Sood, A.K.; Ohdar, R.K.; Mahapatra, S.S. Improving dimensional accuracy of Fused Deposition Modelling processed part using grey Taguchi method. *Mater. Des.* **2009**, *30*, 4243–4252. [CrossRef]
44. Jiang, K.Y.; Gu, Y.H. Controlling Parameters for Polymer Melting and Extrusion in FDM. *Key Eng. Mater.* **2004**, *259–260*, 667–671. [CrossRef]
45. Thrimurthulu, K.; Pandey, P.M.; Reddy, N.V. Optimum part deposition orientation in fused deposition modeling. *Int. J. Mach. Tools Manuf.* **2004**, *44*, 585–594. [CrossRef]
46. Biron, M. *Material Selection of Thermoplastic. Practical and Advanced Information for Plastic Engineers*; Elsevier: Oxford, UK, 2014; pp. 391–393.
47. National Center for Biotechnology Information. PubChem Substance Record for SID 134996936, 14GUK8I73Z. Available online: https://pubchem.ncbi.nlm.nih.gov/substance/134996936 (accessed on 9 December 2021).

materials

MDPI

Article

Stain Susceptibility of 3D-Printed Nanohybrid Composite Restorative Material and the Efficacy of Different Stain Removal Techniques: An In Vitro Study

Nawal Alharbi [1,*], Amal Alharbi [2] and Reham Osman [3]

[1] Department of Prosthetic Dental Sciences, College of Dentistry, King Saud University, Riyadh 12372, Saudi Arabia
[2] Operative Dentistry, AlNakheel Medical Centre, Riyadh 11564, Saudi Arabia; amalmarshed@gmail.com
[3] Prosthodontics Department, Faculty of Dentistry, Cairo University, Cairo 11311, Egypt; rehambosman@gmail.com
* Correspondence: nalharbi@ksu.edu.sa or nawalmurshed@gmail.com

Abstract: Recent burgeoning development in material science has introduced a 3D-printable, nanohybrid composite resin restorative material. However, its performance has not yet been investigated. This study evaluates the stain susceptibility and efficacy of different stain removal techniques. A total of 120 labial veneers were fabricated using milling ($n = 60$) and SLA 3D-printing ($n = 60$). Based on the immersion media: coffee, tea and artificial saliva, each group was divided into three sub-groups ($n = 20$). Stain susceptibility was evaluated by calculating color difference (ΔE_{00}) at 12 and 24 days using a spectrophotometer against black and white backgrounds. Collected data were analyzed with ANOVA and Tukey's post hoc test ($p < 0.05$). A significant interaction effect was found between the staining mediums and fabrication methods in both black and white backgrounds ($p < 0.001$). 3D-printed restorations showed significantly higher stain susceptibility than milled restorations ($p < 0.001$). Prolonged immersion time increased the color difference in both groups. In-office bleaching was more effective in stain removal in both 3D-printed and milled restoration groups. The susceptibility of the presented novel 3D-printed restorative material to color changes in different immersion mediums was clinically not-acceptable. The clinicians might expect the need to replace the restoration after 1–2 years and thus, recommendation for the use of such a material as a permanent restoration cannot be made but rather as a long-term temporary restoration.

Keywords: 3D-printing; additive manufacturing; SLA; restorations; CAD/CAM

1. Introduction

Rapid advancements of digital tools and biomaterials has resulted in the development of an increased number of diagnostic tools, manufacturing technologies and material alternatives to conventional resin restorative techniques [1–3]. The additive manufacturing technique (AM) is the process of building the object by stacking one layer on top of another until the desired object is completed [4]. Dental restorations, resin dentures, study models and esthetic mock-up have all been successfully fabricated using AM technology, and the technique is not considered novel anymore [4,5]. Recent developments in the field of biomaterials have resulted in the introduction of a novel printed nanohybrid composite resin material that has been recommended for use as a definitive restorative material.

One of the main goals of using either a permanent or a provisional restorative material is to offer the patients an esthetic substitute to lost tooth structure. However, the complex harsh intra-oral environment may affect the physical and mechanical properties of the used restorative material. Color stability of restorative materials is known to be influenced by different types of stains to which the material is exposed, composition and surface roughness of the restorative material, as well as the frequency and duration of exposure time. Frequent exposure to coloring beverages is reported to significantly influence the color stability of the conventional resin restorative materials. Another factor that may be influential on the color stability of any restorative material is the manufacturing technique that is used. The stair-stepping phenomena which is commonly observed with 3D-printing technology, especially on curved surfaces, may be of significant importance when considering the color stability and consequently the esthetics provided by 3D- printed resin materials used for anterior esthetic restorations [4,6]. Furthermore, the post-polymerization procedure employed as a part of the AM technique influences the final structure of the material and hence can have a direct effect on the color stability of the printed material [7].

Recent studies have shown that the color stability of the 3D-printed resin restorative materials is significantly lower when compared to that of the milled CAD/CAM materials [8–10]. On the other hand, water sorption is higher and also differs among the different available printed materials [9]. A novel nano-composite 3D-printed material has been introduced in the market and recommended for use as a definitive long-term restorative material. However, it is of utmost importance that the mechanical and physical properties of such a material be tested to enable evidence-based recommendations and not solely relying on marketing information.

Several methods have been proposed to remove the stains from resin restorative materials [11–14]. In-office bleaching has been shown to be a more conservative method in stain removal when compared to surface polishing. The effectiveness of the bleaching technique on stain removal is dependent on the type of stain and the composition of the used material [14]. Whether the same applies to newly introduced printed resin restorative material or not is yet to be investigated.

Therefore, the aim of this in vitro study was to evaluate stain susceptibility and the color stability of the novel introduced 3D-printed, nanohybrid composite resin, permanent restorative material, and furthermore, to evaluate and compare the efficacy of in-office bleaching and surface polishing techniques on stain removal.

2. Materials and Methods

An incisal-wrap labial veneer of an upper central incisor was digitally designed using 3-Shape Dental System™ CAD solution version 2015. The thickness of the veneer was 1 mm, as measured at the mid-labial surface. The digital design file was exported in a Standard Tessellation Language (STL) format and used to fabricate the test specimens (n = 120) using both milling and 3D-printing techniques. Sixty veneers were 3D-printed using a SLA-printer (DFAB; DWS; Thiene, Italy) with a nano-composite resin material (Shade A2; Irix Max; DWS; Thiene, Italy) [15]. Layer thickness was 0.05 mm and maximum laser speed was 5000 mm/s at a printing angle of 180°, where the layers were stacked along the height of the specimen [6,16]. All specimens were cleaned with 95% ethanol for 1 min and post-processed in an ultraviolet light-curing unit (Dcure; DWS; Thiene, Italy) for 5 min following the manufacturer's instructions. In the milling group, 60 veneers were milled from Cerasmart composite resin material (Cerasmart® shade A2; GC, Tokyo, Japan) using a 5-axis milling machine (Ceramill motion 2; Amann Girrbach, Koblach, Austria). All specimens were visually inspected for manufacturing defects and were subsequently polished using Soflex® discs from medium to superfine (SofLEX; 3M; USA) by one trained examiner (A.A.).

All the specimens in both groups (n = 60 milled and n = 60 3D-printed) were cleaned using distilled water in an ultrasonic cleaner. Specimens in each group were randomly divided into 3 subgroups (n = 20) depending on the immersion medium: artificial saliva (Glandosane®, Helvepharm AG), black tea (Lipton®) and coffee (Arpeggio; Nespresso®; Switzerland). In each subgroup, the specimens were immersed for 12 and 24 days and stored in an incubator at 37 °C. Artificial saliva was used as delivered, tea was prepared by dissolving a tea bag in 100 mL of boiling water and coffee was prepared as an espresso coffee using an Arpeggio coffee capsule.

The immersing mediums were refreshed every week to avoid bacterial or yeast contamination. Figure 1 shows a complete flowchart of the experimental setup.

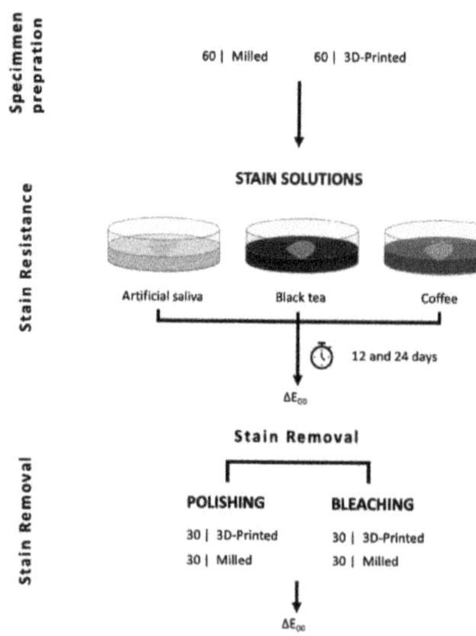

Figure 1. Experiment flowchart.

2.1. Color Measurement

Color stability/stain susceptibility was evaluated by calculating the color difference (ΔE_{00}) using the formula developed by the International Commission on Illumination (CIEDE2000) against both a black and a white background. An average of three measurements was obtained from each specimen at each timepoint using a calibrated spectrophotometer clinical device (VITA Easyshade®V; VITA Zahnfabrik, Germany) [17,18]. All measurements were taken at the mid-labial surface, and the device tip was positioned 3 mm apical to the incisal edge. Measurements were taken at baseline 24 h after specimens' preparation, and at 12 and 24 days after immersion in different staining mediums against black and white backgrounds. The color changes were calculated according to the CIEDE2000 (ΔE_{00}) formula [9,19,20]:

$$\Delta E00 = \sqrt{\left(\frac{\Delta L}{K_L S_L}\right)^2 + \left(\frac{\Delta C}{K_C S_C}\right)^2 + \left(\frac{\Delta H}{K_H S_H}\right)^2 + R_T\left(\frac{\Delta C}{K_C S_C}\right)\left(\frac{\Delta H}{K_H S_H}\right)} \quad (1)$$

Values of ΔE_{00} (perceptibility threshold) ≤ 0.8 denote that the color difference is not perceptible/noticeable by the human eye. Values of $\Delta E_{00} \leq 1.8$ are perceptible but are still clinically acceptable. Values of $\Delta E_{00} \leq 3.6$ are considered moderately unacceptable, $\Delta E_{00} \leq 5.4$ are considered clearly unacceptable and $\Delta E_{00} > 5.4$ are extremely unacceptable [20]. Bleaching effectiveness were considered excellent effectiveness if $\Delta E_{00} > 5.4$, very good effectiveness if $\Delta E_{00} \leq 5.4$, good effectiveness if $\Delta E_{00} \leq 3.6$ and moderately effective if $\Delta E_{00} \leq 1.8$ [20].

2.2. Stain Removal

The stained specimens in each immersion subgroup were randomly divided to receive either of two surface treatments: in-office bleaching group (n = 30) or surface polishing (n = 30). The in-office bleaching was performed using 40% hydrogen peroxide (Opalescence® Boost PF 40%; Ultradent products, Inc., UT) for one hour [14]. Bleaching coat of ~1 mm thickness was refreshed after 30 min, rinsed with water for 30 s and then was dried with tissue paper. Color changes were measured following the above-described technique. In the polishing group ($n = 30$), the labial surface of the specimens was polished for 60–80 s using a sequenced grit roughness Soflex® disc from medium to superfine (3M, USA) following a previously reported polishing protocol [21].

2.3. Statistical Analysis

The results were analyzed using SPSS statistics (IBM SPSS statistics for MAC, v28; IBM Corp). The data were checked for normality of distribution and equivalence of variance using the Schapiro–Wilk test. Analysis of variance (ANOVA) was used to evaluate the effect of the material and staining medium on the color difference, and the efficacy of stain removal methods was evaluated with Tukey's post hoc test. Statistical significance was set at $p < 0.05$. The null hypothesis was that there is no difference between printed and milled material in susceptibility to stains. The second hypothesis was that there is no difference in efficacy of stain removal between polishing and in-office bleaching techniques.

3. Results

Mean and standard deviation of the color difference values (ΔE_{00}) among different staining mediums are presented in Table 1. Two-way ANOVA revealed a statistically significant interaction between the effect of staining mediums and fabrication methods in both black and white backgrounds, $p < 0.001$ (Table 2). Simple main effects analysis showed that ΔE_{00} was significantly higher in printed restorations compared to milled restorations in all test mediums in both black and white backgrounds ($p < 0.001$). Color changes observed after immersion in coffee and tea staining mediums were clinically unacceptable (Figure 2).

Table 1. Mean (SD) of ΔE_{00} of 3D-printed and milled specimens after immersion in artificial saliva, tea and coffee for 12 and 24 days.

		Mean ΔE_{00} (±SD)			
	Time	**Immersion 12 Days**		**Immersion 24 Days**	
Fabrication	**Background / Stain**	**Black**	**White**	**Black**	**White**
3D-Printing	Artificial saliva	0.64 (±26)	0.63 (±0.26)	1.15 (±0.26)	1.34 (±0.25)
	Tea	9.61 (±0.68)	9.36 (±0.84)	14.83 (±0.84)	14.79 (±1.07)
	Coffee	19.65 (±1.35)	19.66 (±1.11)	32.47 (±1.29)	32.68 (±1.51)
	Total	9.97 (±7.88)	9.88 (±7.88)	16.15 (±12.96)	16.27 (±12.99)
Milling	Artificial saliva	1.43 (±0.33)	1.53 (±0.34)	1.41 (±0.71)	1.48 (±0.74)
	Tea	3.83 (±1.33)	3.85 (±1.27)	7.80 (±1.78)	7.61 (±1.89)
	Coffee	3.95 (±1.02)	3.62 (±0.73)	5.42 (±0.71)	5.33 (±0.58)
	Total	3.07 (±0.52)	3.00 (±1.36)	4.88 (±2.90)	4.81 (±2.82)
Total	Artificial saliva	1.03 (±0.5)	1.08 (±0.54)	1.28 (±0.55)	1.41 (±0.55)
	Tea	6.72 (±3.11)	6.60 (±2.99)	11.31 (±3.82)	11.20 (±3.94)
	Coffee	11.80 (±8.04)	11.64 (±8.18)	18.95 (±13.73)	19.01 (±13.89)
	Total	6.52 (±6.63)	6.44 (±6.61)	10.51 (±10.93)	10.54 (±10.99)

Table 2. Results of two-way ANOVA, interaction effect in black and white background for 12 and 24 days.

	Source—Background	Type III Sum of Squares	df	Mean Square	F	Sig
12 days	Fabrication * Stain—Black	1378.51	2	689.25	786.23	<0.001
	Fabrication * Stain—White	1462.95	2	731.48	1022.98	<0.001
24 days	Fabrication * Stain—Black	3998.87	2	1999.44	1809.49	<0.001
	Fabrication * Stain—White	4052.27	2	2026.13	1524.09	<0.001

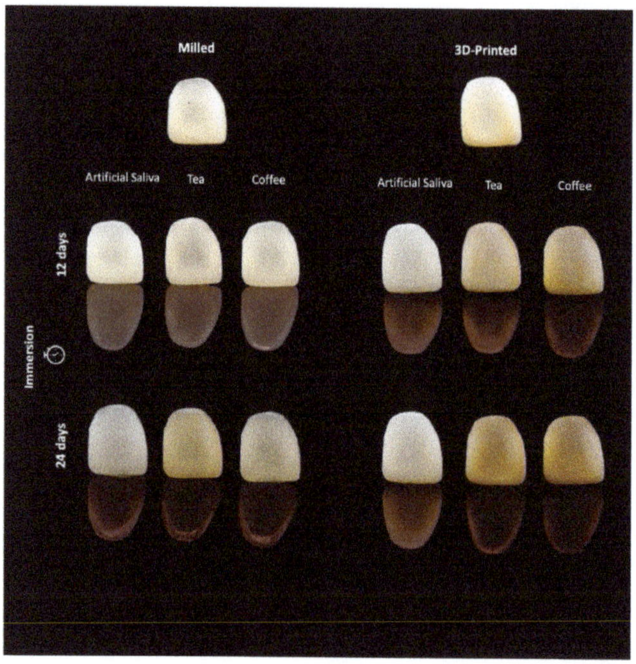

Figure 2. Photograph of ΔE_{00} of stained milled and 3D-printed specimens after 12 and 24 days of immersion in staining mediums.

ANOVA with repeated measurements revealed a significant interaction effect for both fabrication time and staining mediums ($F = 247.73$, $p < 0.001$). Prolonged immersion in tea and coffee for 24 days resulted in significantly higher ΔE_{00} in printed restorations ($p = 0.001$) for both black and white backgrounds. Prolonged immersion in artificial saliva showed no significant difference in ΔE_{00} between milled ($F = 0.01$, $p = 0.938$) and printed restorations ($F = 3.51$, $p = 0.064$). A similar observation was noticed with the white background for milled restorations ($F = 0.41$, $p = 0.839$), whereas for 3D-printed restorations, the values were $F = 7.109$, $p = 0.009$.

The efficacy of in-office bleaching and surface polishing on stain removal is shown in Table 3 and Figure 3. One-way ANOVA revealed a significant interaction effect between fabrication methods, staining mediums and type of treatment ($F = 71.39$, $p < 0.001$). Pairwise comparison revealed that surface polishing resulted in lower ΔE_{00} values compared to the bleaching technique ($F = 189$, $p < 0.001$). Tukey's post hoc test showed no statistically significant difference in ΔE_{00} in coffee-stained milled restorations ($p = 0.443$), and artificial saliva in milled (p = 0.945) and 3D-printed restorations (p = 0.524) between surface polishing and bleaching treatments. Bleaching revealed excellent effectiveness in stain removal for 3D-printed restorative material (ΔE_{00} = 7.87) and good effectiveness with milled material (ΔE_{00} = 3.33) [20]. Figure 4 shows the effect of in-office bleaching in stain removal for both 3D-printed and milled restorations.

Table 3. Mean and SD of ΔE_{00} after subjecting stained specimens to in-office bleaching and surface polishing techniques.

Fabrication	Stain	Treatment	Mean ΔE_{00} (±SD)
3D-Printing	Artificial saliva	Bleaching	1.46 (±0.27)
		Polishing	1.19 (±0.56)
		Total	1.33 (±0.45)
	Tea	Bleaching	8.53 (±0.56)
		Polishing	5.17 (±0.76)
		Total	6.85 (±1.84)
	Coffee	Bleaching	13.67 (±1.10)
		Polishing	4.25 (±1.08)
		Total	8.96 (±4.95)
	Total	Bleaching	7.89 (±5.14)
		Polishing	3.53 (±1.90)
		Total	5.71 (±4.42)
Milling	Artificial saliva	Bleaching	1.60 (±0.65)
		Polishing	1.63 (±0.80)
		Total	1.62 (±0.71)
	Tea	Bleaching	5.37 (±1.79)
		Polishing	3.69 (±1.50)
		Total	4.53 (±1.82)
	Coffee	Bleaching	3.00 (±0.50)
		Polishing	3.33 (±0.74)
		Total	3.17 (±0.64)
	Total	Bleaching	3.33 (±1.93)
		Polishing	2.88 (±1.38)
		Total	3.11 (±1.67)
Total	Artificial saliva	Bleaching	1.53 (±0.49)
		Polishing	1.41 (±0.71)
		Total	1.47 (±0.60)
	Tea	Bleaching	6.95 (±2.07)
		Polishing	4.43 (±1.38)
		Total	5.69 (±2.16)
	Coffee	Bleaching	8.33 (±5.53)
		Polishing	3.79 (±1.02)
		Total	6.06 (±4.55)
	Total	Bleaching	5.61 (±4.48)
		Polishing	3.21 (±1.68)
		Total	4.41 (±3.58)

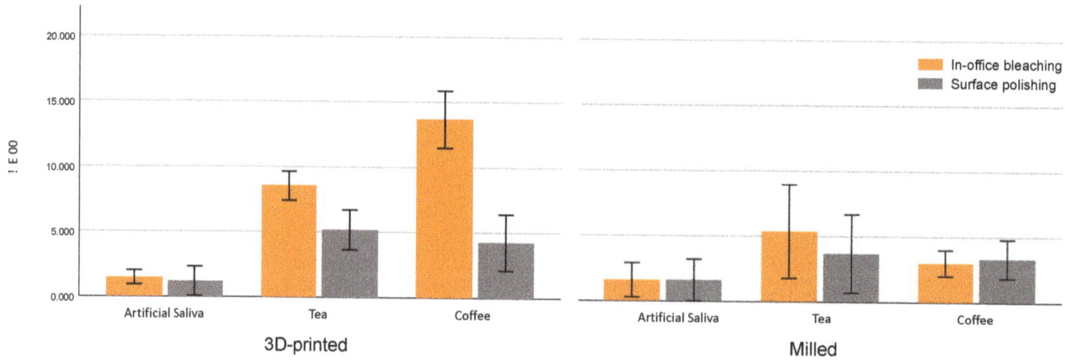

Figure 3. ΔE_{00} of stained milled and 3D-printed specimens after in-office bleaching and polishing techniques after immersion in coffee, tea and artificial saliva.

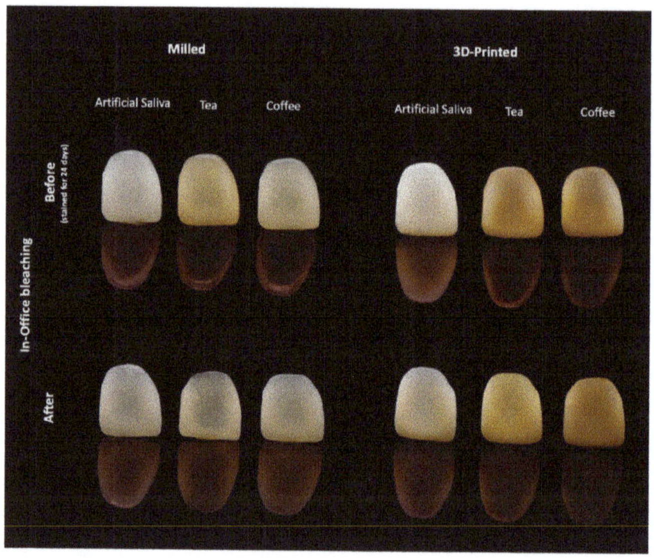

Figure 4. Photograph showing the effect of in-office bleaching in both 3D-printed and milled restoration groups.

4. Discussion

Based on the results of the present in vitro study, the null hypothesis that there would be no difference in color changes of 3D-printed and milled composite restorative material immersed in different staining mediums was rejected. The second hypothesis that there would be no difference between the efficacy of the bleaching and polishing techniques on stain removal was also rejected.

Acknowledging the fact that the color measurement is influenced by the surrounding conditions as well as the geometry and thickness of the tested specimens, the design of a labial veneer restoration was selected for this study to best simulate clinical conditions compared to standard disc-shaped specimens commonly used in other color detection studies [8,9,14,19,22–24]. Furthermore, when the 3D-printing technique is used to fabricate anterior restorations, stair-stepping phenomena is anticipated, especially with the characteristic curved contour of such restorations [3]. This phenomenon will influence surface roughness and subsequently the physical properties of the restoration [6]. All restorations were printed at a 180° build angle, which is shown to offer better dimensional accuracy and less surface roughness [4,6,16].

All measurements were taken against both black and white backgrounds to simulate light reflectance on several clinical conditions, CIV, CV, CII and CI [19,25]. The results revealed that the influence of the background was minimal, and differences in the results between white and black backgrounds after immersion in artificial saliva might be explained by the difference in the translucency of the milled and 3D-printed materials [19] (Tables 1 and 2). Several methods are available and are used to detect color difference in dental restorations, among which, the clinical spectrophotometer is a calibrated and well-established device for quantitative color measurement [17,18]. Color difference was calculated based on the formula CIEDE2000 (ΔE_{00}), which is recommended for better representation of human perceptions of color difference when compared to the CIELAB formula [19,20].

Clinically, dental restorations are expected to be exposed to various staining beverages. The choice of beverages used in this study was based on their frequent use in real life among different cultures, their availability, as well as the fact that their staining ability is widely studied in the literature. All specimens were immersed for 12 and 24 days in staining mediums, time periods which are equivalent to one and two years of intraoral exposure, respectively.

The findings of our study are in agreement with previous studies [23,25,26]. Coffee showed more color difference compared to tea and artificial saliva in the 3D-printed material at both time intervals. Tannin and chlorogenic acid in coffee have been shown to diffuse within the structure of the immersed material and consequently cause its discoloration. Further, the pH of coffee ranges from 4.9 to 5.2, a range of values which has been reported to accelerate the staining capacity of material [12,27,28] (Table 1, Figure 2). In this experiment, all tested materials were immersed in coffee and tea, and showed ΔE_{00} values higher than the acceptability threshold, which is reported to be $\Delta E_{00} \leq 1.8$ in the literature [20]. Therefore, the color changes which were observed in this study for both material groups upon immersion in tea and coffee are considered clinically unacceptable for permanent long-term use, and restoration replacement may be required after a time interval of 1 or 2 years. Patients who do not consume tea or coffee might still experience changes in the color of their restorations, as revealed by color changes of materials upon immersion in saliva, however the range of color change is considered to be clinically acceptable.

In accordance with previous studies on temporary printed restorative materials [8,9,29], the results of the current in vitro experiment revealed that the tested 3D-printed material exhibited higher stain susceptibility compared to the milled material ($p < 001$). Higher stain susceptibility of 3D-printed material may be attributed to the manufacturing technique, which results in multiple layers one stacked on top of the other. Possible incomplete polymerization at the layer interface and presence of microporosities and residual monomers can definitely contribute to increased discoloration potential of printed materials [9].

CAD/CAM blocks used for milled restorations are industrially polymerized at high pressure and temperature to optimize the polymerization process, which results in a more compact structure with improved mechanical and physical properties. The resin matrix composition in the tested milled CAD/CAM material is urethane dimethacrylate (UDMA), and this can explain the higher color stability observed in this group when compared to the 3D-printed material (Figure 2, Table 1). Though no information was provided or available regarding the material composition in 3D-printed material, we can speculate that the resin matrix of material is composed of BIS-GMA. BIS-GMA exhibits low viscosity, a quality which is needed for printable materials using any of the available vat photo-polymerized AM technologies to facilitate the manufacturing process and the flow of the material through the nozzle of the printer without any clogging during the printing process. It is thus of great importance that parallel to and in line with burgeoning advancements in the field of biomaterials, basic information about the novel marketed materials should be provided to enable better evidence-based decisions by the dental practitioners. Furthermore, improving the material structure and filler content are factors that are yet to be evaluated and tested by the manufacturer in close collaboration with clinical research centers to improve the physical and mechanical properties of the newly introduced 3D-printed materials.

The difference in color stability between the tested materials can also be related to the difference in the materials' composition and the microstructure of the resin material involving the type of resin matrix and the filler content of the material. Susceptibility to color change may result from sorption of the stains into the organic matrix. The bisphenol A glycol dimethacrylate (BIS-GMA) matrix is known to have a high water-absorption rate. On the other hand, absence of the hydroxyl side group in urethane dimethacrylate (UDMA) results in a less hydrophilic, more viscous matrix, which results in increased color stability of the milled material and is widely used in hybrid composite resin restorative materials [30,31]. The mechanism of coffee staining depends on the adsorption and sorption of the staining medium within the organic matrix of the material. Thus, the higher susceptibility of milled restoration with UDMA matrix to tea stains can be explained by the fact that the tea is adsorbed to the surface whereas coffee is not able to diffuse to the matrix, hence the increased susceptibility to color changes with tea, whereas coffee resulted in more staining and color change of the printed restorative material, probably owing to the BIS-GMA matrix content of the material. However, such an explanation could not be critically ascertained as the exact filler and matrix content of novel 3D-printed material was not disclosed by the manufacturer.

Oxidation of unreacted residual monomers in the matrix is another factor that may contribute to color changes of material, even without subjecting the material to colorant stains. Polymerization rate and the post-polymerization process have been reported to influence the accuracy of the printed parts [7]. This highlights the importance of proper execution of the post-processing step of any printed restorative material as per manufacturers' recommendations to prolong the survival of restorative material.

Various methods are employed to remove the stains from teeth and dental restorative materials [13, 25,27,32]. Bleaching is shown to be a more conservative and effective method to remove the stains [14]. The peroxide in the bleaching agent will decompose into free radicals that will diffuse into the material and breakdown the pigmentation molecule, and therefore remove or decrease stains [12,32]. On the other hand, surface polishing is based on surface abrasion of the treated surface of the material [22]. The results of the current study showed that in-office bleaching was more effective in both material groups in stain removal than surface polishing ($\Delta E_{00} > 1.8$), which may indicate that the stain was incorporated in the matrix and not only adsorbed on the surface of the specimens (Figures 3 and 4).

The current study is the first to test the stain susceptibility/color stability and efficacy of stain removal techniques in permanent 3D-printed resin material. Though this is an in vitro experimental design, the results provide clinicians with valuable information on the material response to stained beverages. The limitations of the presented in vitro study are associated with the limited number of available materials with similar composition for additional comparisons. Only coffee and tea staining mediums were selected due to their popularity. Whether the materials need replacement after 1–2 years needs to be verified clinically. The lack of detailed information about the composition of the presented material limits our conclusion of the study. Further research should explore the effect of different printing techniques, various materials with different compositions and staining mediums on the color stability of novel introduced 3D-printed materials. The exact degree of conversion of the printed material is still to be explored in future studies, as well as the influence of post-polymerization procedures.

5. Conclusions

The color changes of the presented novel 3D-printed restorative material were very high, and thus at present, with the current composition, recommendation for the use of the material as a permanent restoration cannot be made. The color changes in both milled and 3D-printed material indicate the need for replacement of the material after 1–2 years, and accordingly, the material can be recommended for use as a long-term temporary restoration. The efficacy of stain removal was higher with an in-office bleaching technique compared to surface polishing.

Author Contributions: Conceptualization, N.A. and R.O.; methodology, N.A., R.O. and A.A; writing—original draft preparation, N.A., A.A and O.R; writing—review and editing, N.A., A.A., and O.R; funding acquisition, N.A. All authors have read and agreed to the published version of the manuscript.

Funding: The authors extend their appreciation to the Deputyship for Research & Innovation, "Ministry of Education" in Saudi Arabia for funding this research work through the project number IFKSURG-2020-130.

Institutional Review Board Statement: Not applicable.

Informed Consent Statement: Not applicable.

Data Availability Statement: Data sharing is not applicable for this article.

Acknowledgments: The authors would like to thank DWS for providing the 3D-printed material and Stefano Ardu, Faris Alhabbad for their technical support.

Conflicts of Interest: The authors declare no conflict of interest.

References

1. Van Noort, R. The future of dental devices is digital. *Dent. Mater.* **2012**, *28*, 3–12. [CrossRef] [PubMed]
2. Abduo, J.; Lyons, K.; Bennamoun, M. Trends in computer-aided manufacturing in prosthodontics: A review of the available streams. *Int. J. Dent.* **2014**, *2014*, 783948. [CrossRef]
3. Branco, A.C.; Silva, R.; Santos, T.; Jorge, H.; Rodrigues, A.; Fernandes, R.; Bandarra, S.; Barahona, I.; Matos, A.; Lorenz, K.; et al. Suitability of 3D printed pieces of nanocrystalline zirconia for dental applications. *Dent. Mater.* **2020**, *36*, 442–455. [CrossRef] [PubMed]
4. Alharbi, N.; Wismeijer, D.; Osman, R.B. Additive Manufacturing Techniques in Prosthodontics: Where Do We Currently Stand? A Critical Review. *Int. J. Prosthodont.* **2017**, *30*, 474–484. [CrossRef] [PubMed]
5. Al Mortadi, N.; Eggbeer, D.; Lewis, J.; Williams, R.J. CAD/CAM/AM applications in the manufacture of dental appliances. *Am. J. Orthod. Dentofac. Orthop.* **2012**, *142*, 727–733. [CrossRef]
6. Alharbi, N.; Osman, R. Does build angle have an influence on surface roughness of anterior 3D-printed restorations? An in-vitro study. *Int. J. Prosthodont.* **2021**, *34*, 505–510. [CrossRef] [PubMed]
7. Mostafavi, D.; Methani, M.; Piedra-Cascón, W.; Zandinejad, A.; Att, W.; Revilla-León, M. Influence of the polymerization post-processing procedures on the accuracy of additively manufactured dental model material. *Int. J. Prosthodont.* **2021**. [CrossRef]
8. Kim, J.-E.; Choi, W.-H.; Lee, D.; Shin, Y.; Park, S.-H.; Roh, B.-D.; Kim, D. Color and Translucency Stability of Three-Dimensional Printable Dental Materials for Crown and Bridge Restorations. *Materials* **2021**, *14*, 650. [CrossRef]
9. Shin, J.-W.; Kim, J.-E.; Choi, Y.-J.; Shin, S.-H.; Nam, N.-E.; Shim, J.-S.; Lee, K.-W. Evaluation of the color stability of 3D-printed crown and bridge materials against various sources of discoloration: An in vitro study. *Materials* **2020**, *13*, 5359. [CrossRef]
10. Almejrad, L.; Yang, C.; Morton, D.; Lin, W. The Effects of Beverages and Surface Treatments on the Color Stability of 3D-Printed Interim Restorations. *J. Prosthodont.* **2021**. [CrossRef]
11. Fernandes, B.M.; Tanaka, M.H.; De Oliveira, A.L.B.M.; Scatolin, R.S. Color stability of dental enamel bleached with violet LED associated with or without low concentration peroxide gels. *Photodiagn. Photodyn. Ther.* **2021**, *33*, 102101. [CrossRef]
12. Al-Angari, S.S.; Eckert, G.J.; Sabrah, A.H. Color stability, Roughness, and Microhardness of Enamel and Composites Submitted to Staining/Bleaching Cycles. *Saudi Dent. J.* **2021**, *33*, 215–221. [CrossRef]
13. Sinjari, B.; D'Addazio, G.; Bozzi, M.; Santilli, M.; Traini, T.; Murmura, G.; Caputi, S. SEM Analysis of Enamel Abrasion after Air Polishing Treatment with Erythritol, Glycine and Sodium Bicarbonate. *Coatings* **2019**, *9*, 549. [CrossRef]
14. Alharbi, A.; Ardu, S.; Bortolotto, T.; Krejci, I. In-office bleaching efficacy on stain removal from CAD/CAM and direct resin composite materials. *J. Esthet. Restor. Dent.* **2018**, *30*, 51–58. [CrossRef]
15. DWS. DFAB Performance and Desing. 2019, p. 15. Available online: https://www.dwssystems.com/blog/wp-content/uploads/2019/03/DWS-DFAB_en_low.pdf (accessed on 20 September 2021).
16. Alharbi, N.; Osman, R.B.; Wismeijer, D. Factors Influencing the Dimensional Accuracy of 3D-Printed Full-Coverage Dental Restorations Using Stereolithography Technology. *Int. J. Prosthodont.* **2016**, *29*, 503–510. [CrossRef]
17. Olms, C.; Setz, J.M. The repeatability of digital shade measurement—A clinical study. *Clin. Oral Investig.* **2013**, *17*, 1161–1166. [CrossRef] [PubMed]
18. Dozić, A.; Kleverlaan, C.J.; El-Zohairy, A.; Feilzer, A.J.; Khashayar, G. Performance of five commercially available tooth color-measuring devices. *J. Prosthodont.* **2007**, *16*, 93–100. [CrossRef] [PubMed]
19. Ardu, S.; Duc, O.; Di Bella, E.; Krejci, I.; Daher, R. Color stability of different composite resins after polishing. *Odontology* **2018**, *106*, 328–333. [CrossRef] [PubMed]
20. Paravina, R.D.; Pérez, M.M.; Ghinea, R. Acceptability and perceptibility thresholds in dentistry: A comprehensive review of clinical and research applications. *J. Esthet. Restor. Dent.* **2019**, *31*, 103–112. [CrossRef]
21. Jang, J.-H.; Kim, H.-Y.; Shin, S.-M.; Lee, C.-O.; Kim, D.; Choi, K.-K.; Kim, S.-Y. Clinical Effectiveness of Different Polishing Systems and Self-Etch Adhesives in Class V Composite Resin Restorations: Two-Year Randomized Controlled Clinical Trial. *Oper. Dent.* **2017**, *42*, 19–29. [CrossRef] [PubMed]
22. Al-Nahedh, H.N.; Awliya, W.Y. The effectiveness of four methods for stain removal from direct resin-based composite restorative materials. *Saudi Dent. J.* **2013**, *25*, 61–67. [CrossRef] [PubMed]
23. Peñate, L.; Mercade, M.; Arregui, M.; Roig, M.; Basilio, J.; Cedeño, R. Color Stability of CAD/CAM Interim Material for Long-Term Fixed Dental Prostheses vs. Conventional Materials after Immersion in Different Staining Solutions. *J. Compos. Sci.* **2021**, *5*, 106. [CrossRef]
24. Ardu, S.; Braut, V.; DI Bella, E.; Lefever, D. Influence of background on natural tooth colour coordinates: An in vivo evaluation. *Odontology* **2014**, *102*, 267–271. [CrossRef]
25. Shetty, P.; Purayil, T.-P.; Ginjupalli, K.; Pentapati, K.-C. Effect of polishing technique and immersion in beverages on color stability of nanoceramic composites. *J. Oral Biol. Craniofac. Res.* **2021**, *11*, 53–56. [CrossRef] [PubMed]

26. Sheriff, A.H.; Nasim, I. Effect of different beverages on staining ability of the composite resins. *Drug Invent. Today* **2019**, *12*, 184–188.
27. Alaqeel, S. Effect of Grit-blasting on the Color Stability of Zirconia Ceramics Following Exposure to Beverages. *Cureus* **2020**, *12*, e7170. [CrossRef]
28. Al Amri, M.D.; Labban, N.; Alhijji, S.; Alamri, H.; Iskandar, M.; Platt, J.A. In Vitro Evaluation of Translucency and Color Stability of CAD/CAM Polymer-Infiltrated Ceramic Materials after Accelerated Aging. *J. Prosthodont.* **2021**, *30*, 318–328. [CrossRef]
29. Gruber, S.; Kamnoedboon, P.; Özcan, M.; Srinivasan, M. CAD/CAM Complete denture resins: An in vitro evaluation of color stability. *J. Prosthodont.* **2021**, *30*, 430–439. [CrossRef]
30. Kang, Y.-A.; Lee, H.-A.; Chang, J.; Moon, W.; Chung, S.H.; Lim, B.-S. Color Stability of Dental Reinforced CAD/CAM Hybrid Composite Blocks Compared to Regular Blocks. *Materials* **2020**, *13*, 4722. [CrossRef]
31. Arif, R.; Yilmaz, B.; Johnston, W.M. In vitro color stainability and relative translucency of CAD-CAM restorative materials used for laminate veneers and complete crowns. *J. Prosthet. Dent.* **2019**, *122*, 160–166. [CrossRef]
32. Flaitz, C.M.; Hicks, M.J. Effects of carbamide peroxide whitening agents on enamel surfaces and caries-like lesion formation: An SEM and polarized light microscopic in vitro study. *ASDC J. Dent. Child.* **1996**, *63*, 249–256. [PubMed]

materials

MDPI

Article

Dimensional Accuracy of Dental Models for Three-Unit Prostheses Fabricated by Various 3D Printing Technologies

Soo-Yeon Yoo [1], Seong-Kyun Kim [1,*], Seong-Joo Heo [1], Jai-Young Koak [1] and Joung-Gyu Kim [2]

1 Department of Prosthodontics and Dental Research Institute, Seoul National University Dental Hospital, School of Dentistry, Seoul National University, 101 Daehak-ro, Jongno-gu, Seoul 03080, Korea; sy0502@snu.ac.kr (S.-Y.Y.); 0504heo@snu.ac.kr (S.-J.H.); young21c@snu.ac.kr (J.-Y.K.)
2 Sense Dental Laboratory, 1104, Seoul Soop IT-Valley, 77, Seongsuil-ro, Seongdong-gu, Seoul 04790, Korea; senselab@naver.com
* Correspondence: ksy0617@snu.ac.kr; Tel.: +82-2-2072-3860

Abstract: Previous studies on accuracy of three-dimensional (3D) printed model focused on full arch measurements at few points. The aim of this study was to examine the dimensional accuracy of 3D-printed models which were teeth-prepped for three-unit fixed prostheses, especially at margin and proximal contact areas. The prepped dental model was scanned with a desktop scanner. Using this reference file, test models were fabricated by digital light processing (DLP), Multi-Jet printing (MJP), and stereo-lithography apparatus (SLA) techniques. We calculated the accuracy (trueness and precision) of 3D-printed models on 3D planes, and deviations of each measured points at buccolingual and mesiodistal planes. We also analyzed the surface roughness of resin printed models. For overall 3D analysis, MJP showed significantly higher accuracy (trueness) than DLP and SLA techniques; however, there was not any statistically significant difference on precision. For deviations on margins of molar tooth and distance to proximal contact, MJP showed significantly accurate results; however, for a premolar tooth, there was no significant difference between the groups. 3D color maps of printed models showed contraction buccolingually, and surface roughness of the models fabricated by MJP technique was observed as the lowest. The accuracy of the 3D-printed resin models by DLP, MJP, and SLA techniques showed a clinically acceptable range to use as a working model for manufacturing dental prostheses

Keywords: 3D printing; digital light processing (DLP); multi-jet printing (MJP); stereo-lithography apparatus (SLA); dimensional accuracy

1. Introduction

Digital models can be used to manufacture various dental appliances including fixed prostheses [1]. The impressions made by digital oral scanners enable the three-dimensional (3D) modelling of teeth by a computer and the fabrication of fixed prostheses without conventional working models. It is understood that the fit of fixed prostheses is the most important requirement for its stability and good prognosis. However, this recent development meant that the fit between the abutment and fixed prostheses cannot be determined until a clinician places a restoration in the oral cavity of a patient because it is manufactured only as a digital computer model. Therefore, fabrication of real working models by digital files can be recommended for verifying and correcting ideal fit before delivery.

There are two kinds of new ways to manufacture a dental working model with a scanned digital file; the first is a model fabricated by computer numerical control (CNC) milling machines and the other is by a 3D-printing technique. The previous study showed that the 3D printer could fabricate concave and intricate geometry that is often not achievable by milling [2]. Thus, if resin models are manufactured with oral scanned files by the 3D-printing technique to enhance fit and accuracy of fixed prostheses, the fit of fixed prostheses can be adjusted and confirmed before being delivered. In other words,

3D-printed resin models can be good alternatives to conventional working models in the dental laboratory process.

There are a number of 3D printing technologies—fused filament fabrication (FFF), selective laser sintering (SLS), stereo-lithography apparatus (SLA), digital light processing (DLP), Multi-Jet printing (MJP) technique, and so on. FFF technology was the most common due to relatively inexpensive costs, although the surface was less accurate and blurred rough [3,4]. The SLS method provides design freedom, but the surface created by SLS is rough and material options are limited. SLA and DLP both work with the polymerization of photosensitive resin from the bottom of a tank [1]. The DLP technology works with a plate projector which polymerizes an entire layer, whereas SLA uses a single point laser to polymerize [5]. After the expiry of the patent of SLA technology held by 3D systems (Rock Hill, SC, USA), SLA became one of the most common fabrication methods due to the high resolution, accuracy, clear detail, and smooth surface finish it could produce. DLP techniques have also been extensively used in all kinds of industrial fields. MJP, also known as Multijet (MJ) or PolyJet (PJ), jets photopolymer droplets, and UV light subsequently solidifies the polymer to form a 3D model. MJP is known to be more precise than other 3D-printing techniques, but it is more time consuming and expensive than other fabrication methods [6].

The term 'accuracy' in 3D printing is used when both trueness and precision are achieved, according to ISO 5725-1:1994/Cor 1:1998. The trueness of a measurement method is mentioned when it is possible to conceive of a true value for the property. The need to consider precision arises because tests performed on presumably identical materials under presumably identical circumstances do not, in general, lead to identical results. This is attributed to unavoidable random errors inherent in every measurement procedure. In short, trueness in this study refers to the closest results of the 3D-printed models with the reference model, whereas the precision refers to the closest results under the different replicas by one printing technology [3]. The main outcome for printing accuracy can be shown as the root mean square (RMS) value which is defined as the square root of the mean square (arithmetic mean of the squares of a group of values) between two areas.

The accuracy of a 3D-printed model can be affected by the total errors that occur throughout the overall fabrication process; the model scanning imaging, image segmentation, standard tessellation language (STL) file transition, STL post-processing, slicing of the STL file for 3D printing, 3D printing itself, and post-processing. All these steps are severely dependent on the software, the 3D printer, and after all, the user [7–11]. To reduce errors, digital workflow needed to be simplified, and that was what was done in this present study.

In a previous study that compared the accuracy of intraoral and desktop model scanners, the intraoral scanning method exhibited twice as many 50-µm deviations as the desktop scan method. This may be due to intraoral humidity, patient movement, and limited intraoral spaces [12]. According to Son's study, desktop scanners showed more accurate scanned data than intraoral scanners [13]. Therefore, by using desktop scanner for scanning and producing the STL image file, the comparison of the 3D-printed model itself can be focused on, fabricated by different technologies.

The manual measurements of 3D-printed models are also influenced by the variability of the operator, and there is difficulty in repeatedly selecting the exact landmarks [14]. Although no measurement technique is error-free, computer-aided measurement methods can be beneficial in this case. Through superimposition in computer-aided program with scanned files of 3D-printed resin models and the reference file, errors of measurement can be reduced and the data produced by 3D-printed models can be focused on.

Few studies focused on the 3D-printed models used for fabrication of dental prostheses, such as fixed partial dentures and inlays. These models require higher accuracy than those used for diagnosis or orthodontic uses because the criteria of clinically acceptable marginal discrepancy of fixed prosthesis is only 120 µm [15,16]. Therefore, further studies on the accuracy of digitally-produced models are required. In this study, the aim was to evaluate the differences on the accuracy of 3D-printed models produced by the DLP, MJP, and SLA techniques—which are used for three-unit fixed prosthesis—by comparing RMS values of trueness and precision as well as analyzing marginal deviations and distance to proximal contact on two-dimensional (2D) planes.

2. Materials and Methods

2.1. The Preparation of 3D-Printed Models

In this study, we prepped of molar (#27) with long chamfer margin and premolar (#25) with deep chamfer margin for 3-unit fixed prostheses. This reference model was scanned by industrial 3D scanner (E4 lab scanner, 3Shape, Copenhagen, Denmark) with a resolution of Blue LED and 2 × 5 Mpx, thus, the reference STL file was obtained. The industrial 3D scanner from the manufacturer validated an accuracy of 7 μm according to ISO 12836 [17]. The digital models were replicated 12 times (*n* = 36) using the reference STL file by each of the DLP, MJP, and SLA techniques shown in Figures 1 and 2. The parameters set for the 3D printers in each group are shown in Table 1. Thirty-six 3D-printed models were also scanned with industrial desktop 3D scanner. In previous studies, the surfaces of the DLP, MJP, and SLA casts were lightly dusted with powder to reduce light reflection; however, in the present study, for accuracy of measurements, we used a desktop scanner which does not need a scan spray.

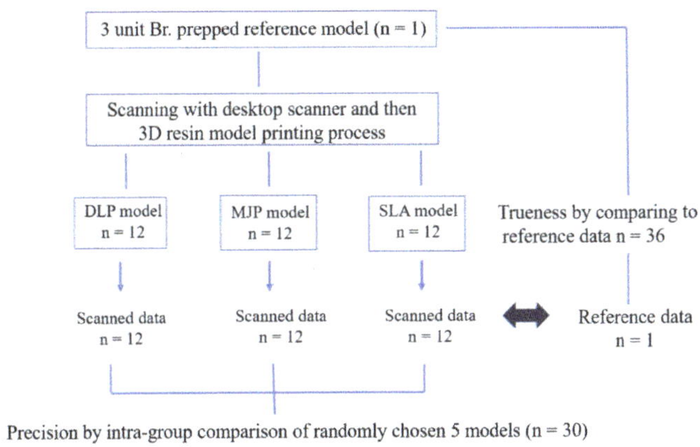

Figure 1. Flow chart of this study. 3D, three-dimensional; DLP, digital light processing; MJP, Multi-Jet printing; SLA, stereo-lithography apparatus.

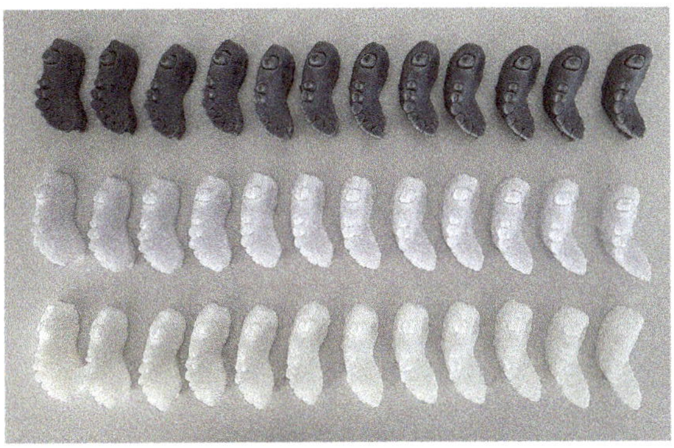

Figure 2. 3D-printed resin models (*n* = 36) of this study. First row; DLP models, second row; MJP models; third row; SLA models.

Table 1. Specifications of the 3D printer and materials used in this study.

3D Printer Model	Technology	Resin Material	Manufacturer of Printers and Resin Materials	Stacking Layer Thickness (μm)	Time	Building Angle (Degree)
Nextdent 5100	DLP	Next Dent model 2.0	3D systems	50	3 h 40 m	0
ProJetMJP 2500+	MJP	Visijet M2R-WT (SL7810)/Visilet M2 Sup	3D systems	32	3 h 42 m	0
ProJetSLA 7000	SLA	Accur ABS white (SL7810)	3D systems	50	43 m	0

2.2. *The Dimensional Accuracy Measurements of 3D-Printed Models*

3D-printed models were analyzed for the accuracy at 4 landmark positions and assessed deviations on margins of prepped teeth and proximal contact area, shown in Figure 3. To measure the accuracy (trueness; inter-printer and precision; intra-printer reliability) of abutment teeth and distances to approximate teeth, the datasets were superimposed through a best-fit alignment method using a 3D inspection software of Geomagic (release 2018, Geomagic control X, 3D Systems, Rock Hill, SC, USA), according to recommendation of ISO-12836 [17]. Since a variety of 3D inspection software are aligned using different protocols, 3D analysis results may differ.

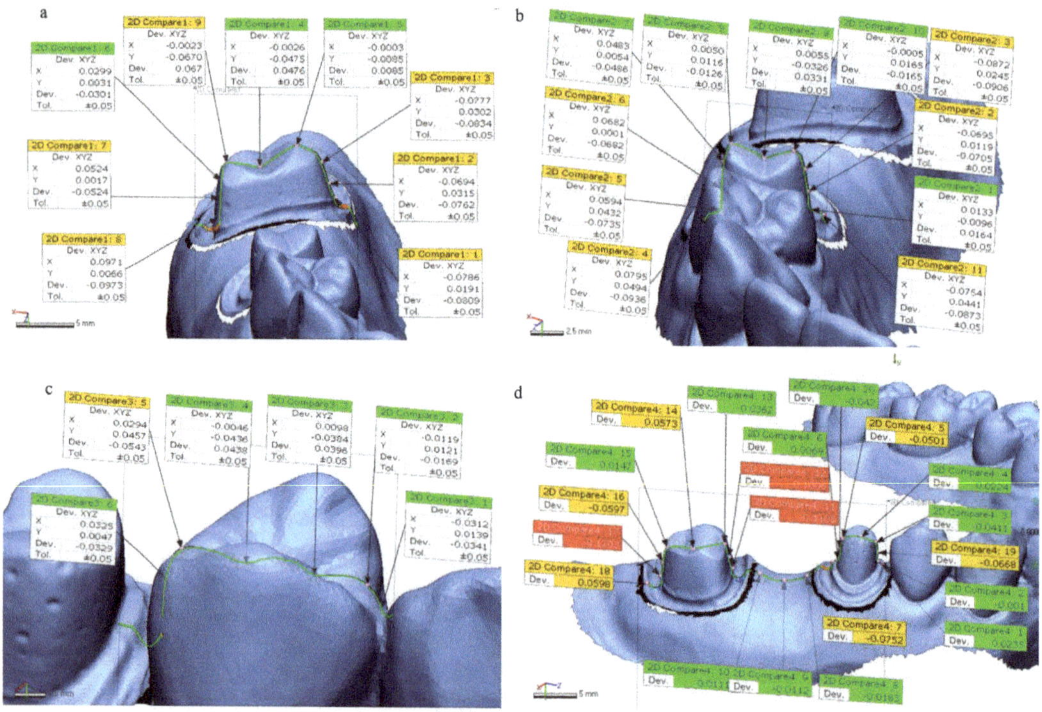

Figure 3. Four landmarks for measurement of trueness on 3D-printed models with the reference file. (**a**) molar tooth at buccolingual section. (**b**) Premolar tooth at buccolingual section. (**c**) Proximal contact to approximate tooth. (**d**) Molar and premolar teeth at mesiodistal section.

Trueness was determined by comparing the measurements on 3D-printed models to those on the original image file (STL file of reference model) (n = 36). The precision of the 3D-printed models was evaluated on 5 randomly chosen samples by superimposing scan data within each group (n = 30) (Figure 1). The quantitative values were automatically calculated by the 3D analysis program based on RMS. The RMS values were used to verify the mean of the positive and negative values using the following formula:

$$\frac{1}{\sqrt{n}} \times \sqrt{\sum\nolimits_{i=1}^{n}} (Xief - Xi)2$$

where n is the sum of the measured points, $Xief$ is the measurement point of i of the reference model, and Xi is the measurement point of i of the dataset of the 3D-printed test models.

We set the tolerance as ±50 μm according to previous studies [18,19]. The percent of points within the tolerance level (inTOL; nominal ±50 μm) were also calculated with respect to accuracy for printed models. A color map expressing visual deviation was set with 20 color segments. The color map showed the amount of deviations between the test model STL file and the reference file [20]. The range of the maximum and minimum nominal values was set at 50 μm, and the range of the maximum and minimum critical values was set at 500 μm (Figure 4).

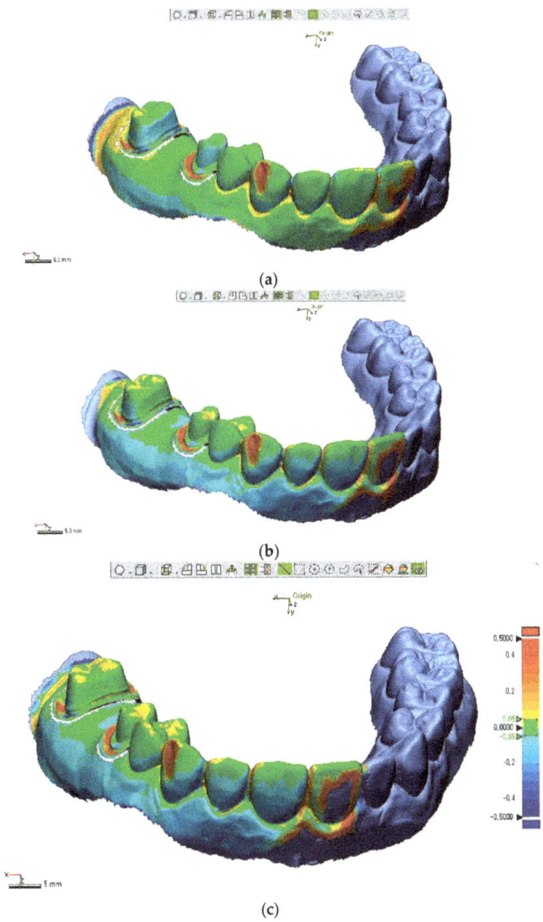

Figure 4. Color maps of 3D model superimpositions of each printed test model STL file with the original reference file. Table 50. μm expressing green colors, and max/min critical range at ±500 μm representing dark red or blue colors. The Scheme 0. to 0.5 mm. (**a**) DLP cast. (**b**) MJP cast. (**c**) SLA cast.

After best fit alignments of the test STL file with reference STL file, we sliced 3D model images to 2D planes (buccolingual and mesiodistal planes). We calculated deviations through Geomagic software at 4 measurement positions: margin of prepped molar and premolar teeth (buccolingual and mesiodistal planes), and proximal contact to an approximate tooth (Figure 5). To assess the deviations at margins and proximal contact of 3D-printed models, the absolute deviation values of 2 marginal points in prepped molar, 4 marginal points of prepped premolar, and 1 point of proximal contact, were analyzed.

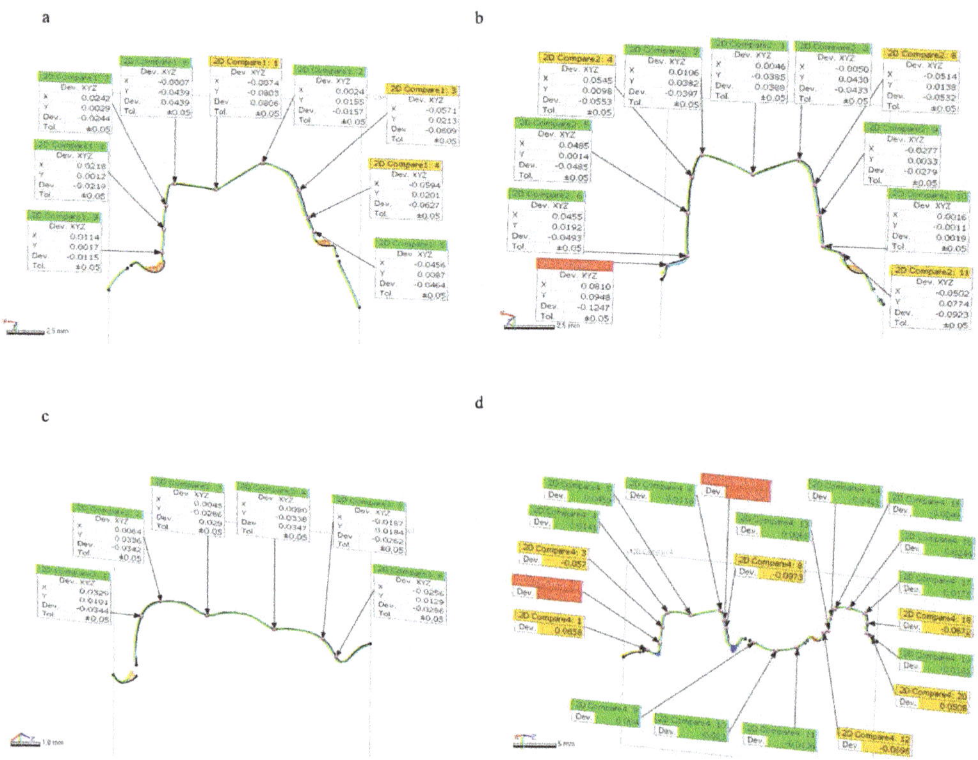

Figure 5. Measurements of deviations in two-dimensional (2D) planes. (**a**) Marginal deviations of molar teeth at a buccolingual plane. (**b**) Marginal deviations of premolar teeth at a buccolingual plane. (**c**) Deviations at proximal contact to approximate tooth. (**d**) Marginal deviations of molar and premolar teeth at a mesiodistal plane.

2.3. *The Measurements of Surface Roughness on 3D-Printed Models*

We measured roughness of 3D-printed models by DLP, MJP, SLA techniques using confocal laser scan microscope (LSM800, ZEISS, 07745 Jena, Germany) because surface roughness could affect the differences of accuracy.

2.4. *Statistical Analyses*

Statistical analyses were conducted using SPSS (IBM Statistics, v.25.0; IBM Corp, Armonk, NY, USA), and significance level was set at 0.05. Normal distribution of all data was examined through the Shapiro–Wilk test and homogeneity of variance with Levene's test. As a result, the deviation values in 2D planes and inTOL (%) for precision between the 3D printer groups were analyzed using one-way ANOVA and Tukey HSD test as post hoc (significance level at $p < 0.05$), while differences of RMS values and inTOL (%) for trueness at 4 landmark 3D areas between printers were analyzed using Kruskal–Wallis H test. The Mann–Whitney U-test and Bonferroni correction were used for post-testing ($p < 0.05/3 = 0.017$).

The Intraclass Correlation Coefficient (ICC) value is the reliability calculated by the raters' measurements. The ICC means reproducibility if the test is repeated several times [21]. The ICC value was also used to show the level of precision, at 95% confidence interval in this study.

3. Results

3.1. *Trueness of 3D-printed Models*

We analyzed accuracy (trueness and precision) through RMS values that are automatically calculated through 3D inspection software at 4 measurement positions (Figure 3). As shown in Table 2, for overall 3D analysis at molar position, there were significant differences in mean RMS values of trueness among all 3 techniques: DLP (0.117 ± 0.007 mm), MJP (0.096 ± 0.029 mm), SLA (0.101 ± 0.004 mm) ($p < 0.001$). For overall 3D analysis at premolar position, MJP (0.054 ± 0.002 mm) technique showed the most accurate result in comparison with DLP (0.064 ± 0.009 mm) and SLA (0.066 ± 0.005 mm) techniques ($p < 0.001$). For overall 3D analysis at proximal contact area, DLP (0.052 ± 0.011 mm) and MJP (0.059 ± 0.012 mm) techniques showed more accurate results than SLA (0.078 ± 0.021 mm) technique ($p < 0.001$). For overall 3D analysis at mesiodistal section (molar to premolar), DLP (0.100 ± 0.022 mm) and MJP (0.098 ± 0.010 mm) techniques showed better results compared to SLA (0.123 ± 0.008 mm) technique ($p < 0.001$).

Table 2. The accuracy (trueness by RMS value (mean ± SD) mm) of 3D-printed models (n = 36).

Positions	DLP (mm)	MJP (mm)	SLA (mm)	p-Value
#27 buccolingul	0.117 ± 0.007 ^{a}	0.096 ± 0.029 ^{b}	0.101 ± 0.004 ^{b}	<0.001
#25 buccolngual	0.064 ± 0.009 ^{c}	0.054 ± 0.002 ^{d}	0.066 ± 0.005 ^{c}	<0.001
Proximal contact	0.052 ± 0.011 ^{e}	0.059 ± 0.012 ^{e}	0.078 ± 0.021 ^{f}	<0.001
#27–25 mesiodistal	0.100 ± 0.022 ^{h}	0.098 ± 0.010 ^{h}	0.123 ± 0.008 ^{g}	<0.001

Different letters indicate statistically significant difference based on Mann-Whitney test at $p < 0.017$.

The inTOL (%) of trueness for 3D-printed models showed significant differences between printing techniques as shown in Table 3 ($p < 0.05$). MJP technique (88.166 ± 5.185%) showed the highest percent within the tolerance 0.05 mm level. Consequently, the 3 different 3D printing techniques in present study showed significant differences in trueness of RMS measurements and inTOL (%).

Table 3. The inTOL (%) of trueness (mean ± SD) for 3D-printed models (n = 36).

Positions	DLP (%)	MJP (%)	SLA (%)	p-Value
#27 buccolingual	81.2405 ± 6.623 ^{a}	84.917 ± 2.874 ^{b}	84.335 ± 2.501 ^{b}	0.037
#25 buccolingual	88.776 ± 8.189 ^{c}	93.661 ± 1.832 ^{d}	88.227 ± 2.537 ^{c}	0.01
Proximal contact	95.488 ± 2.447 ^{e}	92.371 ± 4.106 ^{f}	84.050 ± 5.198 ^{g}	<0.001
#27–25 mesiodistal	85.292 ± 2.799 ^{h}	88.705 ± 0.790 ^{i}	83.086 ± 2.775 ^{j}	<0.001

Different letters indicate statistically significant difference based on Mann-Whitney test at $p < 0.017$.

3.2. *Deviations of 3D-Printed Models at 2D Planes*

We examined the absolute values of deviations, at margins of prepped molar and premolar area, and to proximal contact at 2D planes (Figure 5). For marginal deviations at a buccolingual plane of prepped molar, DLP (0.100 ± 0.022 mm), MJP (0.0291 ± 0.020 mm), SLA (0.070 ± 0.015 mm) groups showed significant differences ($p < 0.001$). For marginal deviations at mesiodistal plane of prepped molar, DLP (0.109 ± 0.015 mm), MJP (0.020 ± 0.012 mm), SLA (0.051 ± 0.044 mm) groups also showed significant differences ($p < 0.001$). However, Table 4 showed marginal deviations of prepped premolar had no significant difference in both buccolingual and mesiodistal planes (p = 0.625, 0.996 respectively). For deviations at proximal contact area on mesiodistal plane, MJP (0.009 ± 0.009 mm) technique showed the lowest value compared to DLP (0.036 ± 0.015 mm) and SLA (0.036 ± 0.015 mm) groups ($p < 0.001$).

Table 4. The absolute values of deviations for 3D-printed models at margins and contact area.

Positions	DLP (mm)	MJP (mm)	SLA (mm)	p-Value
molar (buccolingual)	0.100 ± 0.022 [a]	0.0291 ± 0.020 [b]	0.070 ± 0.015 [c]	<0.001
premolar (buccolingual)	0.074 ± 0.033	0.068 ± 0.029	0.074 ± 0.044	0.625
molar (mesiodistal)	0.109 ± 0.015 [d]	0.020 ± 0.012 [e]	0.051 ± 0.044 [f]	<0.001
premolar (mesiodistal)	0.029 ± 0.028	0.029 ± 0.014	0.029 ± 0.014	0.996
contact to proximal tooth	0.036 ± 0.015 [g]	0.009 ± 0.009 [h]	0.036 ± 0.015 [g]	<0.001

Different letters indicate statistically significant difference based on ANOVA at $p < 0.05$.

Considering the deviation values ((+); expansion, (−); contraction) at each point and 3D color map, the all 3D-printed casts showed contraction buccolingually, and MJP casts showed least change. In posterior regions (molar area), contraction was more than anterior regions (premolar area).

3.3. Precision of 3D-Printed Models

Table 5 showed the DLP (0.244 ± 0.117 mm), MJP (0.272 ± 0.103 mm), and SLA (0.249 ± 0.069 mm) techniques exhibited no significant differences on RMS values of precision (p = 0.381). Table 6 showed the inTOL (%) of precision for 3D-printed models also showed no statistical differences between printing techniques (p = 0.643). Precision of the 3D-printed models was also measured using ICC. The ICC of the three test groups were 0.996 (DLP), 0.955 (MJP), and 0.992 (SLA) as shown in Table 7. All test groups exhibited an excellent level of precision, based on 95% confident interval of the ICC estimation.

Table 5. The accuracy (precision by RMS value (mean ± SD) mm) of 3D-printed models (n = 30).

DLP (mm)	MJP (mm)	SLA (mm)	p-Value
0.244 ± 0.117	0.272 ± 0.103	0.249 ± 0.069	0.381

Table 6. The inTOL (%) of precision (mean ± SD) for 3D-printed models (n = 30).

DLP (%)	MJP (%)	SLA (%)	p-Value
95.596 ± 2.345	95.134 ± 1.726	95.879 ± 0.988	0.643

Table 7. Intraclass Correlation Coefficient (ICC) values of 3D-printed models.

DLP	MJP	SLA
0.996	0.955	0.992

3.4. Surface Roughness of 3D-Printed Models

Table 8 showed the mean surface roughness of 3D-printed models by MJP technique (Ra: 2.345 ± 0.374 μm), which observed the smoothest compared to the DLP (Ra: 4.123 ± 2.531 μm) or SLA (Ra: 7.75 ± 2.478 μm) technique.

Table 8. Mean surface roughness ((mean ± SD) μm) on surface of 3D-printed models.

Measurement	DLP (μm)	MJP (μm)	SLA (μm)
Ra	4.123 ± 2.531	2.345 ± 0.374	7.75 ± 2.478
Sa	56.75 ± 21.132	31.25 ± 14.07	77.3 ± 7.912

4. Discussion

In the analysis process of this study, the analysis software showed 3D deviation data that consisted of automatically calculated RMS, average (+) and average (−) values on 4 measurement sections, and individual deviation values ((+); expansion or (−); contraction) at multiple measurement points of 2D planes (Figures 3 and 5). In this study, only RMS values were used for examining 3D deviations of printed models and absolute deviational values at 2D planes (buccolingual and mesiodistal) because in quantitative evaluation, if the average (+) and average (−) deviations express an equal distribution, the sum values will be close to zero, which make results confusing. In addition to that, the color maps for a qualitative inspection were segmented with 20 colors, showing contraction or expansion at best fit alignment of test STL files with the reference STL file.

Hazeveld et al. concluded that measurement differences of less than 250 μm were clinically acceptable values since the tolerances for manual measurements were almost identical to that value [22]. This study calculated the accuracy of printed models through superimpositions of files with the analyzing program recommended by ISO 12836. With that, the measurement errors were reduced and the true values of 3D-printed models were focused on.

For evaluating RMS and inTOL values between DLP, MJP, and SLA techniques, statistically significant differences in trueness were found. Emir et al. reported that the RMS on the accuracy of complete arch measurements showed significant differences between 3D-printed models: the DLP technique (46.2 μm) showed the most accurate results, followed by SLA (51.6 μm) and MJP (58.6 μm) [23]. On the other hand, Kim et al. reported that the accuracy of full arch models fabricated by the MJP technique (62–106 μm) exhibited the highest accuracy, followed by DLP (76–143 μm) and SLA groups (86–141 μm) [24]. This is consistent with the results from this study, where mean MJP (76 ± 20 μm) printing technology exhibited excellent trueness in 4 measured positions, followed by the mean values of DLP (83 ± 26 μm) and SLA (92 ± 21 μm) printers. It was assumed that Kim's results were also further supported by the measurements of surface roughness from this study. The mean surface roughness in models fabricated by the MJP technique showed the smoothest surface, followed by DLP and SLA.

Although there were significant differences in the RMS of accuracy (trueness), all tested models in this study showed clinically acceptable values based on the standards of previous studies. The previous studies reported that a dimensional difference less than 500 μm in dental models did not affect clinical decision [25], and for orthodontic and diagnostic purposes, less than 300 μm values are known to be clinically acceptable [26]. However, for the fit of the fabrication of prosthesis, when a printed model shows this much discrepancy, it might not be sufficient because other manufacturing processes of prostheses would increase errors, and the fit of prosthesis is one of most important factors for prognosis of treatment. In the same context, Rossini et al. reported that recommended trueness of digital models for clinical setting should be under 200 μm [27], which is twice the results of this study. Consequently, trueness of 3D-printed models by DLP, MJP, and SLA in the present study showed that all casts could be used for fabrication of prosthesis.

All tested models printed by DLP (244 ± 117 μm), MJP (272 ± 103 μm), and SLA (249 ± 69 μm) techniques showed excellent precision according to superimposition data, as well as ICC values above 0.95. According to the study of Kim et al., MJP and DLP techniques were more precise than the SLA techniques [24]. Even though results from this study showed DLP and SLA techniques were more precise than MJP, no statistically significant differences between groups were found ($p = 0.381$). Clinicians can expect that appropriate models for clinical use are printed, regardless of printing order or number under the same conditions.

Deviations of two points in prepped molar, four points of prepped premolar, and one point of intimate tooth contact were also analyzed to assess the deviations of marginal and contact areas. Marginal fit is the most important feature of fixed prostheses, and marginal misfit can lead to secondary caries, pulpitis as well as periodontal problems including gingivitis and bone loss, causing failure of the prosthesis. Therefore, after producing the prostheses using transmitted STL files, they needed to be checked with the working model to reduce errors before the delivery to patients.

The clinically acceptable marginal fit of fixed prostheses has been reported as 90 μm to 200 μm [16,28] and many researchers consider the optimal marginal fit should be within 120 μm [16]. For proximal contact area, 50 μm contact thickness is typically regarded as appropriate [29]. In addition to that, previous studies demonstrated that the linear deviation of printed model regarded acceptable at 200 μm because the measurement error of the plaster model itself is close to this range [22]. Therefore, if the deviation values of 3D-printed models from this study show less than these values at measured points (margins and a proximal contact), clinical use of 3D-printed models for manufacturing prostheses could be considered clinically acceptable.

In the present study, the mean deviation of margins on molars and premolars were all observed within the acceptable range of previous studies (less than 120 μm), and the MJP group showed the fewest deviations (Table 4). For proximal contacts, all deviation values were also less than 50 μm. Therefore, to check the accuracy of fabricated prostheses with the 3D-printed working model, printing by 3D techniques is recommended regardless of the printing methods. Furthermore, Jeong et al. showed 3D-printed models fabricated by SLA techniques (52 μm) were observed to be more accurate than milled models (152 μm) [30]. In other words, to reduce errors of fabrication of prostheses, reproducing digital models by 3D printing, instead of milling, is a good option regardless of the printing materials.

The color map showed contraction (blue) and expansion (orange-red) of 3D-printed models in this study. Prepped tooth (molar or premolar) showed contraction in buccolingual and mesiodistal planes regardless of the 3D techniques (Figure 4). Park et al. suggested that the DLP cast tended to contract, whereas casts in the MJP and SLA groups expanded buccolingually [31]. However, in our study, all casts contracted buccolingually. The differences of those results might be because of the differences in geometry of the measured casts; Park et al. measured deviations on a thin cylinder form of a printed model, while prepped casts for three-unit Br were used in this study, which needs more resin materials (volume). This means more shrinkage could have occurred under polymerization. Similarly, absolute deviation values showed that the posterior region (i.e., molar) deviated more than the anterior region (i.e., premolar) (Table 4). This result can be explained by the presence of a higher density of polymers in the posterior region than in the anterior region; more polymer chains in the resin printing and polymerization process might introduce more deviation [32]. These results might correspond with complaints of dental technicians that adaptation of prostheses to 3D-printed working models is often loose.

The layer thickness setting could be the most decisive factor for accuracy of resin printed models, under the condition in which each printer has a determined x and y resolution [33]. For the stacking layer thickness of 3D resin printing, there was a previous study where part of the printed area deviated from the ideal boundary in each layer, and the chances of potential errors increased with the number of additive layers [34]. In other words, the thinnest layer would not be optimal. Zhang et al. reported that the optimal layer thickness of the DLP technique was 50 μm, showing the best balance between surface accuracy and printing error, while for the SLA technique, optimal layer thickness was 25–50 μm [35]. Accordingly, for most accurate results of different printing techniques, this study used a 50-μm stacking layer in DLP and SLA. However, a 32-μm layer was used for MJP, as recommended by the manufacturer.

A different study concluded that a thinner layer thickness resulted in an increased number of layers, and thus a higher resolution of the z axis [35]. That might explain why MJP (z axis: 790 dpi) showed higher z axis resolution than SLA (z axis: 500 dpi) material used in this study. However, according to the study of Braian et al., high resolution is not equivalent to accuracy [36]. Printers that have high resolution can fabricate models with finer detail; however, other various factors such as layer thickness, number of layers, degree of polymerization shrinkage, polymerizing laser speed and intensity, building direction and angle, thermal changes (expansion or contraction), reference model geometries, supporter design, and post processing can affect the accuracy (trueness and precision) of printed objects on top of the printed materials with different resolutions [22,37–42]. In the present study, the overall resolution of SLA (4000 × 4000 × 500 dpi) was reported to be the highest among DLP (1920 × 1080 dpi), MJP (1600 × 900 × 790 dpi), and SLA, according to a manufacturer. However, MJP showed the smoothest surface (Table 8) and significantly higher accuracy than others (Tables 2 and 5). The building angle, reference model geometries, and supporter design of this study were applied equivalently in DLP, MJP, SLA techniques. Therefore, it was assumed that the degree of polymerization shrinkage of each printing material, as well as the thermal changes of models at printing and post-processing, affected the results of this study. To tackle these effects, further studies are needed.

The cost and printing speeds of devices with different 3D printing technologies vary. In the present study, high-end 3D printers from well-known brands and commercially used 3D printing materials were selected. Even though manufacturing speed was found to be the fastest with the SLA technique in this study, an SLA 3D printer is known to be much more expensive than a DLP printer. Therefore, there need to be consideration about which 3D printing technique is the most cost-effective option to fabricate working digital models with appropriate accuracy. The printing accuracy can also be improved by optimizing the parameter settings. Further studies are needed to reduce deviations and optimize the parameters in various 3D printers.

5. Conclusions

Under the limits of this study, MJP casts showed significantly higher accuracy (trueness) than DLP and SLA casts, and there were no significant differences found in precision. Although all casts contracted buccolingually, the overall 3D accuracy of all the 3D-printed resin models produced by the DLP, MJP, and SLA techniques, showed clinically acceptable ranges. The overall deviation values of printed models at 2D planes also showed clinically acceptable ranges; less than 120 μm for margins and 50 μm for contact areas. It was concluded that dental working models printed by DLP, MJP, and SLA techniques can be used for adjusting and determining the fit of fixed prostheses before delivery.

Author Contributions: Conceptualization, S.-Y.Y.; methodology, S.-K.K. and J.-Y.K.; software, S.-J.H. and J.-G.K.; validation, S.-K.K. and J.-Y.K.; formal analysis, S.-Y.Y. and J.-G.K.; investigation, S.-Y.Y. and J.-G.K.; resources, S.-K.K. and, S.-J.H.; data curation, S.-Y.Y. and S.-J.H.; writing—original draft preparation, S.-Y.Y. and S.-K.K.; writing—review and editing, S.-Y.Y. and J.-Y.K.; visualization, S.-Y.Y. and S.-K.K.; supervision, S.-K.K. All authors gave final approval and agreed to be accountable for all aspects of the work. All authors have read and agreed to the published version of the manuscript.

Funding: This research was supported by Basic Science Research Program through the National Research Foundation of Korea (NRF) funded by the Ministry of Education (NRF-2018R1D1A1B07042333) and by the Korea Medical Device Development Fund grant funded by the Korea government (the Ministry of Science and ICT, the Ministry of Trade, Industry and Energy, the Ministry of Health & Welfare, Republic of Korea, the Ministry of Food and Drug Safety) (Project Number: 202011A02).

Institutional Review Board Statement: Not applicable.

Informed Consent Statement: Not applicable.

Data Availability Statement: Data sharing is not applicable.

Conflicts of Interest: The authors declare no conflict of interest.

References

1. Groth, C.; Kravitz, N.D.; Jones, P.E.; Graham, J.W.; Redmond, W.R. Three-dimensional printing technology. *J. Clin. Orthod.* **2014**, *48*, 475–485.
2. Yau, H.T.; Yang, T.J.; Lin, Y.K. Comparison of 3-D Printing and 5-axis Milling for the Production of Dental e-models from Intra-oral Scanning. *Comput. Aided Des. Appl.* **2015**, *13*, 32–38. [CrossRef]
3. Msallem, B.; Sharma, N.; Cao, S.; Halbeisen, F.S.; Zeilhofer, H.F.; Thieringer, F.M. Evaluation of the Dimensional Accuracy of 3D-Printed Anatomical Mandibular Models Using FFF, SLA, SLS, MJ, and BJ Printing Technology. *J. Clin. Med.* **2020**, *9*, 817. [CrossRef]
4. Kim, G.B.; Lee, S.; Kim, H.; Yang, D.H.; Kim, Y.H.; Kyung, Y.S.; Kim, C.S.; Choi, S.H.; Kim, B.J.; Ha, H.; et al. Three-Dimensional Printing: Basic Principles and Applications in Medicine and Radiology. *Korean J. Radiol.* **2016**, *17*, 182–197. [CrossRef] [PubMed]
5. Reymus, M.; Fotiadou, C.; Kessler, A.; Heck, K.; Hickel, R.; Diegritz, C. 3D printed replicas for endodontic education. *Int. Endod. J.* **2019**, *52*, 123–130. [CrossRef] [PubMed]
6. van Noort, R. The future of dental devices is digital. *Dent. Mater.* **2012**, *28*, 3–12. [CrossRef] [PubMed]
7. El-Katatny, I.; Masood, S.H.; Morsi, Y.S. Error analysis of FDM fabricated medical replicas. *Rapid Prototyp. J.* **2010**, *16*, 36–43. [CrossRef]
8. Salmi, M.; Paloheimo, K.S.; Tuomi, J.; Wolff, J.; Makitie, A. Accuracy of medical models made by additive manufacturing (rapid manufacturing). *J. Cranio Maxillofac. Surg.* **2013**, *41*, 603–609. [CrossRef]
9. Ibrahim, D.; Broilo, T.L.; Heitz, C.; de Oliveira, M.G.; de Oliveira, H.W.; Nobre, S.M.W.; Santos, J.H.G.D.; Silva, D.N. Dimensional error of selective laser sintering, three-dimensional printing and PolyJet (TM) models in the reproduction of mandibular anatomy. *J. Cranio Maxillofac. Surg.* **2009**, *37*, 167–173. [CrossRef]
10. Silva, D.N.; de Oliveira, M.G.; Meurer, E.; Meurer, M.I.; da Silva, J.V.L.; Santa-Barbara, A. Dimensional error in selective laser sintering and 3D-printing of models for craniomaxillary anatomy reconstruction. *J. Cranio Maxillofac. Surg.* **2008**, *36*, 443–449. [CrossRef]
11. Santana, R.R.; Lozada, J.; Kleinman, A.; Al-Ardah, A.; Herford, A.; Chen, J.W. Accuracy of Cone Beam Computerized Tomography and a Three-Dimensional Stereolithographic Model in Identifying the Anterior Loop of the Mental Nerve: A Study on Cadavers. *J. Oral Implantol.* **2012**, *38*, 668–676. [CrossRef] [PubMed]

12. Flugge, T.V.; Schlager, S.; Nelson, K.; Nahles, S.; Metzger, M.C. Precision of intraoral digital dental impressions with iTero and extraoral digitization with the iTero and a model scanner. *Am. J. Orthod. Dentofac. Orthop.* **2013**, *144*, 471–478. [CrossRef]
13. Son, K.; Lee, K.B. Effect of Tooth Types on the Accuracy of Dental 3D Scanners: An In Vitro Study. *Materials* **2020**, *13*, 1744. [CrossRef] [PubMed]
14. Barker, T.M.; Earwaker, W.J.; Lisle, D.A. Accuracy of stereolithographic models of huma anatomy. *Australas. Radiol.* **1994**, *38*, 106–111. [CrossRef] [PubMed]
15. Yeo, I.S.; Yang, J.H.; Lee, J.B. In vitro marginal fit of three all-ceramic crown systems. *J. Prosthet. Dent.* **2003**, *90*, 459–464. [CrossRef] [PubMed]
16. Mclean, J.W.; Fraunhofer, J.A. Estimation of Cement Film Thickness by an in-Vivo Technique. *Br. Dent. J.* **1971**, *131*, 107–111. [CrossRef] [PubMed]
17. *Dentistry—Digitizing Devices for CAD/CAM Systems for Indirect Dental Restorations: Test Methods for Assessing Accuracy*; International Organization for Standardization: Geneva, Switzerland, 2015; pp. 1–19.
18. Sim, J.Y.; Jang, Y.; Kim, W.C.; Kim, H.Y.; Lee, D.H.; Kim, J.H. Comparing the accuracy (trueness and precision) of models of fixed dental prostheses fabricated by digital and conventional workflows. *J. Prosthodont. Res.* **2019**, *63*, 25–30. [CrossRef]
19. Jin, S.J.; Kim, D.Y.; Kim, J.H.; Kim, W.C. Accuracy of Dental Replica Models Using Photopolymer Materials in Additive Manufacturing: In Vitro Three-Dimensional Evaluation. *J. Prosthodont.* **2019**, *28*, e557–e562. [CrossRef]
20. Dong, T.; Wang, X.; Xia, L.; Yuan, L.; Ye, N.; Fang, B. Accuracy of different tooth surfaces on 3D printed dental models: Orthodontic perspective. *BMC Oral Health* **2020**, *20*, 340. [CrossRef]
21. Rungrojwittayakul, O.; Kan, J.Y.; Shiozaki, K.; Swamidass, R.S.; Goodacre, B.J.; Goodacre, C.J.; Lozada, J.L. Accuracy of 3D Printed Models Created by Two Technologies of Printers with Different Designs of Model Base. *J. Prosthodont.* **2020**, *29*, 124–128. [CrossRef]
22. Hazeveld, A.; Slater, J.J.R.H.; Ren, Y.J. Accuracy and reproducibility of dental replica models reconstructed by different rapid prototyping techniques. *Am. J. Orthod. Dentofac. Orthop.* **2014**, *145*, 108–115. [CrossRef]
23. Emir, F.; Ayyildiz, S. Accuracy evaluation of complete-arch models manufactured by three different 3D printing technologies: A three-dimensional analysis. *J. Prosthodont. Res.* **2021**. [CrossRef] [PubMed]
24. Kim, S.Y.; Shin, Y.S.; Jung, H.D.; Hwang, C.J.; Baik, H.S.; Cha, J.Y. Precision and trueness of dental models manufactured with different 3-dimensional printing techniques. *Am. J. Orthod. Dentofac. Orthop.* **2018**, *153*, 144–153. [CrossRef]
25. Liang, Y.M.; Rutchakitprakarn, L.; Kuang, S.H.; Wu, T.Y. Comparing the reliability and accuracy of clinical measurements using plaster model and the digital model system based on crowding severity. *J. Chin. Med. Assoc.* **2018**, *81*, 842–847. [CrossRef] [PubMed]
26. Hirogaki, Y.; Sohmura, T.; Satoh, H.; Takahashi, J.; Takada, K. Complete 3-D reconstruction of dental cast shape using perceptual grouping. *IEEE Trans. Med. Imaging* **2001**, *20*, 1093–1101. [CrossRef]
27. Rossini, G.; Parrini, S.; Castroflorio, T.; Deregibus, A.; Debernardi, C.L. Diagnostic accuracy and measurement sensitivity of digital models for orthodontic purposes: A systematic review. *Am. J. Orthod. Dentofac. Orthop.* **2016**, *149*, 161–170. [CrossRef]
28. Øilo, G.; Fransson, B.; Gjeitanger, R. The fit of metal-ceramic crownsm a clinical study. *Dent. Mater.* **1985**, *1*, 197–199.
29. Daniel, J.A.R.; Kim, S.; Suh, K.-W. An evaluation and adjustment method for natural proximal contacts of crowns using diamond dental strips: A case report. *Oper. Dent.* **2013**, *61*, 60–63.
30. Jeong, Y.G.; Lee, W.S.; Lee, K.B. Accuracy evaluation of dental models manufactured by CAD/CAM milling method and 3D printing method. *J. Adv. Prosthodont.* **2018**, *10*, 245–251. [CrossRef] [PubMed]
31. Park, J.M.; Jeon, J.; Koak, J.Y.; Kim, S.K.; Heo, S.J. Dimensional accuracy and surface characteristics of 3D-printed dental casts. *J. Prosthet. Dent.* **2020**. [CrossRef]
32. Al Sunbul, H.; Silikas, N.; Watts, D.C. Polymerization shrinkage kinetics and shrinkage-stress in dental resin-composites. *Dent. Mater.* **2016**, *32*, 998–1006. [CrossRef]
33. Keating, A.P.; Knox, J.; Bibb, R.; Zhurov, A.I. A comparison of plaster, digital and reconstructed study model accuracy. *J. Orthod.* **2008**, *35*, 191–201; discussion 175. [CrossRef]
34. Favero, C.S.; English, J.D.; Cozad, B.E.; Wirthlin, J.O.; Short, M.M.; Kasper, F.K. Effect of print layer height and printer type on the accuracy of 3-dimensional printed orthodontic models. *Am. J. Orthod. Dentofac. Orthop.* **2017**, *152*, 557–565. [CrossRef] [PubMed]
35. Zhang, Z.C.; Li, P.L.; Chu, F.T.; Shen, G. Influence of the three-dimensional printing technique and printing layer thickness on model accuracy. *J. Orofac. Orthop.* **2019**, *80*, 194–204. [CrossRef]
36. Braian, M.; Jimbo, R.; Wennerberg, A. Production tolerance of additive manufactured polymeric objects for clinical applications. *Dent. Mater.* **2016**, *32*, 853–861. [CrossRef]
37. Revilla-Leon, M.; Meyers, M.J.; Zandinejad, A.; Ozcan, M. A review on chemical composition, mechanical properties, and manufacturing work flow of additively manufactured current polymers for interim dental restorations. *J. Esthet. Restor. Dent.* **2019**, *31*, 51–57. [CrossRef]
38. Alharbi, N.; Osman, R.B.; Wismeijer, D. Factors Influencing the Dimensional Accuracy of 3D-Printed Full-Coverage Dental Restorations Using Stereolithography Technology. *Int. J. Prosthodont.* **2016**, *29*, 503–510. [CrossRef]
39. Alharbi, N.; Osman, R.; Wismeijer, D. Effects of build direction on the mechanical properties of 3D-printed complete coverage interim dental restorations. *J. Prosthet. Dent.* **2016**, *115*, 760–767. [CrossRef]

40. Bugeda, G.; Cervera, M.; Lombera, G.; Onate, E. Numerical analysis of stereolithography processes using the finite element method. *Rapid Prototyp. J.* **1995**, *1*, 13–23. [CrossRef]
41. Hong, W.B.; Lee, Y.T.; Gong, H.Q. A study of the staircase effect induced by material shrinkage in rapid prototyping. *Rapid Prototyp. J.* **2005**, *11*, 82–89.
42. Hong, W.B.; Lee, Y.T.; Gong, H.Q. Thermal analysis of layer formation in a stepless rapid prototyping process. *Appl. Therm. Eng.* **2004**, *24*, 255–268. [CrossRef]

materials

MDPI

Article

Dimensional Accuracy Evaluation of Temporary Dental Restorations with Different 3D Printing Systems

Wonjoon Moon [1], Seihwan Kim [2], Bum-Soon Lim [1], Young-Seok Park [3], Ryan Jin-Young Kim [4,*] and Shin Hye Chung [1,*]

1 Department of Dental Biomaterials Science, Dental Research Institute, School of Dentistry, Seoul National University, 101 Daehak-ro, Jongno-gu, Seoul 03080, Korea; w.moon@snu.ac.kr (W.M.); nowick@snu.ac.kr (B.-S.L.)
2 Department of Aeronautical & Mechanical Engineering, Inha Technical College, 100 Inha-ro, Michuhol-gu, Incheon 22212, Korea; kseihwan@inhatc.ac.kr
3 Department of Oral Anatomy, Dental Research Institute, Center for Future Dentistry, School of Dentistry, Seoul National University, 101 Daehak-ro, Jongno-gu, Seoul 03080, Korea; ayoayo7@snu.ac.kr
4 Department of Dental Science, Dental Research Institute, School of Dentistry, Seoul National University, 101 Daehak-ro, Jongno-gu, Seoul 03080, Korea
* Correspondence: ryankim05@snu.ac.kr (R.J.-Y.K.); den533@snu.ac.kr (S.H.C.); Tel.: +82-2-740-8793 (R.J.-Y.K.); +82-2-740-8693 (S.H.C.)

Abstract: With the advent of 3D printing technologies in dentistry, the optimization of printing conditions has been of great interest, so this study analyzed the accuracy of 3D-printed temporary restorations of different sizes produced by digital light processing (DLP) and liquid crystal display (LCD) printers. Temporary restorations of 2-unit, 3-unit, 5-unit, 6-unit, and full-arch cases were designed and printed from a DLP printer using NextDent C&B or an LCD printer using Mazic D Temp ($n = 10$ each). The restorations were scanned, and each restoration standard tessellation language (STL) file was superimposed on the reference STL file, by the alignment functions, to evaluate the trueness through whole/point deviation. In the whole-deviation analysis, the root-mean-square (RMS) values were significantly higher in the 6-unit and full-arch cases for the DLP printer and in the 5-unit, 6-unit, and full-arch cases for the LCD printer. The significant difference between DLP and LCD printers was found in the 5-unit and full-arch cases, where the DLP printer exhibited lower RMS values. Color mapping demonstrated less shrinkage in the DLP printer. In the point deviation analysis, a significant difference in direction was exhibited in all the restorations from the DLP printer but only in some cases from the LCD printer. Within the limitations of this study, 3D printing was most accurate with less deviation and shrinkage when a DLP printer was used for short-unit restorations.

Keywords: 3D printing; digital dentistry; temporary dental restoration; dimensional measurement accuracy

1. Introduction

Temporary restorations are temporary prostheses used to protect teeth under dental treatment or to replace lost teeth to stabilize the surrounding tissue and maintain esthetics. They protect the teeth from deformation, leakage, chemical irritation, and plaque accumulation before the final prosthesis is prepared [1]. In addition, the incorrect fabrication of temporary restorations may cause inflammation of the gingiva or alter the occlusion due to the movement of adjacent teeth [2], potentially causing serious issues with the placement of the final restoration. Therefore, it is essential to secure the safety and performance of temporary restorations.

Recently, with the rapid introduction of digital dentistry, 3D printing has been newly applied for the fabrication of dental prostheses [3]. Compared to the process of manufacturing temporary restorations through conventional means, 3D printing is considered more comfortable for patients and replaces much of the laboratory work [3]. In terms of efficiency, the digitalization of patient data allows for pre-planning, modification, and simulation during the procedure [4]. As the demand of 3D printing increases, various types of 3D printing techniques are being continuously developed, including digital light processing (DLP) and liquid crystal display (LCD).

The DLP technique is a method of producing a prosthesis through photo-polymerization by irradiating UV light to a tank containing acrylic or epoxy-based light-curing resin that reacts to ultraviolet rays (UV). The DLP technique is fast in printing and guarantees high precision. Therefore, it is used in the manufacturing of medical devices with complex or delicate shapes [5]. However, its biggest disadvantage is that it is expensive and limited to small-sized models. On the other hand, the LCD technique is also based on photo-polymerization but uses liquid crystals in imaging, rather than a light projector in DLP [6]. Compared to the other 3D printing techniques, the LCD technique is cheap and has good resolution, but has been known to have a short service life [7].

Although producing precise temporary restorative materials through 3D printing is critical, there have been a lack of studies regarding its accuracy. Few studies have been performed on 3D-printed temporary restorations, including the cytocompatibility of 3D-printed temporary restorations [8] and fabrication of highly viscous temporary crowns with fast building speed [9]. In addition, comparisons on the products of DLP and LCD-type printers have hardly been made. One study showed that DLP and LCD-type printers could print products of similar mechanical and biological properties if several adjustments in polymerization time and intensity were performed [6]. Therefore, it may be necessary to print temporary restorations using commonly used DLP and LCD techniques and study their accuracy. As the accuracy may vary according to size, variations in sizes may also be needed.

Composite resins have been widely used as restorative materials as they possess good physical, mechanical, and thermal properties [10]. To utilize them, extensive research has been performed on their reinforcement mechanisms [11–14]. In addition, there have been various successful methods to adjust for their esthetic properties such as translucency [15,16], staining [17], and shade [18]. In short, composite resins have various advantages and have been sufficiently studied for a long period of time. Thus, as long as the risk of cytotoxicity due to residual monomers is strictly controlled in the oral cavity [19], the use of composite resins for precise 3D printing may have numerous potential advantages.

Considering the importance of temporary restorations and the convenience of 3D printing technologies, the optimization of printing conditions may offer great advantages in the clinical environment. The accuracy analysis of 3D-printed restorations is one of the essential steps to expand the clinical use of 3D printers in the field of dentistry. Therefore, the purpose of this study was to analyze the accuracy of 3D-printed temporary restorations of different sizes produced by DLP and LCD 3D printers.

The null hypothesis was that the dimensional accuracy of 3D-printed temporary dental restorations would not be affected by their sizes and the type of printer.

2. Materials and Methods

2.1. 3D Model Fabrication and Scanning

Temporary restorations of 2-unit, 3-unit, 5-unit, 6-unit, and full-arch cases were virtually designed from patient models in modeling software (Exocad DentalDB 2.2 Valletta, Exocad GmbH, Darmstadt, Germany) to produce reference STL files. Based on those models, each type of restoration was printed on a DLP-type printer (DLP; NextDent 5100, 3D Systems, Soesterberg, The Netherlands) and an LCD-type printer (LCD; Ka;rv LP550, Shinwon Dental, Seoul, Korea). The DLP printer utilized NextDent C&B (NextDent, Soesterberg, The Netherlands) and the LCD printer used Mazic D Temp (Vericom, Chuncheon, Korea) (Table 1). The DLP printer had a resolution of 1920 × 1080 pixels, build volume of 125 mm × 70 mm × 196 mm, 5 base layers, and post-polymerization time of 30 min (UV-A 315–400 nm; 72 W). The LCD printer had a resolution of 1440 × 2560 pixels, build volume of 68 mm × 121 mm × 140 mm, 5 base layers, and post-polymerization time of 20 min (UV-A 315–400 nm; 72 W). The printed restorations without any defects were selected by visual inspection (*n* = 10 each), washed with isopropanol, sonicated for five minutes, and dried at room temperature, according to the manufacturer's instructions. The restorations were then post-polymerized (LC-3DPrint Box, 3D Systems, Soesterberg, The Netherlands) for 30 min (DLP) or 20 min (LCD), according to the manufacturer's instructions. All the printed restorations were scanned using an optical scanner (MD-ID0300, Medit, Seoul, Korea) to obtain restoration STL files (Figure 1). The entire process was performed by an experienced single operator. Examples of the printed restorations are shown in Figure 2.

Table 1. Printing materials used in the study.

	NextDent C&B	Mazic D Temp
Printer	DLP	LCD
Shade	A3.5	A2
Chemical composition	Methacrylic oligomer, phosphine oxide	Methacrylic oligomer, phosphine oxide
Lot. Number	WY364N04	TP0961A2

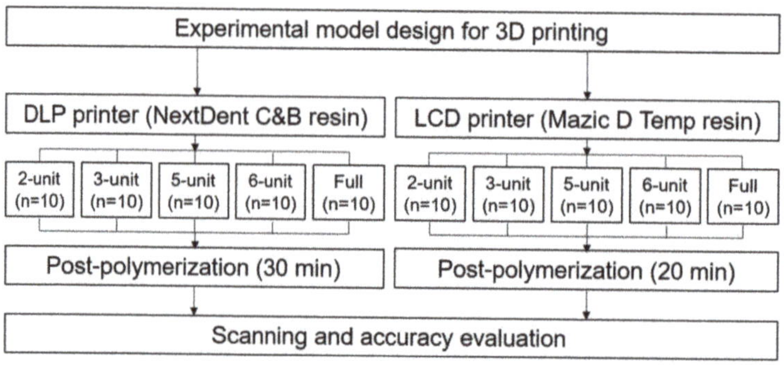

Figure 1. Flowchart of the experimental process.

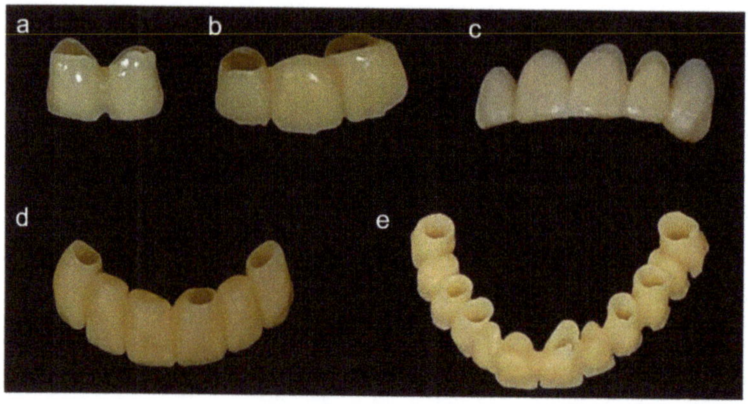

Figure 2. Representative printed restorations. (**a**) 2-unit, (**b**) 3-unit, (**c**) 5-unit, (**d**) 6-unit, and (**e**) full-arch restorations.

2.2. *Superimposition and 3D Deviation Evaluation*

The entire three-dimensional external surface of the restorations was obtained using a 3D scanner that generated a point cloud (set of data points in space) for each restoration. Each restoration STL file was superimposed on the reference STL file to evaluate the trueness of the 3D-printed restorations using metrology software (PointShape Inspector v2.16, DREAMTNS, Seongnam, Korea). Superimposition was performed by "initial alignment" followed by "automatic alignment" functions. The deviation between the datasets of each restoration and the corresponding reference was calculated for all data points that consist of XYZ coordinates. The whole deviation was obtained to evaluate the displacement of the entire external surface and to generate an overall color map that indicates the direction of deviation with blue and red colors indicating negative and positive deviations compared to the reference, respectively. The sampling rate was set at 100%. With regard to the exclusion factor, the software evaluated the reference dataset and automatically set a "maximum distance value" above which it was excluded in the calculation. In addition to the whole-deviation analysis, specific measuring points were located on each reference restoration for point deviation analysis with 6 points on each unit—3 points on the buccal and 3 points on the lingual aspects of the unit, and an additional 3 points were assigned at the distal end of each restoration. Three points of each aspect were at the center of the coronal, middle, and cervical thirds, respectively (Figure 3). The median and interquartile range of the root-mean-square (RMS) and deviation values were calculated for trueness evaluation.

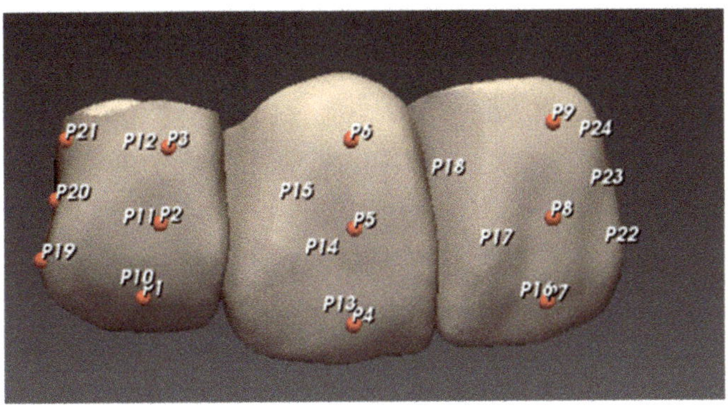

Figure 3. Representation of measuring points on 3-unit restoration: P1–P9 for buccal, P10–P18 for lingual, and P19–P24 for distal.

2.3. *Statistical Analysis*

For the whole-deviation analysis, a comparison among different restorations was performed by the nonparametric Kruskal–Wallis test followed by the Mann–Whitney test with Bonferroni's correction. On the other hand, a comparison between different printers was performed by either the Student's t-test or Mann–Whitney test depending on the normality test by the Kolmogorov–Smirnov test and Shapiro–Wilk test. For the point deviation analysis, a comparison among buccal, lingual, and proximal points was performed by the nonparametric Kruskal–Wallis test followed by the Mann–Whitney test with Bonferroni's correction. The analysis was performed using statistical software (SPSS version 26.0, IBM, Armonk, NY, USA) under a significance level of 0.05.

3. Results

3.1. *Whole-Deviation Analysis and Color Map*

In the whole-deviation analysis, compared to 2-unit restorations, the RMS values were significantly higher in the 6-unit (0.17 mm) and full-arch (0.21 mm) cases for the DLP printer. On the other hand, they were significantly higher in the 5-unit (0.18 mm), 6-unit

(0.17 mm), and full-arch (0.23 mm) cases for the LCD printer. A significant difference between the DLP and LCD printers was observed in the 5-unit and full-arch cases, where the DLP printer exhibited lower RMS values of 0.14 and 0.21 mm, respectively, compared to the LCD printer RMS values of 0.18 and 0.23 mm, respectively (Figure 4). Representative 3D images of the whole deviation are shown in Figure 5 as color maps. DLP restorations tended to exhibit less shrinkage (negative deviation) than LCD restorations, with the shrinkage being most remarkable on the occlusal surfaces.

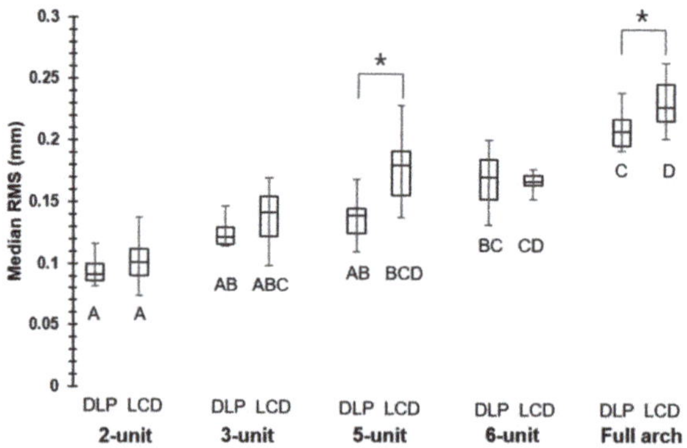

Figure 4. Median RMS of whole deviation; asterisks show significant difference within the same unit, whereas different uppercase letters (A–D) show significant difference within the same printers ($p < 0.05$).

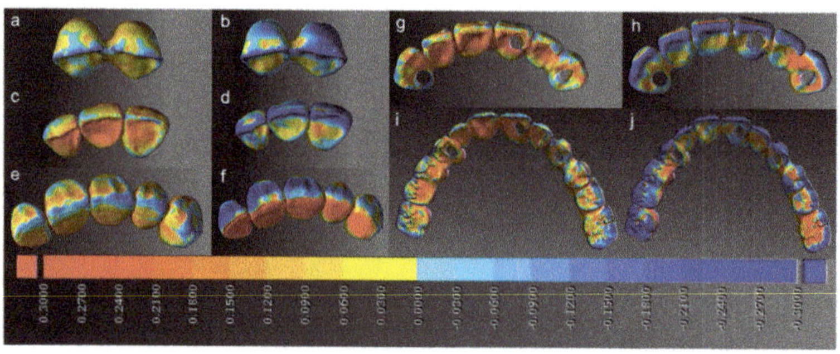

Figure 5. Color maps showing whole deviation; the blue and red colors indicate negative and positive deviations compared to the reference, respectively. (**a**) 2-unit DLP, (**b**) 2-unit LCD, (**c**) 3-unit DLP, (**d**) 3-unit LCD, (**e**) 5-unit DLP, (**f**) 5-unit LCD, (**g**) 6-unit DLP, (**h**) 6-unit LCD, (**i**) full-arch DLP, and (**j**) full-arch LCD restorations.

3.2. Point Deviation Analysis

In the point deviation analysis, significant differences among the buccal, lingual, and proximal points were shown in all the restorations in DLP printing. Proximal deviations (0.06 mm) in the 2-unit cases, buccal and proximal deviations (0.11 and 0.07 mm) in the 3-unit cases, buccal and proximal deviations (0.06 and 0.14 mm) in the 5-unit cases, lingual deviations (0.13 mm) in the 6-unit cases, and proximal deviations (0.20 mm) in the full-arch cases were significantly higher within the same restorations. For LCD printing, significant differences were exhibited in the 5-unit, 6-unit, and full-arch cases, but not in the 2-unit and 3-unit cases. Lingual deviations (0.26 mm) in the 5-unit cases, proximal deviations (0.14 mm) in the 6-unit cases, and buccal and proximal deviations (0.13 and 0.18 mm) in the full-arch cases were significantly higher within the same restorations (Table 2).

Table 2. Median point deviation at the buccal, lingual, and palatal points.

		Median Point Deviation (mm)	
		DLP	LCD
2-unit	Buccal	0.04 [0.02, 0.07] A	0.05 [0.03, 0.08] A
	Lingual	0.04 [0.02, 0.06] A	0.07 [0.03, 0.13] A
	Proximal	0.06 [0.03, 0.12] B	0.06 [0.03, 0.09] A
3-unit	Buccal	0.11 [0.04, 0.17] B	0.05 [0.02, 0.11] A
	Lingual	0.04 [0.02, 0.09] A	0.05 [0.02, 0.12] A
	Proximal	0.07 [0.04, 0.13] B	0.07 [0.02, 0.12] A
5-unit	Buccal	0.06 [0.02, 0.12] B	0.08 [0.03, 0.23] A
	Lingual	0.04 [0.02, 0.07] A	0.26 [0.09, 0.39] B
	Proximal	0.14 [0.04, 0.21] C	0.15 [0.11, 0.19] A
6-unit	Buccal	0.08 [0.03, 0.16] A	0.07 [0.02, 0.13] A
	Lingual	0.13 [0.05, 0.23] B	0.06 [0.03, 0.10] A
	Proximal	0.08 [0.03, 0.17] A	0.14 [0.05, 0.22] B
Full arch	Buccal	0.09 [0.04, 0.17] A	0.13 [0.05, 0.23] B
	Lingual	0.10 [0.04, 0.19] A	0.10 [0.04, 0.18] A
	Proximal	0.20 [0.11, 0.28] B	0.18 [0.12, 0.26] B

Note: Absolute values were used for statistical analysis. Interquartile ranges [first quartile, third quartile] are shown in parentheses. Different uppercase letters indicate significant difference within the same restoration ($p < 0.05$).

4. Discussion

The null hypothesis that the dimensional accuracy of 3D-printed temporary dental restorations would not be affected by their sizes and type of printers was rejected. According to the whole-deviation analysis, the RMS increased with the restoration size. A significant increase in RMS value started to become noticeable in the 6-unit cases in DLP printing, whereas it began to appear in the 5-unit cases in LCD printing. Based on these results, it can be stated that DLP and LCD printing were both inaccurate in larger restorations. This might be attributed to the intrinsic limitation of DLP and LCD printers as they share the same basic operating mechanism. DLP and LCD printing can be used for small restorations, but 3D printers based on other technologies may be considered for the more accurate printing of larger restorations.

The performance of DLP and LCD printing differed in larger restorations such as the 5-unit and full-arch cases. In those cases, DLP printing exhibited lower RMS values, indicating that DLP printing showed better accuracy than LCD printing. However, in DLP and LCD printing, the important parameters are exposure time, wavelength, and amount of power supply [20]. As those parameters were not completely set to be the same for both printers, not enough evidence is available to evaluate the performance of DLP and LCD printing simply based on the results of this study. A comparison between DLP and LCD printing, as seen in this study, is very rare possibly due to their similar backgrounds. Previous studies have compared different 3D printing technologies such as stereolithography apparatus (SLA), DLP, fused filament fabrication (FFF), PolyJet technique, and fused deposition modeling (FDM) [21,22]. The analysis of DLP and LCD printing can be critical as the identification of advantages or disadvantages of one technique may allow for the complete replacement of one with another. This can be an important factor in terms of the efficiency of the research.

On the other hand, according to the point deviation, DLP printing exhibited differences in the direction of deviation in all the restorations. The deviation did not occur uniformly but in a skewed direction. However, LCD printing showed uniform deviation in all directions in the 2- and 3-unit cases but began to exhibit skewed deviations for larger restorations. As this result was not shown in the whole deviation analysis, it was found that the point deviation analysis was capable of revealing obscured data in the whole deviation analysis.

The present study utilized the 3D volumetric analysis in XYZ coordinates. In the past, however, linear measurement was widely used to determine the accuracy of dental models [23,24]. Linear measurement, while mostly based on limited measuring points, had an intrinsic limitation that it varied depending on the reference markers [25] and could not capture the 3D morphological changes [26].

3D deviation measurement with color mapping as in this study was based on the point cloud in XYZ coordinates and was thereby expected to overcome the limitations of linear measurement.

As previously known, shrinkage is one of the challenges of DLP printers [27]. In the color map, such shrinkage was well-presented in both printers, and it was more prominent in LCD restorations. Although DLP and LCD printing are operated under similar mechanisms, their conditions for proper operation are different. For LCD printers to have similar mechanical properties to DLP printers, more powerful or longer post-polymerization processes are required [6]. In this study, there was no specific control on the post-polymerization scheme, so the LCD restorations may not have acquired sufficient mechanical properties to endure shrinkage. In addition, the shrinkage was more concentrated on the occlusal surfaces, and this was consistent with the previous studies that confirmed the occlusal surfaces to be more error-prone [28]. To use the printed restorations by DLP and LCD printing in the clinical environment, chairside adjustments of internal adaptions or designing larger STL files may be considered.

Shrinkage can also be analyzed in terms of the used materials. The shrinkage of composite resins is one of the most widely known characteristics. Numerous factors have been reported to be involved in the shrinkage of composite resins. For example, the differences in filler particles [29], degree of conversion [30], and curing methods [31] resulted in different shrinkage rates. Therefore, optimization of such conditions through changes in the printing parameters and printing materials may be needed to adjust for shrinkage. Moreover, as the printing materials used in this study were both based on methacrylic oligomers, the synthesis of low-shrinkage methacrylate monomers [32] to replace the original monomers may be another option.

Regarding dental models and surgical guides, there have been reports on their clinically acceptable accuracies [33–35]. In particular, less than 100 μm of difference from the reference was suggested as an acceptable value in dental models [36]. However, these results were based on a linear measurement of distances, so they may still have limitations. For the 3D-printed temporary restorations, such information is absent, so it is difficult to determine whether the inaccuracy that occurred in this study is within threshold values. Further studies are required to suggest clinically acceptable levels of inaccuracy.

This study had a limitation as an in vitro study. The accuracy of 3D-printed restorations should eventually be evaluated inside the oral cavity where additional considerations on temperature, moisture, and pH are required. For example, the current experimental conditions might be tested in vivo. Moreover, this study was confined to a limited number of printing techniques, printing materials, and build direction, and factors such as aging were also not considered. Although the printing materials in this study had the same overall chemical composition, they were from different manufacturers. As these factors are known to influence the accuracy of 3D-printed restorations [37,38], further studies are necessary to discuss the accuracy in more detail.

5. Conclusions

The 3D printing of temporary restorations was more inaccurate for larger restorations in both DLP and LCD printers. Differences between DLP and LCD printing were observed in larger restorations, where the degree of inaccuracy was smaller in DLP printing. The restorations by DLP printing were less prone to shrinkage, which was prominent on the occlusal surfaces. The direction of deviation was always skewed to one side in DLP printing, but was uniform in LCD printing for smaller restorations. Within the limitations of this study, 3D printing was most accurate with less deviation and shrinkage when a DLP printer was used for short-unit restorations. However, further studies to improve the degree of deviation, direction of deviation, shrinkage, and actual adaptation in the oral cavity are necessary.

Author Contributions: Conceptualization, methodology, software, writing—original draft, W.M.; data curation, B.-S.L. and Y.-S.P.; supervision, B.-S.L. and S.K.; writing—review and editing, W.M. and S.H.C.; investigation, validation, Y.-S.P. and S.K.; project administration, visualization, funding acquisition, S.H.C. and R.J.-Y.K. All authors have read and agreed to the published version of the manuscript.

Funding: This research was funded by the National Research Foundation of Korea (NRF), grant numbers 2019-R1G1A1004813 and 2020-R1A2C1102316.

Institutional Review Board Statement: Not applicable.

Informed Consent Statement: Not applicable.

Data Availability Statement: Data sharing is not applicable to this article.

Conflicts of Interest: The authors declare no conflict of interest.

References

1. Tjan, A.H.; Castelnuovo, J.; Shiotsu, G. Marginal fidelity of crowns fabricated from six proprietary provisional materials. *J. Prosthet. Dent.* **1997**, *77*, 482–485. [CrossRef]
2. Karlsen, K. Gingival reactions to dental restorations. *Acta Odontol. Scand.* **1970**, *28*, 895–904. [CrossRef]
3. Dawood, A.; Marti, B.M.; Sauret-Jackson, V.; Darwood, A. 3D printing in dentistry. *Br. Dent. J.* **2015**, *219*, 521–529. [CrossRef]
4. Vasamsetty, P.; Pss, T.; Kukkala, D.; Singamshetty, M.; Gajula, S. 3D printing in dentistry–Exploring the new horizons. *Mater. Today* **2020**, *26*, 838–841. [CrossRef]
5. Rahman, M.M. Statistical Analysis of the Digital Micromirror Devices Hinge Sag Phenomenon. Ph.D. Thesis, Texas Tech University, Lubbock, TX, USA, 2002.
6. Chen, H.; Cheng, D.-H.; Huang, S.-C.; Lin, Y.-M. Comparison of flexural properties and cytotoxicity of interim materials printed from mono-LCD and DLP 3D printers. *J. Prosthet. Dent.* **2020**, in press. [CrossRef]
7. Quan, H.; Zhang, T.; Xu, H.; Luo, S.; Nie, J.; Zhu, X. Photo-curing 3D printing technique and its challenges. *Bioact. Mater.* **2020**, *5*, 110–115. [CrossRef] [PubMed]
8. Park, J.-H.; Lee, H.; Kim, J.-W.; Kim, J.-H. Cytocompatibility of 3D printed dental materials for temporary restorations on fibroblasts. *BMC Oral Health* **2020**, *20*, 1–9. [CrossRef] [PubMed]
9. Li, X.; Xie, B.; Jin, J.; Chai, Y.; Chen, Y. 3D printing temporary crown and bridge by temperature controlled mask image projection stereolithography. *Procedia Manuf.* **2018**, *26*, 1023–1033. [CrossRef]
10. Yadav, R.; Kumar, M. Dental restorative composite materials: A review. *J. Oral Biosci.* **2019**, *61*, 78–83. [CrossRef] [PubMed]
11. Dafar, M.O.; Grol, M.W.; Canham, P.B.; Dixon, S.J.; Rizkalla, A.S. Reinforcement of flowable dental composites with titanium dioxide nanotubes. *Dent. Mater.* **2016**, *32*, 817–826. [CrossRef]
12. Noushad, M.; Ab Rahman, I.; Husein, A.; Mohamad, D. Nanohybrid dental composite using silica from biomass waste. *Powder Technol.* **2016**, *299*, 19–25. [CrossRef]
13. Kumar, S.R.; Patnaik, A.; Bhat, I. Development and characterization of marble dust-filled dental composite. *J. Compos. Mater.* **2017**, *51*, 1997–2008. [CrossRef]
14. Altaie, A.; Bubb, N.L.; Franklin, P.; Dowling, A.H.; Fleming, G.J.; Wood, D.J. An approach to understanding tribological behaviour of dental composites through volumetric wear loss and wear mechanism determination; beyond material ranking. *J. Dent.* **2017**, *59*, 41–47. [CrossRef]
15. Ryan, E.-A.; Tam, L.E.; McComb, D. Comparative translucency of esthetic composite resin restorative materials. *J. Can. Dent. Assoc.* **2010**, *76*, a84.
16. Awad, D.; Stawarczyk, B.; Liebermann, A.; Ilie, N. Translucency of esthetic dental restorative CAD/CAM materials and composite resins with respect to thickness and surface roughness. *J. Prosthet. Dent.* **2015**, *113*, 534–540. [CrossRef]
17. Ardu, S.; Braut, V.; Gutemberg, D.; Krejci, I.; Dietschi, D.; Feilzer, A.J. A long-term laboratory test on staining susceptibility of esthetic composite resin materials. *Quintessence Int.* **2010**, *41*, 695–702. [PubMed]
18. Romero, M.F. Esthetic anterior composite resin restorations using a single shade: Step-by-step technique. *J. Prosthet. Dent.* **2015**, *114*, 9–12. [CrossRef]
19. Pagano, S.; Coniglio, M.; Valenti, C.; Negri, P.; Lombardo, G.; Costanzi, E.; Cianetti, S.; Montaseri, A.; Marinucci, L. Biological effects of resin monomers on oral cell populations: Descriptive analysis of literature. *Eur. J. Paediatr. Dent.* **2019**, *20*, 224–232.
20. Shahrubudin, N.; Lee, T.C.; Ramlan, R. An overview on 3D printing technology: Technological, materials, and applications. *Procedia Manuf.* **2019**, *35*, 1286–1296. [CrossRef]
21. Kim, S.-Y.; Shin, Y.-S.; Jung, H.-D.; Hwang, C.-J.; Baik, H.-S.; Cha, J.-Y. Precision and trueness of dental models manufactured with different 3-dimensional printing techniques. *Am. J. Orthod. Dentofac. Orthop.* **2018**, *153*, 144–153. [CrossRef] [PubMed]
22. Fiorenza, L.; Yong, R.; Ranjitkar, S.; Hughes, T.; Quayle, M.; McMenamin, P.G.; Kaidonis, J.; Townsend, G.C.; Adams, J.W. The use of 3D printing in dental anthropology collections. *Am. J. Phys. Anthropol.* **2018**, *167*, 400–406. [CrossRef]
23. Caputi, S.; Varvara, G. Dimensional accuracy of resultant casts made by a monophase, one-step and two-step, and a novel two-step putty/light-body impression technique: An in vitro study. *J. Prosthet. Dent.* **2008**, *99*, 274–281. [CrossRef]
24. Martorelli, M.; Gerbino, S.; Giudice, M.; Ausiello, P. A comparison between customized clear and removable orthodontic appliances manufactured using RP and CNC techniques. *Dent. Mater.* **2013**, *29*, e1–e10. [CrossRef] [PubMed]
25. Hazeveld, A.; Slater, J.J.H.; Ren, Y.; Orthopedics, D. Accuracy and reproducibility of dental replica models reconstructed by different rapid prototyping techniques. *Am. J. Orthod. Dentofac. Orthop.* **2014**, *145*, 108–115. [CrossRef] [PubMed]
26. Brosky, M.; Major, R.; DeLong, R.; Hodges, J.S. Evaluation of dental arch reproduction using three-dimensional optical digitization. *J. Prosthet. Dent.* **2003**, *90*, 434–440. [CrossRef]

27. Nejadebrahim, A.; Ebrahimi, M.; Allonas, X.; Croutxé-Barghorn, C.; Ley, C.; Métral, B. A new safranin based three-component photoinitiating system for high resolution and low shrinkage printed parts via digital light processing. *RSC Adv.* **2019**, *9*, 39709–39720. [CrossRef]
28. Wang, W.; Yu, H.; Liu, Y.; Jiang, X.; Gao, B. Trueness analysis of zirconia crowns fabricated with 3-dimensional printing. *J. Prosthet. Dent.* **2019**, *121*, 285–291. [CrossRef]
29. Labella, R.; Lambrechts, P.; Van Meerbeek, B.; Vanherle, G. Polymerization shrinkage and elasticity of flowable composites and filled adhesives. *Dent. Mater.* **1999**, *15*, 128–137. [CrossRef]
30. Silikas, N.; Eliades, G.; Watts, D. Light intensity effects on resin-composite degree of conversion and shrinkage strain. *Dent. Mater.* **2000**, *16*, 292–296. [CrossRef]
31. Sakaguchi, R.L.; Berge, H.X. Reduced light energy density decreases post-gel contraction while maintaining degree of conversion in composites. *J. Dent.* **1998**, *26*, 695–700. [CrossRef]
32. Ge, J.; Trujillo, M.; Stansbury, J. Synthesis and photopolymerization of low shrinkage methacrylate monomers containing bulky substituent groups. *Dent. Mater.* **2005**, *21*, 1163–1169. [CrossRef]
33. Sherman, S.L.; Kadioglu, O.; Currier, G.F.; Kierl, J.P.; Li, J. Accuracy of digital light processing printing of 3-dimensional dental models. *Am. J. Orthod. Dentofac. Orthop.* **2020**, *157*, 422–428. [CrossRef]
34. Brown, G.B.; Currier, G.F.; Kadioglu, O.; Kierl, J.P. Accuracy of 3-dimensional printed dental models reconstructed from digital intraoral impressions. *Am. J. Orthod. Dentofac. Orthop.* **2018**, *154*, 733–739. [CrossRef] [PubMed]
35. Kim, T.; Lee, S.; Kim, G.B.; Hong, D.; Kwon, J.; Park, J.-W.; Kim, N. Accuracy of a simplified 3D-printed implant surgical guide. *J. Prosthet. Dent.* **2020**, *124*, 195–201.e192. [CrossRef] [PubMed]
36. Rungrojwittayakul, O.; Kan, J.Y.; Shiozaki, K.; Swamidass, R.S.; Goodacre, B.J.; Goodacre, C.J.; Lozada, J.L. Accuracy of 3D printed models created by two technologies of printers with different designs of model base. *J. Prosthodont.* **2020**, *29*, 124–128. [CrossRef]
37. Reymus, M.; Stawarczyk, B. In vitro study on the influence of postpolymerization and aging on the Martens parameters of 3D-printed occlusal devices. *J. Prosthet. Dent.* **2020**, in press. [CrossRef]
38. Reymus, M.; Fabritius, R.; Keßler, A.; Hickel, R.; Edelhoff, D.; Stawarczyk, B. Fracture load of 3D-printed fixed dental prostheses compared with milled and conventionally fabricated ones: The impact of resin material, build direction, post-curing, and artificial aging—An in vitro study. *Clin. Oral Investig.* **2020**, *24*, 701–710. [CrossRef] [PubMed]

materials

MDPI

Article

The Role of Solvents in Lithography-Based Ceramic Manufacturing of Lithium Disilicate

Malte Hartmann *, Markus Pfaffinger and Jürgen Stampfl

Institute of Materials Science and Technology, Faculty of Mechanical and Industrial Engineering, Technische Universität Wien, Getreidemarkt 9, 1060 Vienna, Austria; markus.pfaffinger@cubicure.com (M.P.); juergen.stampfl@tuwien.ac.at (J.S.)
* Correspondence: malte.hartmann@fau.de

Abstract: Digital dentistry is increasingly replacing conventional methods of manually producing dental restorations. With regards to computer-aided manufacturing (CAM), milling is state of the art. Additive manufacturing (AM), as a complementary approach, has also found its way into dental practices and laboratories. Vat photo-polymerization is gaining increasing attention, because it enables the production of full ceramic restorations with high precision. One of the two predominantly used ceramic materials for these applications is lithium disilicate, $Li_2Si_2O_5$. This glass ceramic exhibits a substantial fracture toughness, although possesses much lower bending strength, than the other predominantly used ceramic material, zirconia. Additionally, it shows a much more natural optical appearance, due to its inherent translucency, and therefore is considered for anterior tooth restorations. In this work, an optimized formulation for photo-reactive lithium disilicate suspensions, to be processed by vat photo-polymerization, is presented. Following the fundamental theoretical considerations regarding this processing technique, a variety of solvents was used to adjust the main properties of the suspension. It is shown that this solvent approach is a useful tool to effectively optimize a suspension with regards to refractive index, rheology, and debinding behavior. Additionally, by examining the effect of the absorber, the exposure time could be reduced by a factor of ten.

Keywords: refractive index; debinding; glass ceramics; digital dentistry; additive manufacturing; vat photo-polymerization

1. Introduction

In dentistry, the development of computer-aided design/computer-aided manufacturing (CAD/CAM) systems in the 1980s brought a significant change to the field [1]. Continuous automatization and computerization finally led to the formation of a so-called digital dentistry, where the whole workflow—from assessment of the dentition situation by modern scan methods, via modelling of the restoration by adapted software, to the automated production of the restoration by CAM—is completed digitally. All necessary data is recorded virtually, so that, ideally, the manual preparation of impressions or models can be discarded.

The CAM method that has been developed primarily for this case is milling. This technique is now state of the art. In recent years, additive manufacturing (AM) has gained increasing attention as a complementary approach and, for certain cases, has found its way into dental laboratories and practices [2]. To enable a successful restoration, like a crown or bridge, high precision and good surface quality are necessary. Vat photo-polymerization is an AM method that excels in these categories. By combining this technology with the colloidal processing route, the production of full ceramic parts is possible [3].

This work focuses on lithography-based ceramic manufacturing (LCM) with regards to the technology and lithium disilicate with regards to the material. Lithium disilicate is one of the materials used predominantly for full ceramic restorations (the other one being zirconia) [4]. In LCM, suspensions or pastes are used, whose formulation can be rather complex. Changing one constituent or the fractions of the composition can easily result in a negative influence on other properties of the formulation. Here an approach was chosen that includes a change of the solvent composition. The aim was to change certain properties of the suspension, such as refractive index, rheology, and debinding behavior, without interfering too much with the polymerization mechanism. Table 1 lists typical components for such a suspension. In the following, these components and considerations of importance regarding their selection are discussed.

Table 1. Typical formulation for a photo-reactive suspension used in lithography-based ceramic manufacturing (LCM).

Component	Mass Fraction (%)
Solvent	10–20
Monomer	10–20
Photoinitiator	<0.5
Dispersant	<5
Absorber	<0.1
Ceramic filler	60–80

The starting point for the formulation is the filler. Amount of solid loading, particle size, particle size distribution, shape of the powder particles, and chemical constitution are factors that must be evaluated when developing a formulation. Amount of solid loading, particle size, and particle shape mainly determine the rheological behavior of the suspension. The viscosity, for example, increases with increasing solid loading and deviation from spherical particle shape [5,6].

The chemical constitution of the powder is pivotal for the strategy of stabilizing the suspension against agglomeration and sedimentation. Colloidal suspensions are divided into lyophilic and lyophobic colloids. In lyophilic colloids, the solvent has a strong affinity to the dispersed particles. In this case, the liquid is strongly adsorbed on the surface, and the system is stable by itself, because the free Gibbs energy is decreased during the process of dispersing. On the other hand, lyophobic colloids show no affinity between liquid and particle surface. The free Gibbs energy increases during the process of dispersing and attractive forces between the particles are active, which is the reason for quick agglomeration. In most cases, ceramic suspensions are lyophobic colloids [7]. Therefore, it is useful to acquire knowledge about what kind of attractive forces appear during dispersing and how they can be overcome by purposefully introducing repulsive forces to create suspensions with the desired stability.

A meaningful tool with regards to these considerations is the dispersing agent. By binding to the particle surface, it allows one to specifically introduce repulsive forces. In general, the following strategies are used for this purpose: electrostatic stabilization, steric stabilization, or electrosteric stabilization. In the case of suspensions in organic liquids, as they come into use in, for example, slip casting or tape casting, mostly steric stabilization is applied, where unloaded polymer chains are adsorbed on the particle surface [8]. Stable suspensions have the advantage that, in LCM, they enable higher homogeneity with regards to the solid loading of green bodies. In the case of unstable suspensions, over the course of the printing process, segregation and sedimentation take place, which leads to a different solid loading of the green bodies, depending on the height of the printed object [9].

Thixotropy is an effective instrument to prevent sedimentation and, at the same time, enables a good processability. It is defined as: "A time dependency of the flowing properties of non-Newtonian fluids, whose viscosity is decreased by continuous external influences and returns to starting viscosity only after the ceasing of load [10]". It is important to stress that in addition to shear-thinning behavior, thixotropic materials exhibit a time dependency of the viscosity recovery (i.e., after a mechanical load has been removed for a certain time period, the viscosity returns to its initial state).

In LCM, this is extensively practical. As long as no shearing forces are applied to the suspension (e.g., during storage), the suspension is ideally highly viscous and stable. When shearing forces are applied by the doctor blade during coating, the structural strength of the suspension is decreased. This way, the suspension yields to the load and enables easy processing. After the coating process, thixotropy leads to an increase of structural strength and therefore to the stability of the suspension after a given time period. This way, introducing a thixotropic additive enables the stabilization during storage and processing of an otherwise unstable suspension [11].

Since the basic mechanism for layer generation in LCM is based on photo-polymerization, optical properties like the refractive index are especially relevant for this method. When the difference in refractive index between dispersing phase and dispersed phase is high, the penetration depth of light is low and the widening, due to scattering, is high. When the difference in refractive index is low, penetration depth is high and widening low. To enable a high precision in LCM, it is necessary to target a small difference in refractive index (refractive index matching). The penetration depth can afterwards be decreased by utilizing an appropriate concentration of absorber [12].

Absorbers are chemical substances, which, ideally, are inert with regards to the polymerization and, by absorbing photons, reduce the penetration depth of light into the material. In vat photo-polymerization, the penetration depth determines the z-resolution. This is significant, for example, in the case of overhanging features of the part to be built. As the currently built part is always surrounded by redundant photo-reactive suspension, overhangs will inevitably be filled with cured material if the penetration (cure depth) is considerably higher than the layer thickness. Therefore, the cure depth should be of the same magnitude as the layer height. By varying the concentration of absorber, the cure depth can be adjusted for a given exposure. Therefore, it is essential that an absorbing agent efficiently absorbs at the emission wavelength of the light source. If the substance absorbs in the visible wavelength spectrum, it is called a dye [13]. Using an absorber leads to a higher conversion of double bonds at the same cure depth [14]. Understanding this is essential for the additive manufacturing process. The cure depth can also be decreased by reducing the exposure, but layers generated in this manner possess only insufficient mechanical stability and easily rupture (e.g., when detached from the vat or, in the worst case, when only gelled).

Being another main constituent of typical photo-reactive suspensions, the solvent has several functions. Firstly, it dissolves the solid organic constituents (photo-initiator and absorber). Secondly, it reduces the viscosity of the suspension. Thirdly, it assists the debinding process. Thermal debinding is by far the most implemented method. In this case, the binder is removed by heating, typically at atmospheric pressure and in oxidizing or non-oxidizing atmosphere. The mechanisms and physico-chemical factors that are fundamental to this process have been examined intensively in the literature. The debinding is controlled by heat transfer into the green body and mass transport of volatile substances and waste products, through the filled and unfilled pores, to the outside of the green body. It is important to mention that ceramic particles can influence the degradation process of the pure polymer [15].

As mentioned, debinding often takes place in oxidizing atmosphere (in many cases ambient air). It was shown that the oxidizing atmosphere at first hinders the chemical degradation of poly(methyl methacrylate) at low temperatures (200–300 °C), but accelerates it at higher temperatures later. In any case, it is a core property of the oxidizing atmosphere to reduce the amount of residual carbon in ceramic bodies [16].

In general, the debinding process can be divided into three phases. In phase one, warming takes place until the softening of the binder starts (lower than 200 °C). The chemical degradation is limited in this phase, but volatile lower-molecular-weight species (e.g., solvents) must diffuse through binder-filled pores and convert into the gas phase.

The rapid generation of these species and the presence of dissolved air or captured air bubbles can lead to defects in the ceramic body [17]. In phase two (200–300 °C), higher-molecular-weight products are quickly degraded, and the diffusion and degassing of the resulting degradation products takes place. If the softened/molten binder possesses enough mobility, a redistribution of binder can happen, and therefore a non-planar debinding front can appear. This can ease and accelerate the exit of volatile species. Lower-molecular-weight species, like plasticizers or waxes, can leave a concentration gradient behind [18]. In phase three (300–400 °C), the rest of the binder is slowly removed by degradation and degassing. This process is now alleviated by the high porosity of the brown body, but a residual amount of carbon is still present. Often, temperatures up to 600 °C or higher are necessary to significantly reduce this residual amount of carbon.

2. Materials and Methods

2.1. Materials

2.1.1. Solvent

Since preliminary experiments with phthalates showed promising results, this group of solvents was used for further investigation [9]. From the group of phthalates, dimethyl (DMP), diethyl (DEP), dibutyl (DBP), diallyl (DAP), and benzyl butyl phthalate (BBP) were used. All of them were obtained from Sigma-Aldrich (Merck KGaA, Darmstadt, Germany). The structural formulas of the phthalates are shown in Figure 1.

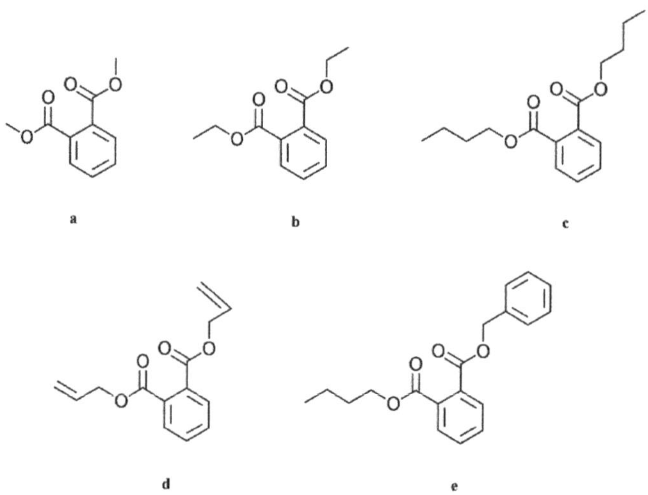

Figure 1. Chemical structures of the respective phthalates: (**a**) dimethyl phthalate, (**b**) diethyl phthalate, (**c**) dibutyl phthalate, (**d**) diallyl phthalate, (**e**) benzyl butyl phthalate.

2.1.2. Monomers

Two monomers under the denotations SR348C and SR833S were used exclusively. They were obtained from the company Sartomer (Arkema, Colombes, France). SR348C is a difunctional ethoxylated bisphenol-A dimethacrylate with a high viscosity (550–1700 mPa·s at 25 °C). SR833S is a difunctional tricyclodecane dimethanole diacrylate with a low viscosity (120–160 mPa·s at 25 °C). Both structural formulas are given in Figure 2.

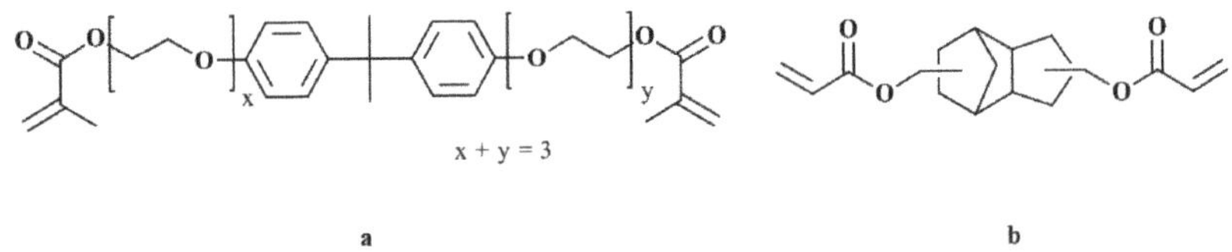

Figure 2. Chemical structures of (**a**) SR348C and (**b**) SR833S.

2.1.3. Dispersant

The dispersant is a commercially available substance called Solplus K500, produced by the company Lubrizol (Wickliffe, OH, USA). It is a brown, highly viscous, completely polymeric additive, which, according to the producer, is suitable for inorganic fillers in plasticizer suspensions. The chemical structure is not listed. The producer recommends an addition of 1–3% with regards to the mass of the filler.

2.1.4. Photo-Initiator

For this work, the photo-initiator Ivocerin was used exclusively. It was provided by our project partner Ivoclar Vivadent AG (Schaan, Liechtenstein). The chemical structure is shown in Figure 3. A specialty of this molecule is its considerable absorbance in the visible wavelength spectrum [19].

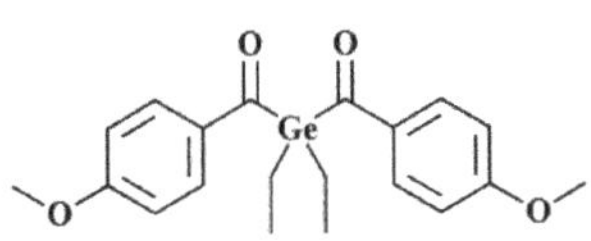

Figure 3. Chemical structure of the photo-initiator Ivocerin.

2.1.5. Absorber

The two azo-dyes Sudan IV and Disperse Orange 3 served as absorbers. They were obtained from Sigma-Aldrich (Merck KGaA, Darmstadt, Germany). The structural formulas are given in Figure 4.

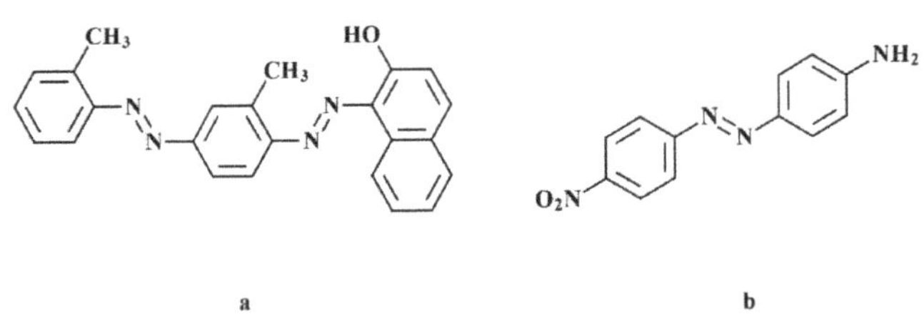

Figure 4. Chemical structures of (**a**) Sudan IV and (**b**) Disperse Orange 3.

2.1.6. Filler

As filler, the glass precursor for lithium disilicate was used. After green part production, during sintering, the crystalline phase is generated. The glass precursor has the denotation PU GM e.max LT Transpa and was provided by our project partner Ivoclar Vivadent AG (Schaan, Liechtenstein). The chemical composition is stated in Table 2.

Table 2. Chemical composition of the cast blanks.

Component	Mass Fraction (%)
SiO_2	57–80
Li_2O	11–19
K_2O	0–13
P_2O_5	0–11
ZrO_2	0–8
ZnO	0–8
Al_2O_3	0–5
MgO	0–5
Coloring Oxides	0–8

2.2. *Methods*

2.2.1. Sample Preparation

Firstly, the respective organic materials were merged according to the composition given in Table 3. The glass powder was added in two steps, after each of which a mixing time of one minute at 2350 rpm was applied. A solid loading of 72.55% with regards to the mass was utilized. Afterwards, for complete dispersion and degassing, an additional mixing program was applied, which is given in Table 4. The machine software allows the combination of several steps into one program. For the program shown in Table 4, the total mixing time is 10 min.

Table 3. Composition of the photo-reactive suspensions.

Component	Mass Fraction (%)
Solvent	11.61
Monomers	14.53
Dispersant	1.08
Photoinitiator	0.20
Absorber	0.03
Glass powder	72.55

Table 4. Program for preparing and degassing glass suspensions.

Program Step	Mixing Duration (min)	Rotational Speed (rpm)	Pressure (mbar)
1	2	2350	1000
2	3	800	500
3	5	800	100

Suspensions were prepared using a wall mixer DAC 600.2 VAC-P from the company Hauschild & Co.KG (Hamm, Germany). This model allows degassing during mixing by applying a vacuum. The range of rotational speed is 800–2350 rpm, and the maximum mixing capacity is 500 g.

2.2.2. Lithography-Based Ceramic Manufacturing

LCM is a modified version of vat photo-polymerization—a modified version of the DLP(digital light processing)-based bottom-up vat photo-polymerization, to be exact. The machine used in this work was a prototype based on the patent WO2010045951 called Blueprinter 5 (built in-house). Figure 5 shows a schematic setup, and Table 5 shows certain specifications of this machine. Exposure happens through the transparent vat. The distinctiveness of this system is the rotating material vat, which enables coating by combination with the stationary doctor blade. Additionally, the vat can be tilted to ease the process of detaching the part from the vat surface. The main difference of LCM compared to conventional vat photo-polymerization is the use of ceramic suspensions. In this regard, LCM is a shaping method within the ceramic processing route [20]. If not stated otherwise directly in the respective paragraph, a layer height of 50 μm was used in every printing process described in this work.

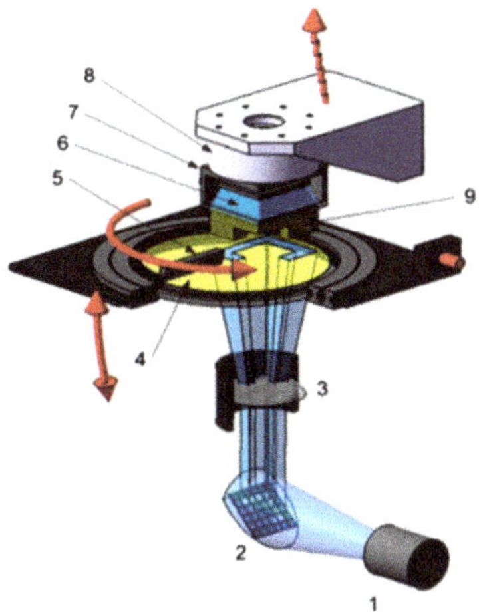

Figure 5. Schematic representation of an LCM machine: LED light source (1), DMD chip (2), optical lens (3), material vat (4), doctor blade (5), backwards exposure (6), building platform (7), load cell (8), part (9) [21]. Reproduced with permission from Passakorn Tesavibul; Ruth Felzmann; Simon Gruber; Robert Liska; Ian Thompson; Aldo R. Boccaccini; Jürgen Stampfl, Materials Letters; published by Elsevier, 2012.

Table 5. Specifications of the LCM prototype.

Specification	BP5
Exposure system	DLP
Emission wavelength (nm)	460
Resolution (pixels)	1920 × 1200
Pixel size (μm)	40
Vat diameter (mm)	150
Building volume (wxdxh) (mm)	77 × 43 × 110

2.2.3. Debinding

The thermal debinding is executed in a HRF 7/22 convection oven from Carbolite Gero GmbH & Co.KG (Neuhausen, Germany). The temperature program (E-MP/9) is shown in Figure 6 [9]. For the debinding process, green bodies are embedded in a zirconia sand (Ø = 1 mm) from the company Powdercon (Biebbertal, Germany).

2.2.4. Sintering

Sintering is performed in a Programat P700 dental oven from the company Ivoclar Vivadent AG (Schaan, Liechtenstein). This model is a small vacuum oven, which is appropriate for sintering lithium disilicate glass ceramics of the product group IPS e.max. The temperature program (RG_Lisi2_7_mod.6) is shown in Figure 7 [22].

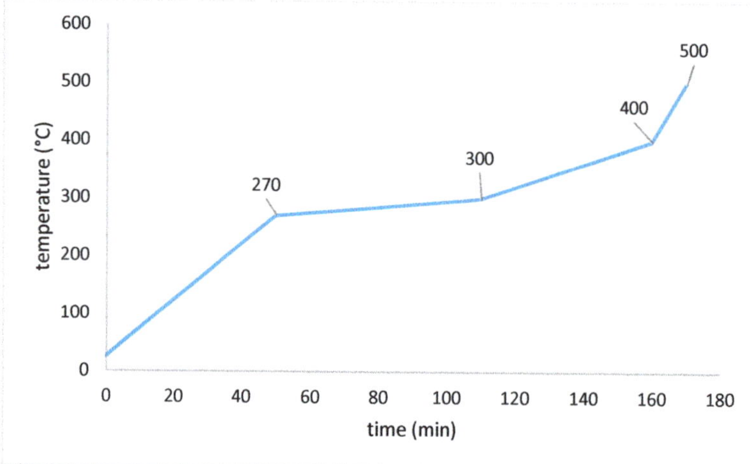

Figure 6. Debinding program E-MP/9.

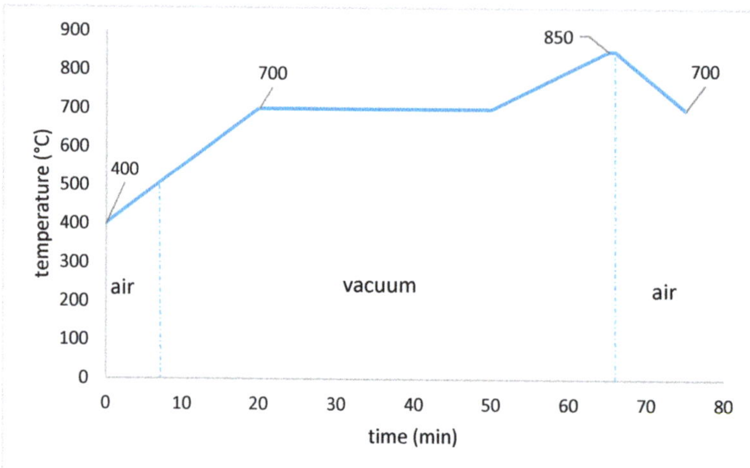

Figure 7. Sintering program RG_Lisi2_7_mod.6.

2.3. *Analyses*

2.3.1. Refractive Index

The refractive index of liquid substances was determined by using an Abbe refractometer. The temperature can be adjusted by a flow heater. In most cases in the literature, the n_D^{20} is measured, meaning the refractive index at a temperature of 20 °C and at the wavelength of the D-line of a sodium vapor lamp ($\lambda = 589$ nm). In this work, the refractive index at a temperature of 23 °C (at $\lambda = 589$ nm) was measured to reproduce the conditions in the LCM machine.

2.3.2. Exposure Tests

Exposure tests were conducted to determine the penetration depth D_p and the critical polymerization energy E_c. D_p is the penetration depth of light into the measured material, at which the irradiance has decreased to 1/e (e being Euler's constant). E_c is the exposure at which the material solidifies at least partially, meaning it is at the transition point from liquid to solid (gel point) [23].

They were performed by the following procedure: A plastic template with quadratic notches (edge length = 10 mm, depth = 3 mm) was put on a thin transparent polyethylene foil. Four notches were filled with the material to be measured. The filled template was put on the exposure area of the LCM machine, and each notch was subjected to a circular exposure field with a diameter of 6 mm. (The parameters of exposure were varied accordingly.) The (partially) cured objects were taken from the notches and their thickness was determined by using an outside micrometer. The average thickness of four specimens served as a value for the cure depth C_d at the chosen exposure (E_{max}). Determining the border between solidified and residual material can be difficult, especially for specimens with a high refractive index difference, where the specimens tend to be gelled rather than cured. This leads to a relatively high uncertainty and an imperfect fitting of the linear models in some cases. Nevertheless, the data is essential for determining the behavior of the material during the LCM process.

Subsequently, the values for C_d, depending on the exposure, were plotted in a half-logarithmical scale (Jacobs working curve). According to Equation (1), D_p is the slope of the resulting curve and E_c is the point of intersection with the x-axis. E_{max} is the maximum exposure (i.e., the exposure chosen for each measurement).

$$C_d = D_p \ln\left(\frac{E_{max}}{E_c}\right) \quad (1)$$

2.3.3. Rheology

Viscosity measurements were performed with a MCR 300 oscillation rheometer from the company Anton Paar (Graz, Austria) at room temperature (25 °C) and by utilizing a CP50-1 cone-plate system with a diameter of 50 mm and a gap height of 100 µm. Samples consisted of all the constituents of the suspension formulation (solvent, monomer, dispersing agent, filler), except for photoinitiator and absorbing agent, to avoid rheological effects in case of undesired light exposure/polymerization.

2.3.4. Thermal Analyses

Thermogravimetric analyses (TGA) were performed with a TGA Q500 from the company TA Instruments (New Castle, DE, USA). Cylindrical bodies with a height and diameter of 6 mm, produced by LCM, were measured. A heating rate of 1 K/min and a maximum temperature of 600 °C were chosen. Alumina crucibles with a low wall served as sample holders.

Thermo-mechanical analyses (TMA) were practical to determine the change of length of a specimen, depending on the temperature, and were conducted at a TMA Q400 of TA Instruments (New Castle, DE, USA). Cylindrical bodies with a height and diameter of 6 mm, produced by LCM, were measured. A heating rate of 1 K/min and a maximum temperature of 600 °C was chosen. Alumina crucibles with a high wall served as sample holders.

3. Results

3.1. Refractive Index

Halloran et al. showed that a small difference between the refractive index of the organic and the inorganic phase leads to a high precision of parts produced by AM based on photo-polymerization [12, 13]. Therefore, it was one of the core considerations of this work to reduce this difference by choosing appropriate solvents. Accordingly, the refractive indices of the pure phthalates were first determined. The component BBP shows by far the highest refractive index of the solvents. Figure 8 compares these values to the refractive indices of the monomers and to the target value of the glass precursor. Only BBP shows a higher value than the glass precursor.

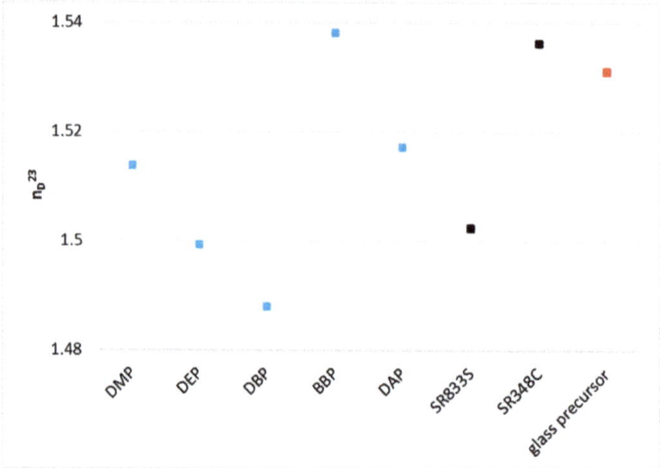

Figure 8. Comparison of the refractive indices of pure substances with the target value of the glass filler (value taken from literature [18]).

As the next step, it was necessary to determine the refractive indices of the whole organic composition for each solvent. As could be anticipated, the composition with BBP came closest to the target value, as can be seen in Figure 9. The reference was a mixture without any solvent. In conclusion, from this group of solvents, the utilization of the component BBP is to be considered when a refractive index matching is desired.

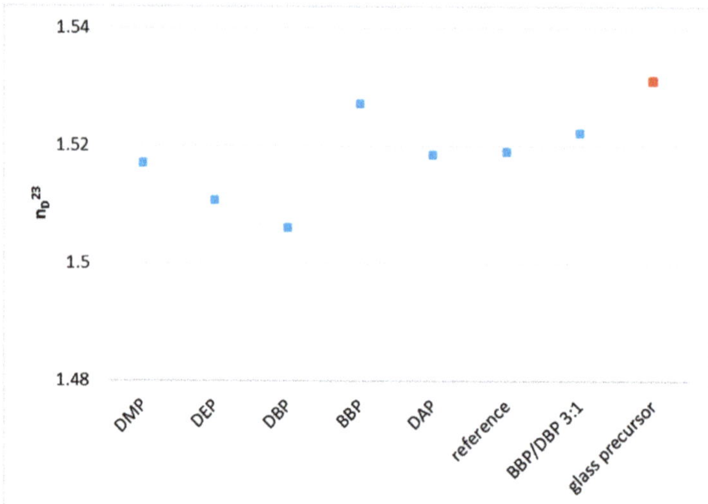

Figure 9. Refractive indices of the respective mixtures of each phthalate, the dispersing agent Solplus K500, and the monomer mixture of SR348C and SR833S.

3.2. *Rheology*

The utilization of one of the mentioned phthalates significantly reduced the viscosity, especially in the range of low shear rates, as can be seen in Figure 10. Emphasis is to be put on the composition with DBP, which showed the lowest viscosity in the range from 0–65/s and was different from the other compositions in that it showed very low viscosity at low shear rates. This resulted in the composition being flowable, but not stable against sedimentation.

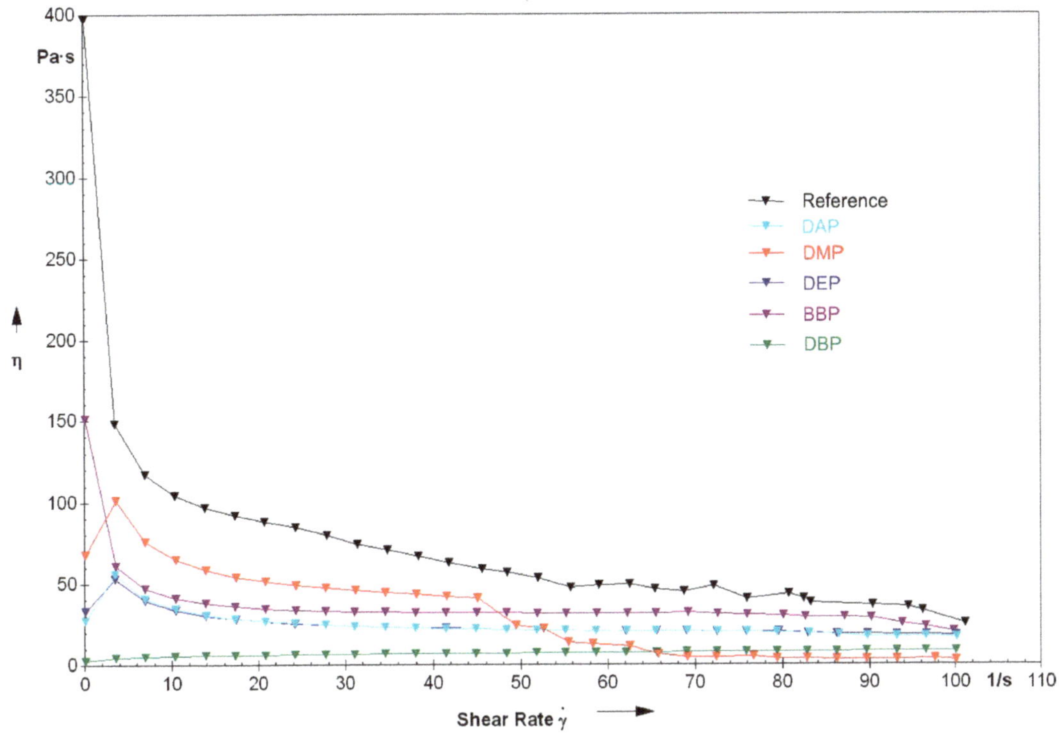

Figure 10. Viscosity in relation to shear rate for lithium disilicate suspensions prepared by using various phthalates.

Figure 11 shows the measurements for compositions with BBP and DBP, together with a composition with a 3:1 mixture of the two solvents. On the one hand, the flowability of the DBP suspension is advantageous, because it allows an uncomplicated processing. On the other hand, the rise of viscosity at low shear rates is advantageous, because it increases resistance to sedimentation. The mixture of those two phthalates makes a good compromise. On the one hand, the viscosity, compared to BBP, is decreased, and a certain flowability is present. On the other hand, the viscosity is high enough to enable stability against sedimentation, especially because of the increase of viscosity at low shear rates.

3.3. Debinding

Figure 12 shows the TGA results. In the case of the phthalate suspensions, we can see a two-step process, with the first step being the evaporation of solvents in a temperature range from 75 to 250 °C. The weight loss for the reference, about 1% in this temperature range, is negligible. The second step is the degradation of the polymer network in a temperature range from 250 to 450 °C. Compared to the reference, we can see that this step is completed at lower temperatures for the phthalate suspensions when the solid loading of 72.5 wt% is reached (DMP: 290 °C, DEP: 300 °C, DBP: 360 °C, BBP: 390 °C, DAP: 410 °C, reference: 425 °C).

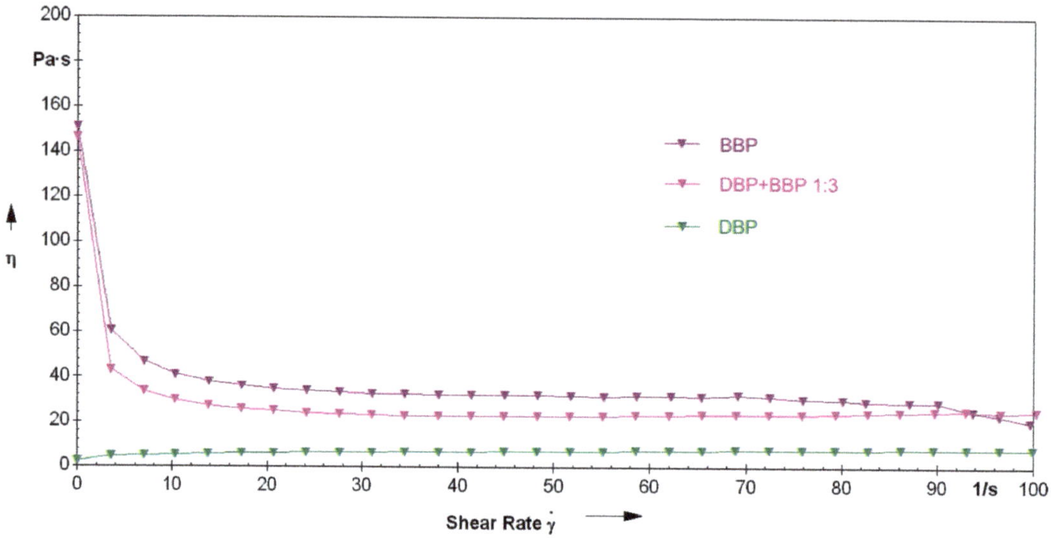

Figure 11. Direct comparison of the rheological properties of the formulations with either BBP, DBP, or a 3:1 mixture of the two.

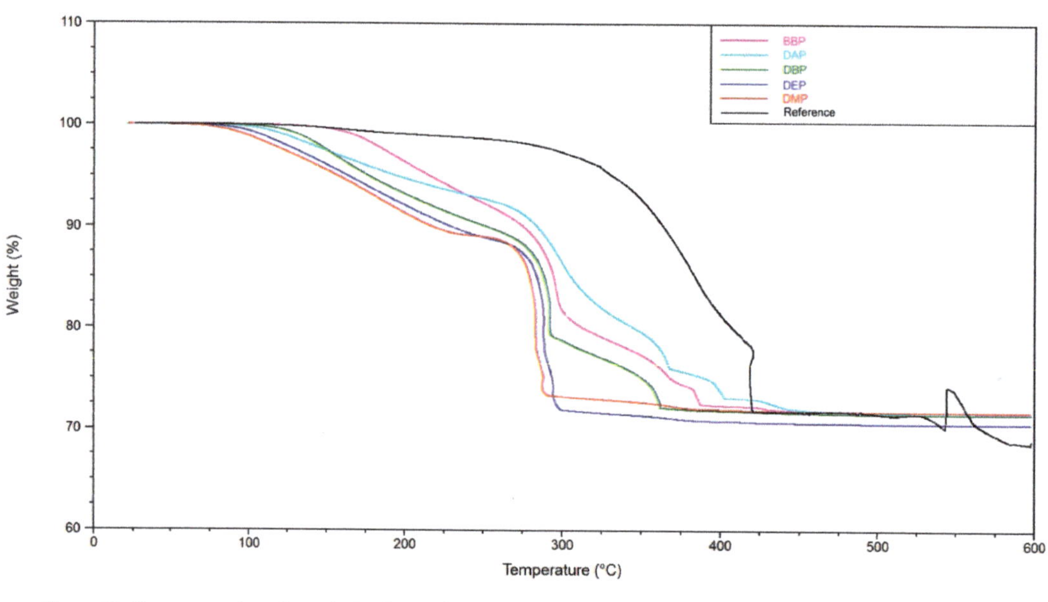

Figure 12. Thermo-gravimetric analysis of green bodies produced by LCM using suspensions with varying solvents.

In TMA measurements (Figure 13), a positive influence of the phthalates can be recognized as well. The maximum expansion for the various phthalate suspensions is under 10%, while the reference shows a maximum expansion of 50%. Together with several spikes showing rapid expansion, this means complete destruction of the part, as can be seen in Figure 15a.

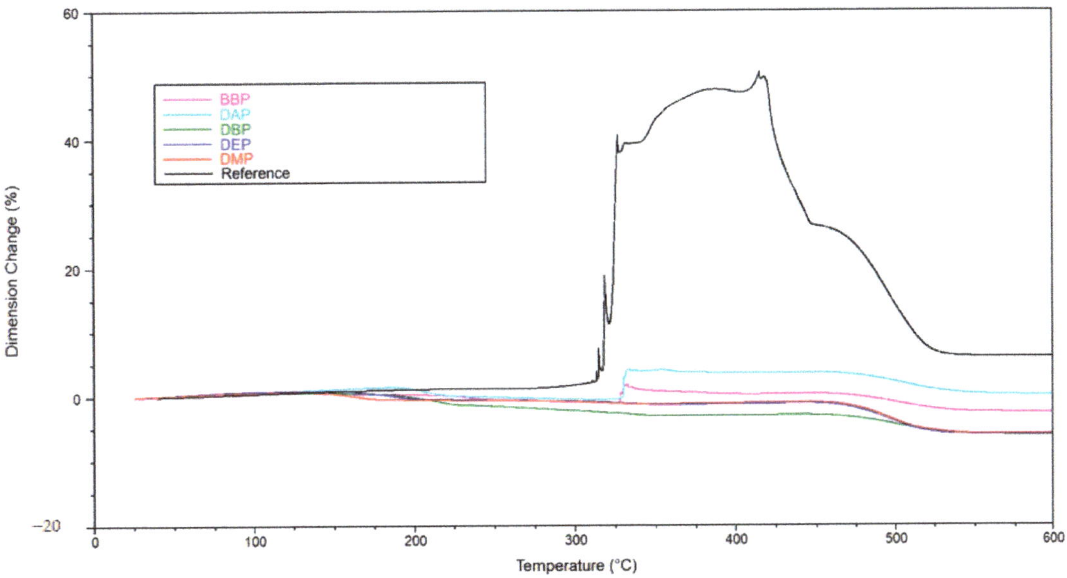

Figure 13. Thermomechanical analysis of green bodies produced by LCM using different phthalate suspensions.

In Figure 14, the reference curve is removed, and a detailed depiction of the phthalate suspensions is shown. It allows one to see that in the case of DAP and BBP, rapid expansion occurs at temperatures between 325 and 350 °C. As mentioned, this means crack extension, as can be verified in Figure 15b,c. The DBP sample is shown as an opposite example. In this case, no crack extension could be observed (Figure 15d).

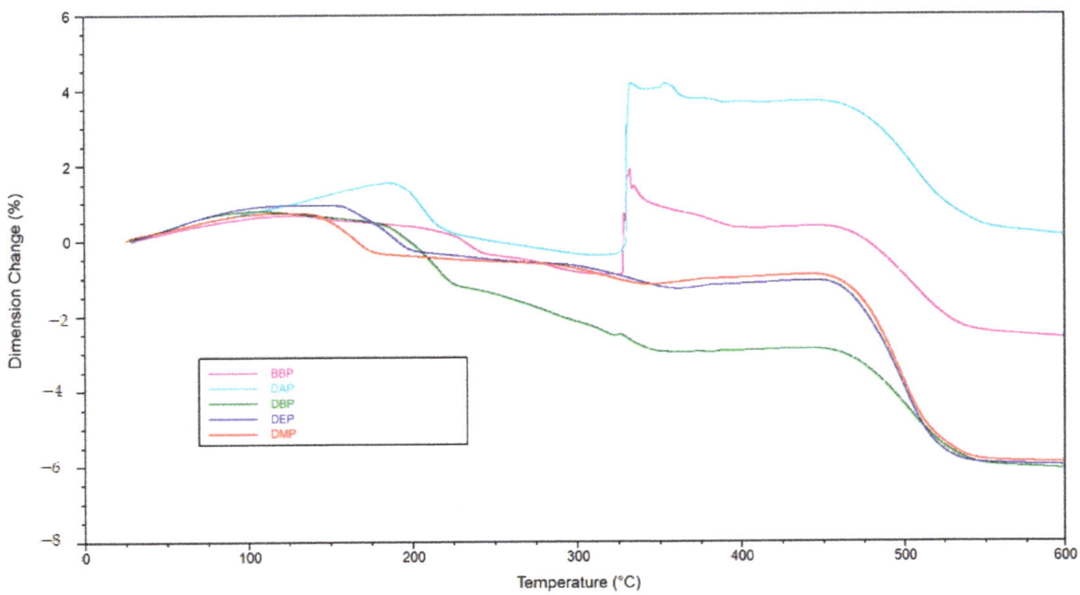

Figure 14. Detailed depiction of the thermomechanical analysis from Figure 13.

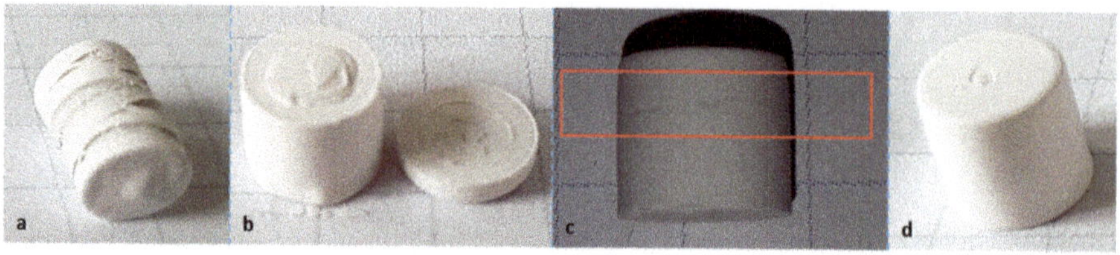

Figure 15. Specimens after the thermomechanical analysis from Figure 13; (**a**) reference, (**b**) DAP, (**c**) BBP, (**d**) DBP.

As mentioned previously, the component BBP is necessary when a refractive index matching is desired. Should crack extension be unavoidable during debinding (at considerably low heating rates of 1 K/min), this component needs to be discarded. To allow at least a partial utilization of BBP, it was attempted to specifically mix in a certain amount of DBP, since it showed the lowest expansion during TMA measurements, and additionally, had a positive influence on the rheological properties (increase of flowability).

Figure 16 shows the direct comparison of the TMA measurements of green bodies produced by LCM using suspensions with either BBP, DBP, or a 3:1 mixture of the two solvents. To make sure the results are reproducible, two single measurements were performed in each case. For the mixture of BBP/DBP, there is no crack extension observable. Even the small peak at 325 °C, in the case of DBP, could be avoided. A possible explanation is that DBP exits the green body slightly earlier (bp. 340 °C) than BBP (bp. 370 °C) and leaves open porosity, which facilitates the exit of BBP and of degradation products of the polymer network later.

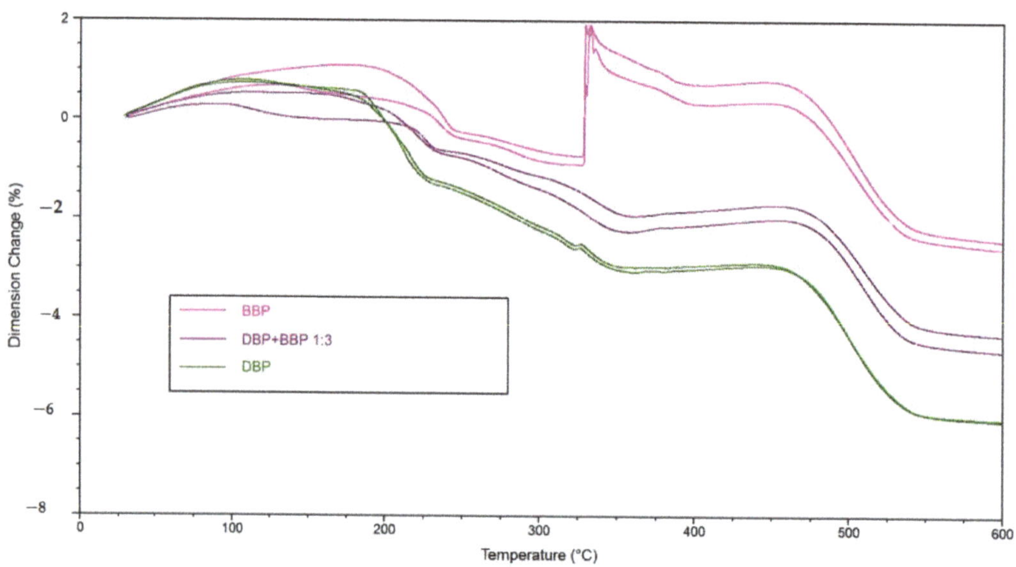

Figure 16. Direct comparison of the thermomechanical measurements (two each) of green bodies, produced by LCM with BBP, DBP, and 3:1-mixture of both, respectively.

3.4. Exposure Tests

To characterize the behavior of the different phthalate suspensions during the exposure in the AM process, exposure tests were performed. Figure 17 shows the Jacobs working curve for the especially relevant suspensions with BBP, DBP, and a 3:1 mixture of the two. Table 5 lists the parameters calculated from the working curves.

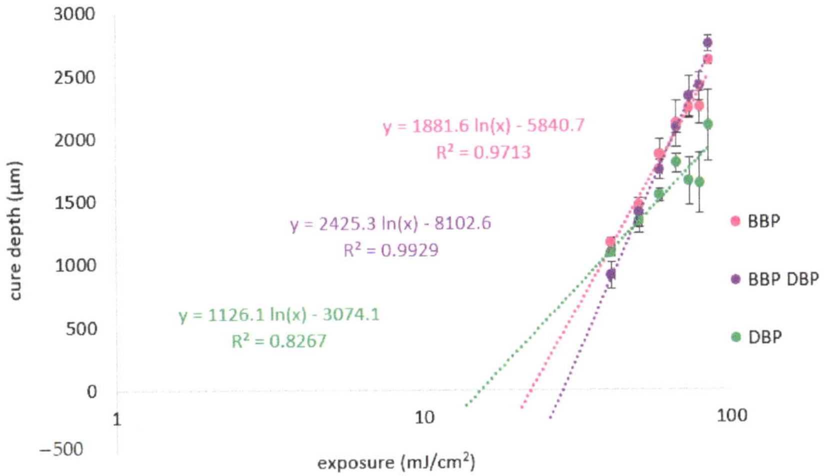

Figure 17. Jacobs working curve for lithium disilicate suspensions prepared by using various phthalates and no absorbing agent.

According to theory, D_p should increase with decreasing difference of refractive index between organic mixture and filler of the suspension. The results for DBP and BBP fit well to this expectation (Table 6). The refractive index difference is comparatively high for the DBP suspension, therefore D_p is low. The refractive index difference is low for the BBP suspension, therefore D_p is high. Opposingly, it is surprising that the highest value is achieved for the mixture of the two phthalates. Previously, we have seen that the refractive index matching is best for the BBP suspension. Therefore, the highest value was expected for the BBP sample.

Table 6. Penetration depth and critical polymerization energy, calculated from Figure 17.

Suspension	D_p (µm)	E_c (mJ/cm^2)
DBP	1126	15
BBP	1882	22
BBP/DBP 3:1	2425	28

Two explanations are possible. On the one hand, the refractive index of the material rises during polymerization. Should this rise in refractive index lead to a better matching, this could explain the higher D_p. On the other hand, the target value of the glass filler is a literature value. In the literature, it is already noted that the refractive index (depending on the batch) can vary between 1.528 and 1.534. Consequently, the exact target value for this batch is not known and should be determined experimentally.

The high penetration depths of the phthalate suspensions lead to the necessity for high concentrations of absorbing agents to effectively decrease D_p. In this work, two substances were examined for this purpose: Disperse Orange 3 (DO3) and Sudan IV (S4). Figure 18 shows the Jacobs working curves for the suspensions with a 3:1 mixture of BBP/DBP, with a concentration of 0.03% with regards to the total mass of the suspension for DO3 and S4, respectively.

Both absorbing agents lead to similar values for D_p, as can be seen in Table 6. It is noticeable that in the case of DO3, E_c is increased by a factor of four, compared to the version without absorbing agent (Table 7). In the case of S4, E_c remains nearly unchanged.

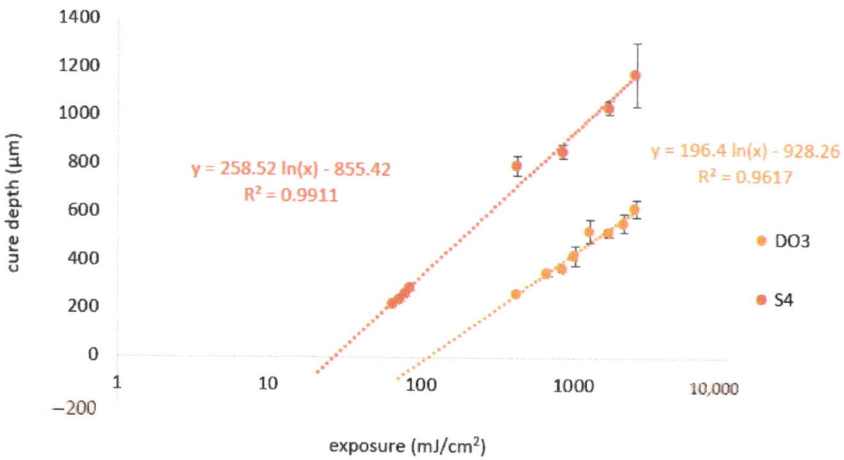

Figure 18. Jacobs working curve for lithium disilicate suspensions prepared by using a 3:1-mixture of BBP and DBP and either Sudan IV or Disperse Orange 3 as absorber.

Table 7. Penetration depth and critical polymerization energy, calculated from Figure 18.

Suspension	D_p [µm]	E_c [mJ/cm^2]
Disperse Orange 3	196	113
Sudan IV	259	27

These perceptions are relevant for the exposure time in the AM process. Figure 19 shows two siemens stars, produced by LCM using a suspension with a 3:1 mixture of BBP/DBP with either DO3 (a) or S4 (b) in the same concentration (0.03%). In the case of DO3, an exposure time of 10 s was needed. In the case of S4, an exposure time of 1 s was needed. In both cases, an exposure of 85 mW/cm^2 was applied.

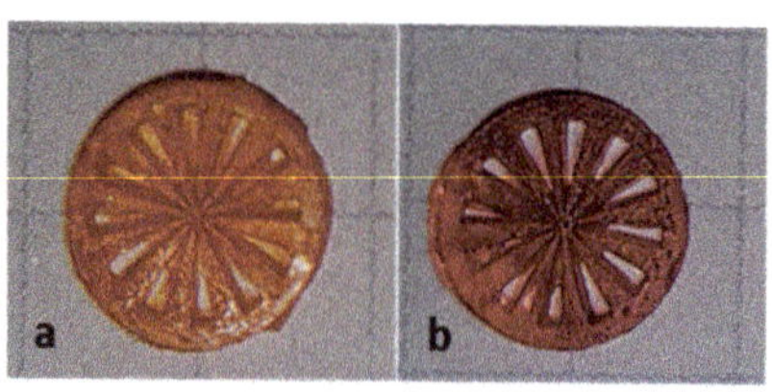

Figure 19. Green bodies of Siemens stars produced by LCM, using Disperse Orange 3 (**a**) and Sudan IV (**b**).

4. Discussion

4.1. Refractive Index

Using phthalates, the refractive index of the organic fraction can be increased significantly and therefore matched closely to the refractive index of the inorganic phase. By choosing a 3:1 mixture of BBP/DBP, the difference between organic and inorganic phase is $\Delta n = 0.0089$.

Some issues persist with regards to a perfect refractive index matching. Firstly, the target value is a literature value. The refractive index of the filler varies according to the producer, with a relatively big margin ($n = 1.531 \pm 0.003$). The experimental determination of the refractive index of the glass powder batch at hand should give a more exact and reliable value. Secondly, the refractive indices of all the components of the formulation should be determined at processing temperature and processing wavelength to reach the target value precisely. The presented solvents are an appropriate tool for that.

4.2. Debinding

The TGA and TMA experiments clearly show two things. On the one hand, the utilization of a solvent enables a debinding procedure without crack extension (see reference without solvent). On the other hand, the choice of solvent is a deciding factor for the speed that can be applied to this procedure. At a heating rate of 1 K/min, the application of BBP and DAP leads to crack extension. In the case of DMP, DEP, and DBP, this heating rate could be used without crack extension. An additional observation is that by adding a component that is easily debindable (in this case DBP), the crack extension can effectively be avoided. Accordingly, a 3:1 mixture of BBP/DBP leads to a successful debinding procedure at the same heating rate.

A possible explanation is that the DBP molecules, due to their chemical constitution, possess a weaker intermolecular interaction with the other components inside the green body, for example BBP, and exit the green body at lower temperatures (TGA, Figure 12). An interesting subject for future work would be to determine the intermolecular interactions by quantum mechanical calculations. We estimate that, consequently, more open porosity is present in the green body that facilitates the exit of polymer degradation products at a later stage of the procedure. If both mechanisms happen chronologically separated, a successful debinding is to be expected. In the case of BBP, the exit of the solvent molecules happens at a higher temperature/later in time, which is the reason why, presumably, not enough open porosity is present when the degradation of the polymer network starts. Consequently, a higher pressure builds up inside the green body, which eventually leads to fracture of the sample, as shown in the TMA measurements (Figures 13 and 14). Therefore, it is necessary to choose an easily debindable component that establishes enough open porosity early on, before the degradation of the polymer network begins.

4.3. Rheology

Likewise, regarding rheology, the choice of the solvent is of major significance. Accordingly, the viscosity of a suspension prepared without a solvent is at 100–75 Pa·s for a shear rate range of 15–45 s^{-1}. Opposingly, the viscosity of the suspension prepared with the 3:1 mixture of BBP/DBP is at 30 Pa·s for the same shear rate range.

An explanation for the different rheological behavior of the DBP suspension could be the already mentioned weaker intermolecular forces. Due to the lipophile character of DBP (compared to, for example, DMP), the non-covalent network structure of the suspension is not as pronounced. This network structure seems to be significant for the buildup of stability.

4.4. Absorbing Agent

The results of the exposure tests could identify a deciding disadvantage of DO3: at a concentration that is necessary to reduce the penetration depth to an appropriate extent, the critical polymerization energy is increased by a factor of four. This shows an inhibition of the polymerization by the mono azo dye. We assume that the reason for this is the nitro function on the phenyl ring, which acts as a radical quencher by mesomeric effect. With Sudan IV, an alternative option was presented that can reduce D_p effectively without increasing E_c. With this alternative, the exposure time could be reduced from 10 s to 1 s.

Conclusively, it was shown that by changing the solvent, many important properties of a photoreactive suspension for the additive manufacturing of glass ceramics can be influenced, and by combination, those properties can be adapted according to requirements.

Future investigations should focus on other groups of solvents to improve the refractive index matching even further, and to see if shown benefits can be reproduced with other chemical substances. Additionally, it should be investigated if these considerations regarding the formulation of a photoreactive suspension are also valid for other types of glasses or glass ceramics, and how these changes affect the final properties of the ceramics, like translucency/transparency or mechanical strength.

Author Contributions: Conceptualization, M.H. and M.P.; methodology, M.H. and M.P.; validation, M.H. and J.S.; formal analysis, M.H.; investigation, M.H.; resources, J.S.; data curation, M.H.; writing—original draft preparation, M.H.; writing—review and editing, M.H.; visualization, M.H.; supervision, J.S.; project administration, J.S.; funding acquisition, J.S. All authors have read and agreed to the published version of the manuscript.

Funding: Financial support from the Austrian Federal Ministry for Digital and Economic Affairs; the National Foundation for Research, Technology, and Development; and the Christian Doppler Research Association is gratefully acknowledged (Christian Doppler Laboratory for Digital and Restorative Dentistry).

Institutional Review Board Statement: Not applicable.

Informed Consent Statement: Not applicable.

Data Availability Statement: The data presented in this study are available on request from the corresponding author. The data are not publicly available due to a retention period.

Conflicts of Interest: The authors declare no conflict of interest.

References

1. Duret, F.; Blouin, J.-L.; Duret, U.B. CAD-CAM in Dentistry. *J. Am. Dent. Assoc.* **1998**, *117*, 715–720. [CrossRef] [PubMed]
2. Hartmann, M.; Stampfl, J. Additive Fertigung in der digitalen Zahnheilkunde. *BHM Berg-Hüttenmänn. Mon.* **2019**. [CrossRef]
3. Gebhardt, A.; Kessler, J.; Thurn, L. *3D-Drucken: Grundlagen und Anwendungen des Additive Manufacturing (AM)*; Aufl. München: Hanser, München, 2016.
4. Baltzer, A. *Oxidkeramiken und CAD/CAM-Technologien: Atlas für Klinik, Labortechnik und Werkstoffkunde*; Deutscher Ärzteverlag: Köln, Germany, 2007.
5. Choi, G.N.; Krieger, I.M. Rheological studies on sterically stabilized model dispersions of uniform colloidal spheres: II. Steady-shear viscosity. *J. Colloid Interface Sci.* **1986**, *113*, 101–113. [CrossRef]
6. Farris, R.J. Prediction of the Viscosity of Multimodal Suspensions from Unimodal Viscosity Data. *Trans. Soc. Rheol.* **1968**, *12*, 281–301. [CrossRef]
7. Hunter, R.J. *Foundations of Colloid Science*; Oxford University Press: Oxford, UK, 2001.
8. Napper, D.H. *Polymeric Stabilization of Colloidal Dispersions*; Academic Press: New York, NY, USA, 1983.
9. Pfaffinger, M. Entwicklung und Optimierung Photopolymerisierbarer Schlicker für den Lithography-Based Ceramic Manufacturing (LCM) Prozess. Ph.D. Thesis, Technische Universität Wien, Vienna, Austria, 2017.
10. Fundamental Technical Standards Committee. *Nicht newtonsche Flüssigkeiten. Viskosität—Teil 3*; DIN 1342-3; Beuth Verlag GmbH: Berlin, Germany, 2011.
11. Pfaffinger, M.; Hartmann, M.; Schwentenwein, M.; Stampfl, J. Stabilization of tricalcium phosphate slurries against sedimentation for stereolithographic additive manufacturing and influence on the final mechanical properties. *Int. J. Appl. Ceram. Technol.* **2017**, *14*, 499–506. [CrossRef]
12. Gentry, S.P.; Halloran, J.W. Light scattering in absorbing ceramic suspensions: Effect on the width and depth of photopolymerized features. *J. Eur. Ceram. Soc.* **2015**, *35*, 1895–1904. [CrossRef]
13. Halloran, J.W. Ceramic Stereolithography: Additive Manufacturing for Ceramics by Photopolymerization. *Annu. Rev. Mater. Res.* **2016**, *46*, 19–40. [CrossRef]
14. Hofstetter, C.; Orman, S.; Baudis, S.; Stampfl, J. Combining cure depth and cure degree, a new way to fully characterize novel photopolymers. *Addit. Manuf.* **2018**, *24*, 166–172. [CrossRef]
15. Lewis, J.A. Binder removal from Ceramics. *Annu. Rev. Mater. Sci.* **1997**, *27*, 147–173. [CrossRef]
16. Kashiwagi, T.; Hirata, T.; Brown, J.E. Thermal and oxidative degradation of poly(methyl methacrylate) molecular weight. *Macromolecules* **1985**, *18*, 131–138. [CrossRef]
17. Dong, C.; Bowen, H.K. Hot-Stage Study of Bubble Formation During Binder Burnout. *J. Am. Ceram. Soc.* **1989**, *72*, 1082–1087. [CrossRef]
18. Cima, M.J.; Lewis, J.A.; Devoe, A.D. Binder Distribution in Ceramic Greenware During Thermolysis. *J. Am. Ceram. Soc.* **1989**, *72*, 1192–1199. [CrossRef]
19. Hirt, T.; Moszner, N. *Report aus Forschung und Entwicklung*; F&E Ivoclar Vivadent AG: Schaan, Liechtenstein, 2013.
20. Euroceram-Bottom-UP Process. Available online: https://www.euroceram.org/en/technologies/photopolymerization/bottom-up-process.html (accessed on 28 August 2019).
21. Tesavibul, P. Processing of 45S5 Bioglass® by lithography-based additive manufacturing. *Mater. Lett.* **2012**, *74*, 81–84. [CrossRef]
22. Gmeiner, R. Stereolithographic Ceramic Manufacturing (SLCM) of Lithium Disilicate and Bioactive Glass Ceramics for Dental and Medical Applications. Ph.D. Thesis, Technische Universität Wien, Vienna, Austria, 2016.
23. Jacobs, P.F. Fundamentals of Stereolithography. *Int. Solid Free. Fabr. Symp.* **1992**, *16*. [CrossRef]

materials

MDPI

Article

In Vitro Comparison between Metal Sleeve-Free and Metal Sleeve-Incorporated 3D-Printed Computer-Assisted Implant Surgical Guides

Kyung Chul Oh, June-Sung Shim and Ji-Man Park *

Department of Prosthodontics, Yonsei University College of Dentistry, Seoul 03722, Korea; kyungabc@yuhs.ac (K.C.O.); jfshim@yuhs.ac (J.-S.S.)
* Correspondence: jimarn@yuhs.ac; Tel.: +82-2-2228-3156; Fax: +82-2-312-3598

Abstract: The present study aims to compare the accuracy of metal sleeve-free 3D-printed computer-assisted implant surgical guides (MSF group) ($n = 10$) with metal sleeve-incorporated 3D-printed computer-assisted implant surgical guides (MSI group) ($n = 10$). Implants of diameter 4.0 mm and 5.0 mm were placed in the left second premolars and bilateral first molars, respectively, using a fully guided system. Closed-form sleeves were used in teeth on the left and open-form sleeves on the right. The weight differences of the surgical guides before and after implant placement, and angular deviations before and after implant placement were measured. Weight differences were compared with Student's t-tests and angular deviations with Mann–Whitney tests. Cross-sectional views of the insert parts were observed with a scanning electron microscope. Preoperative and postoperative weight differences between the two groups were not statistically significant ($p = 0.821$). In terms of angular deviations, those along the mesiodistal direction for the left second premolars were significantly lower in the MSF group ($p = 0.006$). However, those along the mesiodistal direction for the bilateral molars and those along the buccolingual direction for all teeth were not significantly different ($p > 0.05$). 3D-printed implant surgical guides without metal sleeve inserts enable accurate implant placement without exhausting the guide holes, rendering them feasible for fully guided implant placement.

Keywords: computer-assisted implant surgical guide; metal sleeve-free implant surgical guide; metal sleeve-incorporated surgical guide; additive manufacturing; angular deviation; fully guided implant placement

1. Introduction

Prosthetically driven implant placement has long been considered fundamental for the long-term success of dental implants [1,2]. However, it was not until the 1990s that this protocol was clinically implemented. The emergence of cone-beam computed tomography (CBCT) scanning and the development of dental implant planning software have significantly contributed to achieving this goal [3,4]. Currently, additive manufacturing or 3D printing is commonly used in dentistry, with its most extensive application being the fabrication of computer-assisted surgical stents or guides [5,6]. Compared to milling technology, it decreases the laboratory time and reduces material consumption [7].

Surgical stents help clinicians locate the initial entry point of implants and partially navigate the direction and angulation of the implants [8,9]. In contrast, surgical guides differ from surgical stents as they aim to accurately navigate the direction, depth, and angulation of implants [9,10]. Several comparative in vitro and in vivo studies evaluating the accuracy of surgical stents and guides have been performed. These studies reported that the mean angular deviation of dental implants placed with the aid of surgical stents and surgical guides ranged from 4.65° to 7.79° and 2.30° to 4.16°, respectively, indicating the superior accuracy of fully guided implant placement system [9,11–13].

Sleeves play an important role in achieving this purpose. These are equipped as prefabricated metal forms (i.e., metal sleeve) or their information is incorporated in the designing software of the surgical guide so that they can be manufactured simultaneously during additive manufacturing of surgical guides (i.e., metal sleeve-free) [14]. Studies that compared the accuracy of implant placement in relation to the pre-planned implant positions with the use of surgical guides commonly used surgical guides that required metal sleeve insertion; industrial 3D printers were used to fabricate the body of the surgical guides, and the metal sleeves were inserted [12,15–22]. As in-office 3D printers are becoming more popular and their accuracy is being reported as comparable to that of industrial printers, metal sleeveless surgical guides are becoming a major trend [23–25].

However, the diameter of the sleeves in metal sleeveless surgical guides may be prone to distortion and may cause variations in the inner diameter of the sleeves, depending on the build-angle condition during additive manufacturing [26]. In addition, debris may easily accumulate around the surgical sites [27]. In contrast, metal sleeves may be fabricated with a larger tolerance to allow the rotation of the guide drills, as these sleeves are more resistant to trimming [28]. It can be hypothesized that these characteristics may affect both the safety and accuracy of implant placement.

Hence, the present study aimed to compare the safety and accuracy of metal sleeve-free 3D-printed computer-assisted implant surgical guides with metal sleeve-incorporated 3D-printed computer-assisted implant surgical guides in a fully guided implant placement system. The loss of any material component was measured by the weight difference, and the accuracy of the implant placement was evaluated by measuring the angular deviation. The null hypothesis was that the weight difference of the surgical guides and the angular deviation of the implants before and after implant placement would differ between the two types of surgical guides.

2. Materials and Methods

2.1. Preparation of the Typodonts and Classification of the Groups

A total of 20 mandibular typodonts (CIBM01, Osstem, Busan, Korea) with missing right first molars and left second premolars and first molars were used in this study. Radiopaque markers (Tetric N-Ceram, Ivoclar Vivadent, Schaan, Liechtenstein) were attached to the buccal surfaces of the bilateral second molars and the labial surface of the right central incisor (Figure 1). Ten typodonts received implant placement with metal sleeve-free 3D-printed computer-assisted implant surgical guides (n = 10, MSF group) for all implants, whereas the remaining ten received implant placement with metal sleeve-incorporated 3D-printed computer-assisted implant surgical guides (n = 10, MSI group) for all implants.

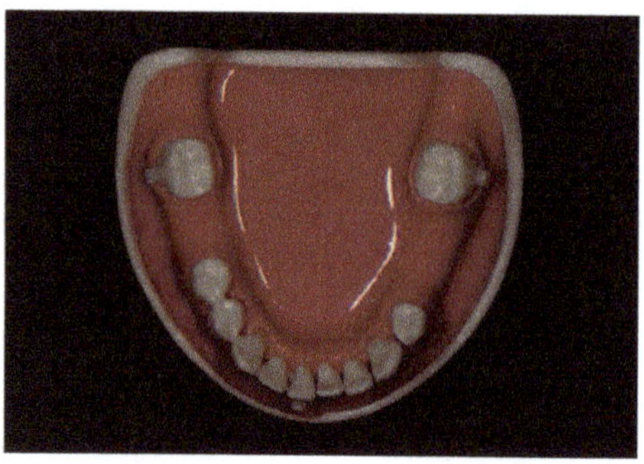

Figure 1. Mandibular typodont (CIBM01, Osstem, Busan, Korea) used in the present study. Radiopaque markers (Tetric N-Ceram, Ivoclar Vivadent, Schaan, Liechtenstein) were attached to the buccal surfaces of the bilateral second molars and the labial surface of the right central incisor.

2.2. Design and Fabrication of the Computer-Assisted Implant Surgical Guides

Each typodont was scanned using a tabletop scanner (T500, Medit Co., Seoul, Korea) and a CBCT scanner (PHT-30LFO, Vatech, Seoul, Korea). The resultant standard tessellation language (STL) file and the Digital Imaging and Communications in Medicine files were imported into an implant planning software program (Implant Studio version 1.7.3.2, 3Shape A/S, Copenhagen, Denmark). The three radiopaque markers served as references to align the surface scan data obtained with the tabletop scanner and the CBCT scan data by a 3-point matching method.

Placement of a 4.0 mm diameter implant (TSIII, Osstem) was planned for the left second premolar, and that of 5.0 mm diameter implants (TSIII) was planned for the bilateral first molars. The guides were designed such that the implants could be placed under complete guidance using a fully guided surgical kit (OneGuide, Osstem). For the left second premolar and first molar, the sleeves were designed in a closed form, whereas for the right first molar, the sleeve was designed in an open form. For the MSI group, an additional step was included within the workflow of the software program to select the metal sleeves before finalizing the guide design.

All surgical guides were fabricated one-by-one by a 3D printer (NextDent 5100, 3D Systems, Rock Hill, SC, USA) that uses a continuous digital light processing technology and a resin material (NextDent SG, 3D Systems). All guides were printed with a 30° build orientation angle and a slicing resolution along the z-axis of 100 μm. The guides were soaked in isopropyl alcohol for 10 min and cured in a post-curing machine for 30 min (LC-3DPrint Box, 3D Systems). Subsequently, the supports were removed, and the guides were polished. For the MSI group, the sleeves were attached to the guides by means of cyanoacrylate glue (Loctite, Düsseldorf, Germany) (Figure 2).

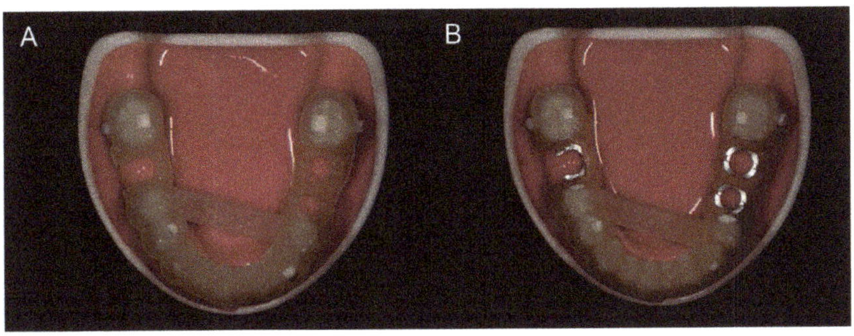

Figure 2. 3D-printed computer-assisted implant surgical guides fabricated with a 3D printer (NextDent 5100, 3D Systems, Rock Hill, SC, USA) and a resin material (NextDent SG, 3D Systems). (**A**) Metal sleeve-free surgical guide (MSF group). (**B**) Metal sleeve-incorporated surgical guide (MSI group).

2.3. Measurement of the Weight Difference of the Surgical Guides before and after Implant Placement

Prior to implant placement, the weight of each surgical guide was measured using an electronic scale (OHAUS Explorer EX324G, OHAUS Corp., Parsippany, NJ, USA). Immediately after implant placement, the weight of the surgical guides was re-measured with the same electronic scale.

2.4. Surgical Procedures

Drilling procedures were performed according to the manufacturer's guidelines by an experienced clinician. Two identical sets of drills were prepared for the drillings and applied separately for each group. After the surgical guide was placed on its corresponding typodont, tissue punch drills were applied to the surgical sites to remove the gingival portion of the typodont. Subsequently, initial drills were applied, and then a tapered drill designated for implants with the corresponding implant diameter and a length of 7 mm was applied. Two additional tapered drills with the same diameter were used to finalize the drilling procedures. The drills were not rotated prior to their insertion into the sleeves to avoid unintentionally damaging the surgical guide surface around the sleeves. The drillings were conducted in a to-and-fro motion, and all drilling procedures were conducted under profound saline irrigation, with the drilling speeds ranging from 800 to 1200 rpm. Finally, the implants were inserted with the surgical guides placed on the typdont. The insertion torques ranged from 30 to 50 N cm.

2.5. *Measurement of the Angular Deviation of the Implants*

Scan bodies (TSSBM and TSBS, Osstem) were connected to the three implants on each typodont, scanned with a tabletop scanner (T500), and saved as an STL file. An extra 4.0 mm diameter implant and an extra 5.0 mm diameter implant were prepared and connected to the corresponding scan body individually and then scanned using the same tabletop scanner. The files were then saved in STL format. The implant-scan body assembly was superimposed over the typodont with scan bodies connected by means of the common part, using the best-fit alignment function in CAD software. This enabled the presentation of implant fixtures on the STL file of the typodont and was saved as another STL file. This STL file was re-imported into the same implant-planning software program [29]. The angulation between the preoperative and postoperative stages of the implant was measured from both the mesiodistal and buccolingual perspectives (Figure 3).

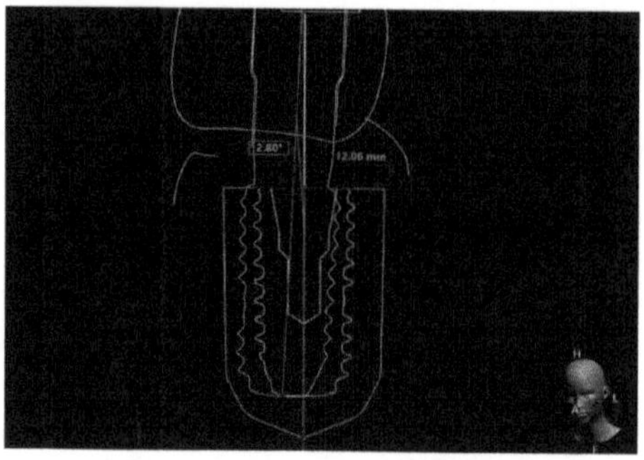

Figure 3. Representative image of the measurement method of the preoperative and postoperative angular deviation of the implant using the implant planning software program (Implant Studio version 1.7.3.2, 3Shape A/S, Copenhagen, Denmark). The green line indicates the contour of the implant in the preoperative stage, whereas the yellow line indicates the postoperative contour.

2.6. *Scanning Electron Microscopic (SEM) Analysis*

Cross-sectional surfaces of the metal sleeve-free insert parts and metal sleeve inserts were obtained before and after the drilling procedures. The surfaces were coated with platinum using a sputter coater (E-1010, Hitachi, Ltd., Tokyo, Japan) with a 100 nm thickness. The specimens were observed with a scanning electron microscope (Hitachi S-3000 N, Hitachi, Ltd.) at an accelerating voltage of 15 kV and under 18× and 80× magnifications.

2.7. *Statistical Analysis*

Student's *t*-test was used to compare the mean weight difference between the two groups, and Mann–Whitney tests were used to compare the mean angular deviations. The data were analyzed using statistical software (IBM SPSS Statistics v23.0, IBM Corp, Armonk, NY, USA), with the level of significance set to $\alpha = 0.05$.

3. Results

All 20 implant surgical guides were successfully fabricated. The mean of the preoperative and postoperative weight differences of the surgical guides in the MSF and MSI groups were 21.09 mg and 21.49 mg, respectively. No statistically significant differences were observed between the two groups ($p = 0.821$) (Figure 4 and Table 1). Statistically significant differences were observed in terms of the angular deviations mesiodistally for the left second premolar area, with the MSF group exhibiting significantly smaller angular deviations ($p = 0.006$), while the differences were not significant buccolingually between the two groups ($p = 0.125$) (Figure 5 and Table 1). There were no statistically significant differences between the two groups either buccolingually or mesiodistally for the right first molar ($p = 0.617$ and $p = 0.294$, respectively) as well as either buccolingually or mesiodistally for the left first molar ($p > 0.999$ and $p = 0.989$, respectively). Pre-drilling, the SEM image of the MSF group appeared layered; however, after drilling, a squeezed area appeared (Figure 6). Pre-drilling, the SEM of the MSI group showed a smooth metal surface. Post-drilling, a significant black area appeared (Figure 7).

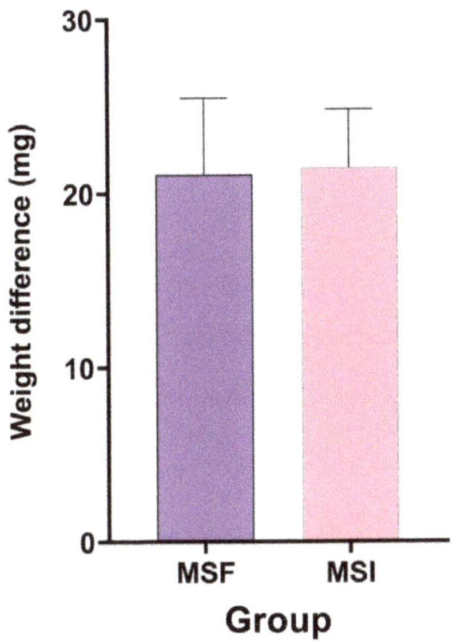

Figure 4. Preoperative and postoperative weight differences of the MSF and MSI groups. No statistically significant differences were observed. Data are expressed as mean ± standard deviations.

Table 1. Weight difference of the surgical guides prior to and following implant placement and angular deviations prior to and following implant placement between the MSF and MSI groups. Data are expressed as mean ± standard deviations. BL, buccolingual. MD, mesiodistal.

Group		MSF	MSI
Weight difference (mg)		21.09 ± 4.38	21.49 ± 3.34
	Measurement location and direction		
Angular deviation (°)	46BL	2.97 ± 2.62	3.52 ± 2.76
	46MD	0.41 ± 0.95	0.84 ± 1.07
	35BL	1.15 ± 1.38	0.49 ± 1.04
	35MD *	0.61 ± 0.65	3.01 ± 1.68
	36BL	1.62 ± 1.65	1.49 ± 1.46
	36MD	0.96 ± 0.57	0.90 ± 0.96

An asterisk indicates the statistically significant difference ($p < 0.05$).

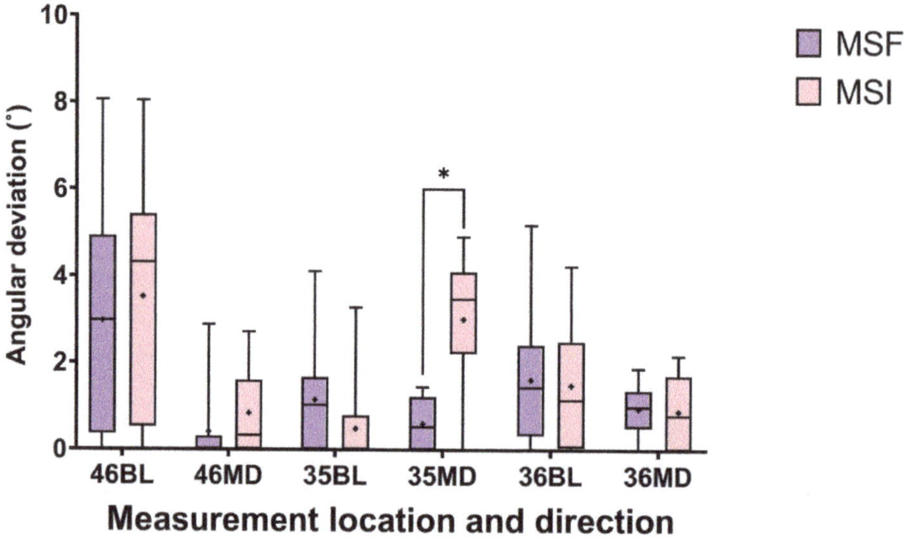

Figure 5. Preoperative and postoperative angular deviations of the MSF and MSI groups. The lines inside the boxes indicate median values, and the cross signs inside the boxes indicate mean values. The borders of the boxes indicate the 25th and 75th percentiles. The whiskers indicate the minimum and maximum values. The statistically significant difference is marked with an asterisk ($p < 0.05$). BL, buccolingual. MD, mesiodistal.

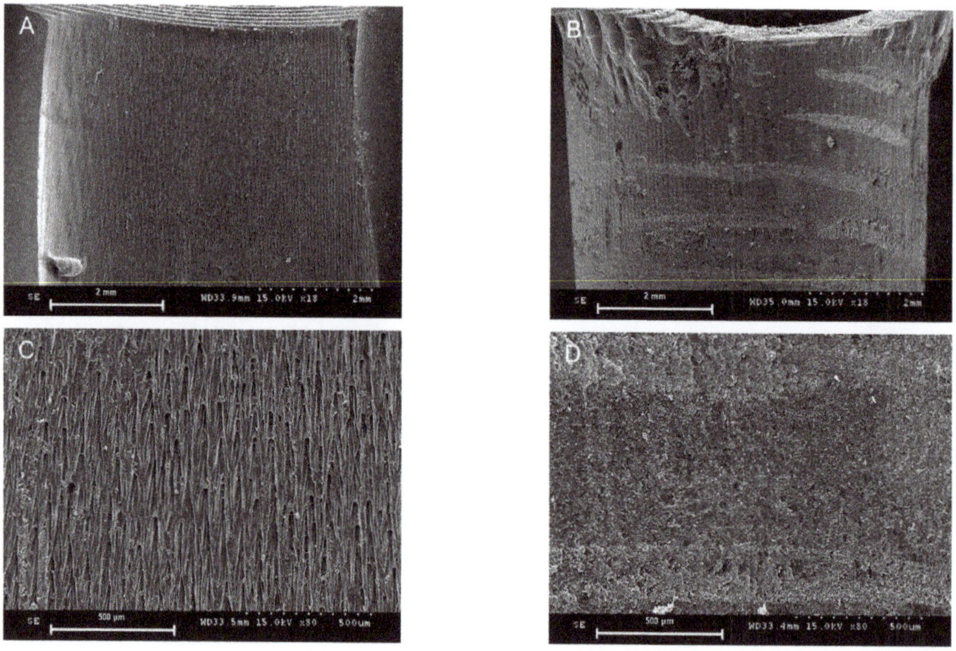

Figure 6. Representative scanning electron microscopic images. Cross-sectional view of a sleeve insert from a preoperative (**A**) and a postoperative (**B**) image from the MSF group in a lower magnification (18×). Cross-sectional view of a sleeve insert from a preoperative (**C**) and a postoperative (**D**) image from the MSF group at a higher magnification (80×).

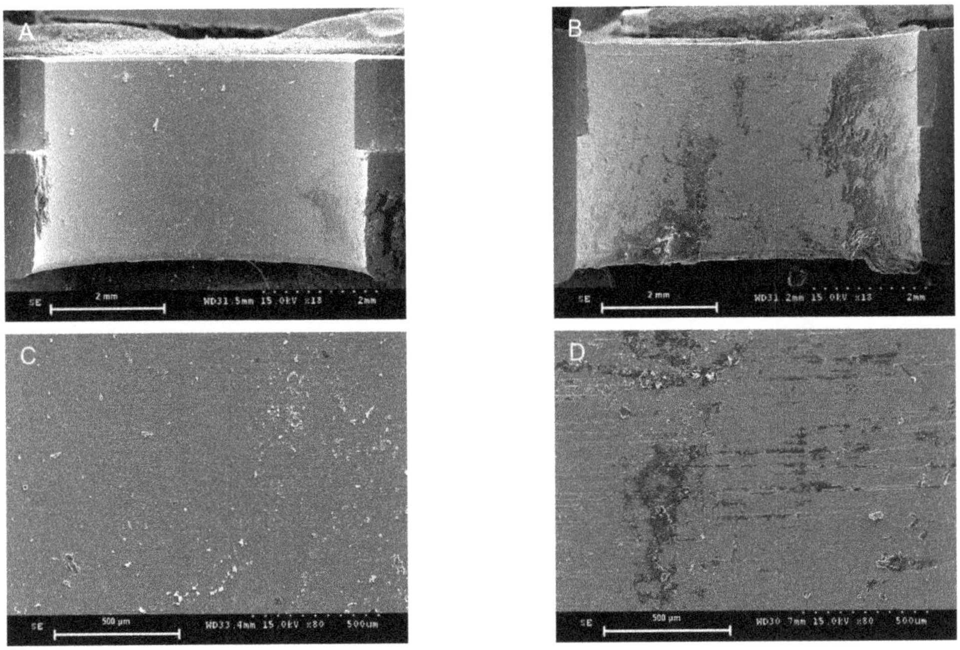

Figure 7. Representative scanning electron microscopic images. Cross-sectional view of a sleeve insert from a preoperative (**A**) and a postoperative (**B**) image from the MSI group at a lower magnification (18×). Cross-sectional view of a sleeve insert from a preoperative (**C**) and a postoperative (**D**) image from the MSI group at a higher magnification (80×).

4. Discussion

3D printing is a key topic in various parts of industry as well as in the medical and dental fields. Nowadays, its application is not only limited to a macroscopic scale but has expanded to the microscopic cellular levels in which the technology can manufacture functional scaffolds for biomedical applications [30,31]. The biggest advantage of this technology is that it enables personalized fabrication of the object from a large variety of materials [32,33]. In the present study, a monomer based on acrylic esters and a digital light processing 3D printer were used to fabricate the surgical guides.

The null hypothesis that the weight difference between the two types of surgical guides before and after implant placement would differ was rejected, whereas the other null hypothesis that the preoperative and postoperative angular deviation of the implants would differ was accepted. The guide drills were prepared individually for the two groups in order to avoid unwanted damage to the surgical sites that may arise from wearing out of the drills. In this study, the guides of both groups were in-office 3D-printed, as this was considered adequate to achieve comparable accuracy to that of industrial 3D printers for clinical purposes.

The three implantation sites in each typodont were designed with different guide holes and implant diameter combinations to represent different clinical situations: an open sleeve with a wide-diameter implant for the right first molar area, closed sleeve with a wide-diameter implant for the left first molar area, and closed sleeve with a narrow-diameter implant for the left second premolar area. Open sleeves can be useful in the molar areas as they can be used with a smaller amount of mouth opening, making it possible to perform implant drilling in cases with an insufficient interarch space. The sleeves are usually C-shaped with the open part facing buccally; therefore, placing an implant with an open sleeve design surgical guide on a premolar was precluded.

Concerns about using surgical guides include the inner surface of the sleeves being trimmed during the drilling procedures and the components of the surgical guides being embedded in the surgical site during the drilling process. It would be best to assess the change on the inner surface of the sleeve. However, this change may be hardly detectable considering the small differences. Alternatively, evaluation of the weight difference pre- and postoperatively can be an indirect, practical method to evaluate this concern.

The weight was measured immediately before and after implant placement to exclude potential distortion of the 3D-printed resin materials. The weight results indicated that the metal sleeves and metal-free sleeves were vulnerable to trimming with a series of guide drills composed of metal components. This was confirmed by the SEM image analyses. In the MSI group, the preoperative SEM images showed a smooth metal surface, in contrast to the layered appearance of the MSF group. This layering occurs due to the principle of additive manufacturing technology in which an object is built-up layer-by-layer. However, both groups showed postoperative signs of depression, as identified through the images. In the MSF group, this appeared as a pressed, flat, and squeezed surface, as if the skin were pressed against a glass window. In the MSI group, the area that experienced friction due to contact with the guide drill was highly polished and appeared as a dark area. This suggests that the tolerance with the guide drill of the MSF group may be tighter than that of the MSI group.

Previous studies have used both preoperative and postoperative CBCT scan datasets for measuring the angular deviation [9,34,35]. However, a limitation exists in this protocol. CBCT scan datasets might differ owing to the different orientation of the patients/objects, and the quality of the postoperative CBCT scan datasets can be affected by the implant-induced metal artifacts. Hence, the superimposition of the two CBCT scan datasets may not be accurate. The method for angular deviation measurement proposed in the present study used a scan body that allowed the addition of two different scan datasets by functioning as a shared common part. A recent study reported comparable outcomes of the scan body and postoperative CBCT methodology when used to evaluate the difference between the position of the implant in the preoperative planning stage and the actual implant position [29]. This protocol may be particularly beneficial in clinical situations, as it does not require additional CBCT scans.

The angular deviation was evaluated because it is a parameter directly related to the attrition of the inner part of the sleeves. The buccolingual angular deviation of the implants placed at the right first molar area exhibited a higher value than the other implants, although the values were not statistically analyzed. This may be attributed to the characteristics of the open sleeve form design per se, which cannot completely guide the drill path. The statistically significant difference observed in the mesiodistal angular deviation of the left second premolar area may be attributed to the intrinsic tolerance of the metal sleeve per se, as well as to the errors during the attachment of the metal sleeves to the surgical guides, leading to incomplete adaptation of the metal sleeves. However, the difference of 2.40° between the two groups may be considered clinically acceptable. It can be assumed that the cross-section of the metal sleeve-free inserts may not conform to a complete circle but an oval form according to the build angle set for 3D printing. However, the results indicate that the build angle used in the present study was suitable for additive manufacturing of the guides. Moreover, in contrast to metal inserts that require additional costs and procedures for attachment, metal sleeve-free inserts are cost-effective. Therefore, metal sleeveless surgical guides may outweigh the metal sleeve-incorporated guides with the 3D printer used in the present study.

However, careful interpretation is mandatory, as the present study has a few limitations. First, the study was in vitro. The model was scanned with a tabletop scanner, the alveolar bone and soft tissue portions were not reproduced as in the clinical situation, and the study did not reflect patient movements or simulate the presence of saliva or blood. Second, only a single 3D printer and a fully guided implant surgery system were evaluated. Third, the angular deviation may differ according to the method of determination of the cross-sectional plane for the angular analysis. Further studies with different 3D printer systems and guided implant surgical kits, and subsequent clinical studies with a split-mouth study design, will be of great value to verify the findings of the present study. Moreover, comparative studies using computer-assisted implant surgical guides, navigation surgery systems, and robots will be crucial to evaluate the digital technology applicability to the field of implant surgery [36].

5. Conclusions

Within the limitations of the present study, the following conclusions can be drawn. First, on combining the two analyses, the performance of the MSF group was comparable to that of the MSI group, demonstrating the feasibility and validity of fabricating the surgical guides with an additive technology alone, that is, without attaching metal sleeves. Second, the sleeve inserts in the MSF and MSI groups exhibited noticeable changes after the drilling procedures with guide drills.

Author Contributions: Conceptualization, K.C.O. and J.-M.P.; methodology, J.-M.P.; software, K.C.O.; validation, J.-S.S. and J.-M.P.; formal analysis, K.C.O.; investigation, J.-S.S. and J.-M.P.; resources, J.-M.P.; data curation, K.C.O.; writing—original draft preparation, K.C.O.; writing—review and editing, J.-S.S. and J.-M.P.; visualization, K.C.O.; supervision, J.-S.S. and J.-M.P.; project administration, J.-M.P.; funding acquisition, J.-M.P. All authors have read and agreed to the published version of the manuscript.

Funding: This work was supported by the Technology Innovation Program (20007888, Development of dental surgery and treatment assistant robot and navigation system technology for high-precision implant surgery) funded by the Ministry of Trade, Industry & Energy (MOTIE, Korea).

Institutional Review Board Statement: Not applicable.

Informed Consent Statement: Not applicable.

Data Availability Statement: Data available on request due to restrictions eg privacy or ethical.

Conflicts of Interest: The authors declare no conflict of interest.

References

1. Handelsman, M. Surgical guidelines for dental implant placement. *Br. Dent. J.* **2006**, *201*, 139–152. [CrossRef] [PubMed]
2. Jung, R.E.; Schneider, D.; Ganeles, J.; Wismeijer, D.; Zwahlen, M.; Hammerle, C.; Tahmaseb, A. Computer technology applications in surgical implant dentistry: A systematic review. *Int. J. Oral Maxillofac. Implants* **2009**, *24*, 92–109. [PubMed]
3. De Vos, W.; Casselman, J.; Swennen, G. Cone-beam computerized tomography (CBCT) imaging of the oral and maxillofacial region: A systematic review of the literature. *Int. J. Oral Maxillofac. Surg.* **2009**, *38*, 609–625. [CrossRef] [PubMed]
4. Tahmaseb, A.; Wismeijer, D.; Coucke, W.; Derksen, W. Computer technology applications in surgical implant dentistry: A systematic review. *Int. J. Oral Maxillofac. Implants* **2014**, *29*, 25–42. [CrossRef] [PubMed]
5. Alharbi, N.; Wismeijer, D.; Osman, R.B. Additive Manufacturing Techniques in Prosthodontics: Where Do We Currently Stand? A Critical Review. *Int. J. Prosthodont.* **2017**, *30*, 474–484. [CrossRef] [PubMed]
6. Revilla-León, M.; Özcan, M. Additive manufacturing technologies used for processing polymers: Current status and potential application in prosthetic dentistry. *J. Prosthodont.* **2019**, *28*, 146–158. [CrossRef] [PubMed]
7. Henprasert, P.; Dawson, D.V.; El-Kerdani, T.; Song, X.; Couso-Queiruga, E.; Holloway, J.A. Comparison of the accuracy of implant position using surgical guides fabricated by additive and subtractive techniques. *J. Prosthodont.* **2020**, *29*, 534–541.
8. Orentlicher, G.; Abboud, M. Guided surgery for implant therapy. *Oral Maxillofac. Surg. Clin.* **2011**, *23*, 239–256. [CrossRef]
9. Smitkarn, P.; Subbalekha, K.; Mattheos, N.; Pimkhaokham, A. The accuracy of single-tooth implants placed using fully digital-guided surgery and freehand implant surgery. *J. Clin. Periodontol.* **2019**, *46*, 949–957. [CrossRef]
10. D'Souza, K.M.; Aras, M.A. Types of implant surgical guides in dentistry: A review. *J. Oral Implantol.* **2012**, *38*, 643–652. [CrossRef]
11. Varga, E., Jr.; Antal, M.; Major, L.; Kiscsatári, R.; Braunitzer, G.; Piffkó, J. Guidance means accuracy: A randomized clinical trial on freehand versus guided dental implantation. *Clin. Oral Implants Res.* **2020**, *31*, 417–430. [CrossRef] [PubMed]
12. Abduo, J.; Lau, D. Accuracy of static computer-assisted implant placement in anterior and posterior sites by clinicians new to implant dentistry: In vitro comparison of fully guided, pilot-guided, and freehand protocols. *Int. J. Implant Dent.* **2020**, *6*, 10. [CrossRef] [PubMed]
13. Younes, F.; Eghbali, A.; De Bruyckere, T.; Cleymaet, R.; Cosyn, J. A randomized controlled trial on the efficiency of free-handed, pilot-drill guided and fully guided implant surgery in partially edentulous patients. *Clin. Oral Implants Res.* **2019**, *30*, 131–138. [CrossRef] [PubMed]
14. Elkomy, M.M.; Khamis, M.M.; El-Sharkawy, A.M. Clinical and radiographic evaluation of implants placed with fully guided versus partially guided tissue-supported surgical guides: A split-mouth clinical study. *J. Prosthet. Dent.* **2020**, in press. [CrossRef]
15. D'haese, J.; Van De Velde, T.; Elaut, L.; De Bruyn, H. A prospective study on the accuracy of mucosally supported stereolithographic surgical guides in fully edentulous maxillae. *Clin. Implant Dent. Relat. Res.* **2012**, *14*, 293–303. [CrossRef]
16. Farley, N.E.; Kennedy, K.; McGlumphy, E.A.; Clelland, N.L. Split-mouth comparison of the accuracy of computer-generated and conventional surgical guides. *Int. J. Oral Maxillofac. Implants* **2013**, *28*, 563–572. [CrossRef]
17. Horwitz, J.; Zuabi, O.; Machtei, E.E. Accuracy of a computerized tomography-guided template-assisted implant placement system: An in vitro study. *Clin. Oral Implants Res.* **2009**, *20*, 1156–1162. [CrossRef]
18. Laederach, V.; Mukaddam, K.; Payer, M.; Filippi, A.; Kühl, S. Deviations of different systems for guided implant surgery. *Clin. Oral Implants Res.* **2017**, *28*, 1147–1151. [CrossRef]
19. Pettersson, A.; Kero, T.; Söderberg, R.; Näsström, K. Accuracy of virtually planned and CAD/CAM-guided implant surgery on plastic models. *J. Prosthet. Dent.* **2014**, *112*, 1472–1478. [CrossRef]
20. Vermeulen, J. The Accuracy of Implant Placement by Experienced Surgeons: Guided vs. Freehand Approach in a Simulated Plastic Model. *Int. J. Oral Maxillofac. Implants* **2017**, *32*, 617–624. [CrossRef]

21. De Santis, D.; Malchiodi, L.; Cucchi, A.; Cybulski, A.; Verlato, G.; Gelpi, F.; Nocini, P.F. The Accuracy of Computer-Assisted Implant Surgery Performed Using Fully Guided Templates versus Pilot-Drill Guided Templates. *BioMed Res. Int.* **2019**, *2019*, 9023548. [CrossRef]
22. Schulz, M.C.; Hofmann, F.; Range, U.; Lauer, G.; Haim, D. Pilot-drill guided vs. full-guided implant insertion in artificial mandibles—A prospective laboratory study in fifth-year dental students. *Int. J. Implant Dent.* **2019**, *5*, 23. [PubMed]
23. Oh, K.C.; Park, J.-M.; Shim, J.-S.; Kim, J.-H.; Kim, J.-E.; Kim, J.-H. Assessment of metal sleeve-free 3D-printed implant surgical guides. *Dent. Mater.* **2019**, *35*, 468–476. [CrossRef] [PubMed]
24. Sarhan, M.M.; Khamis, M.M.; El-Sharkawy, A.M. Evaluation of the accuracy of implant placement by using fully guided versus partially guided tissue-supported surgical guides with cylindrical versus C-shaped guiding holes: A split-mouth clinical study. *J. Prosthet. Dent.* **2020**, in press. [CrossRef] [PubMed]
25. Hromadnik, V.; Pieralli, S.; Spies, B.; Beuer, F.; Wesemann, C. Accuracy of a workflow using sleeveless 3D printed surgical guides made from a cost-effective and biodegradable material: An in vitro study. *Clin. Oral Implant. Res.* **2019**, *30*, 519. [CrossRef]
26. Rubayo, D.D.; Phasuk, K.; Vickery, J.M.; Morton, D.; Lin, W.-S. Influences of build angle on the accuracy, printing time, and material consumption of additively manufactured surgical templates. *J. Prosthet. Dent.* **2020**, in press. [CrossRef]
27. Smith, P.N.; Palenik, C.J.; Blanchard, S.B. Microbial contamination and the sterilization/disinfection of surgical guides used in the placement of endosteal implants. *Int. J. Oral Maxillofac. Implants* **2011**, *26*, 274–281.
28. Zhou, M.; Zhou, H.; Li, S.-Y.; Zhu, Y.; Geng, Y.-M. Comparison of the accuracy of dental implant placement using static and dynamic computer-assisted systems: An in vitro study. *J. Stomatol. Oral Maxillofac. Surg.* **2020**, in press. [CrossRef]
29. Zhou, M.; Zhou, H.; Li, S.; Geng, Y. Dental implant location via surface scanner: A pilot study. *BMC Oral Health* **2020**, *20*, 306. [CrossRef]
30. Nesic, D.; Schaefer, B.M.; Sun, Y.; Saulacic, N.; Sailer, I. 3D printing approach in dentistry: The future for personalized oral soft tissue regeneration. *J. Clin. Med.* **2020**, *9*, 2238.
31. Nesic, D.; Durual, S.; Marger, L.; Mekki, M.; Sailer, I.; Scherrer, S.S. Could 3D printing be the future for oral soft tissue regeneration? *Bioprinting* **2020**, *20*, e00100. [CrossRef]
32. Baron, J.; Hazubski, S.; Otte, A. 3D Multi-Material Printing of an Anthropomorphic, Personalized Replacement Hand for Use in Neuroprosthetics Using 3D Scanning and Computer-Aided Design: First Proof-of-Technical-Concept Study. *Prosthesis* **2020**, *2*, 362–370. [CrossRef]
33. Molinero-Mourelle, P.; Gómez-Polo, M.; Gómez-Polo, C.; Ortega, R.; del Río Highsmith, J.; Celemín-Viñuela, A. Preliminary study on the assessment of the marginal fit of three-dimensional methacrylate oligomer phosphine oxide provisional fixed dental prostheses made by digital light processing. *Prosthesis* **2020**, *2*, 240–245. [CrossRef]
34. Bencharit, S.; Staffen, A.; Yeung, M.; Whitley, D., III; Laskin, D.M.; Deeb, G.R. In vivo tooth-supported implant surgical guides fabricated with desktop stereolithographic printers: Fully guided surgery is more accurate than partially guided surgery. *J. Oral Maxillofac. Surg.* **2018**, *76*, 1431–1439. [CrossRef] [PubMed]
35. Van Assche, N.; Van Steenberghe, D.; Guerrero, M.; Hirsch, E.; Schutyser, F.; Quirynen, M.; Jacobs, R. Accuracy of implant placement based on pre-surgical planning of three-dimensional cone-beam images: A pilot study. *J. Clin. Periodontol.* **2007**, *34*, 816–821. [CrossRef]
36. Park, J.-M.; Kim, J.; Shim, J.-S. Review of computer-assisted implant surgeries: Navigation surgery system vs. computer-guided implant template vs. robot. *Implantology* **2018**, *22*, 50–58.

materials

MDPI

Article

Evaluation of the 3D Printing Accuracy of a Dental Model According to Its Internal Structure and Cross-Arch Plate Design: An In Vitro Study

Seung-Ho Shin, Jung-Hwa Lim, You-Jung Kang, Jee-Hwan Kim, June-Sung Shim and Jong-Eun Kim *

Department of Prosthodontics, Yonsei University College of Dentistry, Yonsei-ro 50-1, Seodaemun-gu, Seoul 03722, Korea; shin506@prostholabs.com (S.-H.S.); erin0313@prostholabs.com (J.-H.L.); kyj@yuhs.ac (Y.-J.K.); jee917@yuhs.ac (J.-H.K.); jfshim@yuhs.ac (J.-S.S.)

* Correspondence: gomyou@yuhs.ac; Tel.: +82-2-2228-3160

Received: 13 November 2020; Accepted: 26 November 2020; Published: 28 November 2020

Abstract: The amount of photopolymer material consumed during the three-dimensional (3D) printing of a dental model varies with the volume and internal structure of the modeling data. This study analyzed how the internal structure and the presence of a cross-arch plate influence the accuracy of a 3D printed dental model. The model was designed with a U-shaped arch and the palate removed (Group U) or a cross-arch plate attached to the palate area (Group P), and the internal structure was divided into five types. The trueness and precision were analyzed for accuracy comparisons of the 3D printed models. Two-way ANOVA of the trueness revealed that the accuracy was 135.2 ± 26.3 μm (mean ± SD) in Group U and 85.6 ± 13.1 μm in Group P. Regarding the internal structure, the accuracy was 143.1 ± 46.8 μm in the 1.5 mm-thick shell group, which improved to 111.1 ± 31.9 μm and 106.7 ± 26.3 μm in the roughly filled and fully filled models, respectively. The precision was 70.3 ± 19.1 μm in Group U and 65.0 ± 8.8 μm in Group P. The results of this study suggest that a cross-arch plate is necessary for the accurate production of a model using 3D printing regardless of its internal structure. In Group U, the error during the printing process was higher for the hollowed models.

Keywords: 3D printing; CAD/CAM; additive manufacturing; internal structure; trueness; precision

1. Introduction

Dental models have been produced to reproduce patient dental information outside the oral cavity for treatment processes such as consultation, diagnosis, and prosthesis fabrication [1]. However, the traditional plaster model produced after making intraoral impressions using alginate or silicone impression material can be damaged, either during the transportation or storage of the impression body, and the plaster model itself [1]. Moreover, the need to store various models made during long-term orthodontic treatment or prosthetic treatment can result in difficulties associated with physical space limitations [2]. Recent improvements in dental computer-aided design/computer-aided manufacturing (CAD/CAM) systems have made it possible to digitize information about the oral cavity using an intraoral scanner or scanning a model using model scanner [3]. The obtained digitized data can be stored, retrieved, transmitted, and analyzed using various types of digital software [4,5]. In the diagnosis process for orthognathic surgery or implant surgery, cone beam computed tomography (CBCT) data and digital model data can be aligned, and this can be used to establish a surgery or treatment plan on digital software as well [6,7]. However, despite these benefits of digital models, physical models are still required in many clinical situations, and so digital data must be manufactured accurately when a physical dental model is needed [3,8].

The methods for producing products from digital data can be broadly divided into additive manufacturing (AM) and subtractive manufacturing (SM) [9]. SM has the following disadvantages: directly milling materials with the milling bur [10] means that precise areas smaller than the diameter of the milling bur cannot be processed [11], and it is wasteful when a large amount of material needs to be discarded [12]. These aspects make SM an unfavorable method for making dental models. AM methods such as digital light processing (DLP) and stereolithography (SLA) have recently been widely used [13], and 3D printing has become widely used in the dental field due to improvements in the accuracy and speed of printing [8]. A 3D printer using AM converts the designed CAD file into slice data, organizes it by layer, and creates the desired shape [14]. AM uses the smallest possible amount of material and can be used to manufacture objects with complex internal shapes [2,15].

When creating a dental model using 3D printing, it is very important that the scanned data are accurately manufactured and reproduced [4]. When using a printed model to evaluate occlusion or fabricate a prosthesis, errors in the model can affect the accuracy of the produced prosthesis [16]. Previous studies of the accuracy of 3D printed dental models have included comparisons and evaluations of the accuracies of conventional gypsum models and models produced using SM [17–19], and comparisons of the accuracy of the produced model have been made according to the 3D printer type [20]. Other studies have investigated parameters that mainly affect the accuracy of printed components, such as the type of resin used, printing angle, layer thickness, and temperature [8,21–26]. It has been reported that DLP and SLA printers are the most suitable for dental 3D printing, since they are more precise than printers based on fused deposition modeling [16,27].

The large amount of photocured resin required to manufacture a dental model is expensive, and so various efforts have been made to reduce the resin material consumed [3]. If a part such as the palate or tongue is unnecessary to the purpose of a diagnosis or treatment, it can be removed during the premodeling process and then not printed, producing a hollow design inside the model [28,29]. Such a modeling strategy can also reduce the printing time required for the 3D printing process [2,30]. A previous study that controlled the internal structure compared hollow and nonhollow models [31]. However, no previous studies have applied various hollowing methods to determine changes according to the amount of hollowing or forming a lattice structure internally, or investigated internal structure changes and interactions with a cross-arch plate.

Therefore, the present study was designed to evaluate the accuracy of 3D printed models according to the presence or absence of a cross-arch plate, the internal filling rate, and the thickness of the shell. The following null hypotheses were established: (1) the accuracy of a 3D printed model does not vary with the presence and absence of a cross-arch plate, and (2) the accuracy does not vary with the shell thickness or interior structure design of a 3D printed model.

2. Materials and Methods

The model design and overall experimental workflow of this study are illustrated in Figure 1. To design the model in each group, a maxillary tooth dentiform model (D85DP-500B.1, Nissin, Kyoto, Japan) was scanned using a tabletop scanner (Identica T500, Medit, Seoul, Korea), with the obtained data exported in the Standard Triangulated Language (STL) digital file format. The converted design file was then imported into the modeling software (Meshmixer, Autodesk, San Rafael, CA, USA), the palate and other unnecessary structures were deleted, and the U-shaped model (Group U) was designed. The cross-arch plate model (Group P) was designed by attaching a 1.5 mm-thick cross-arch plate at the position of the palate in Group U (Figure 2).

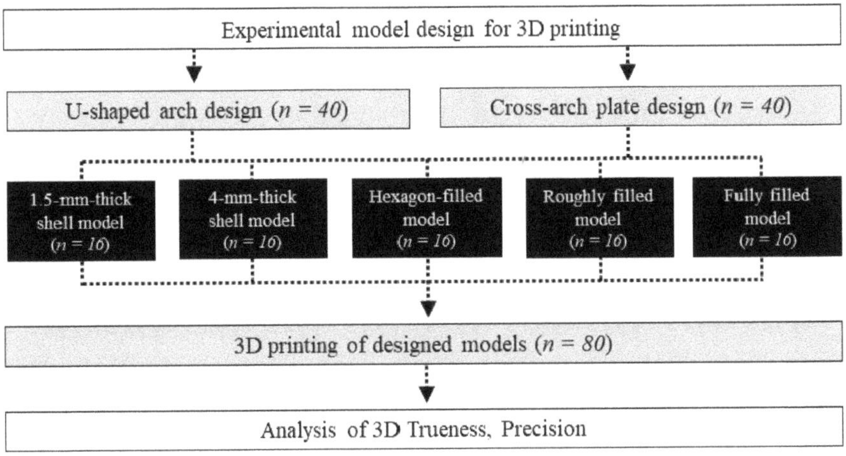

Figure 1. Flowchart of the overall experimental process of this study.

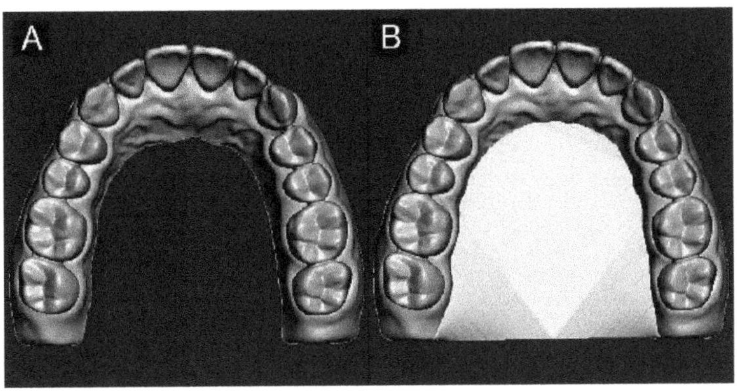

Figure 2. Experimental model designs: (**A**) U-shaped arch and (**B**) cross-arch plate.

Based on the designed files for Groups U and P, 3D modeling software (Meshmixer, Autodesk, San Rafael, CA, USA; Rhino 5, Robert McNeel & Associates, Seattle, WA, USA) was used to model the internal structure of the model area excluding the plate area in various ways (Figure 3). For the 1.5 mm hollow model (Figure 3A), the hollowing function was applied after designating the shell thickness of the model as 1.5 mm (Figure 3A,F). The 4 mm hollow model was the same as the 1.5 mm hollow model except that it had a 4 mm thick shell (Figure 3B,G). For the hexagon-filled model, after designing a hollow model with a shell thickness of 1.5 mm, the hexagon structure was processed and arranged according to the shape of the hollow inner surface of the model (Figure 3C,H). The hexagon structure was produced by designing a hexagon shape with a side length of 2 mm using Adobe Illustrator CS (Adobe, San Jose, CA, USA), and then using the extrude closed planar curve function of CAD software (Rhino 5, Robert McNeel & Associates, Seattle, WA, USA). The roughly filled model used a solid model that completely filled the interior (i.e., no empty space), and a selective pixel application technique was applied during 3D printing by using the pixel-dimming function of slicing open-source software (NanoDLP) to adjust the illuminance of pixels on the liquid crystal display (LCD) screen when 3D printing was applied (Figure 3D,I). A 50% pixel opening setting was applied in the option setting of the selective pixel application. A fully filled model that was completely filled internally with no empty space was then printed in 3D (Figure 3E,J).

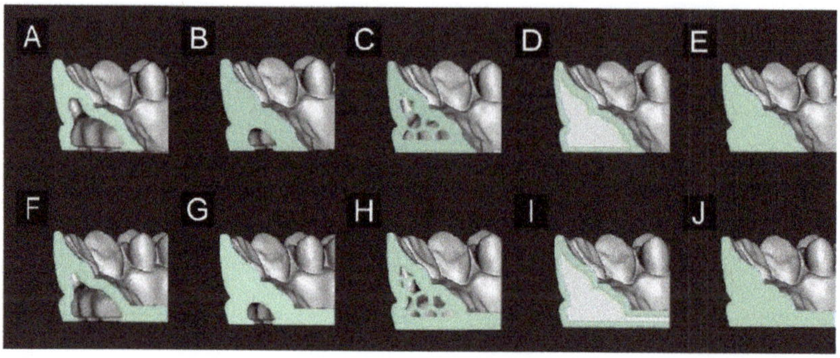

Figure 3. Designs of the 3D printed models: (**A**,**F**) hollow model with a 1.5 mm-thick shell, (**B**,**G**) hollow model with a 4 mm-thick shell, (**C**,**H**) hexagon-filled model, (**D**,**I**) roughly filled model, (**E**,**J**) fully filled model. (**A**–**E**) U-shaped model design; and (**F**–**J**) cross-arch plate model design.

Eight models for each group were printed using the photopolymer resin (MAZIC®D, Vericom, Chuncheon, Korea) and a DLP 3D printer (Phrozen Shuffle, Phrozen, Hsinchu, Taiwan). The thickness of each printing layer was set to 100 μm, and a printing support structure was attached to the bottom of the model. Table 1 lists the amounts of resin consumed for the different printed models.

Table 1. Resin consumption according to model design (units: mL).

Each Name	Cross-Arch Plate (Group P)	U-Shaped Arch Plate (Group U)
Hollow model with 1.5 mm-thick shell	12.28	8.83
Hollow model with 4 mm-thick shell	17.38	13.89
Hexagon-filled model	15.22	13.48
Roughly filled model	19.50	15.59
Fully filled model	19.56	16.07

All of the printed models were washed with 90% isopropyl alcohol in a washing machine (Formwasher, Formlabs, Somerville, MA, USA) and then polymerized using an ultraviolet post-curing unit (CureM D102, Sona Global, Seoul, Korea) according to the manufacturer's instructions.

Each printed model was scanned with a tabletop 3D scanner, and the scanned data were exported as an STL file and sent for 3D inspection software (Geomagic Control X, 3D Systems, Rock Hill, SC, USA). Removing the lower part of the scan data up to the height of the cross-arch plate design, only the tooth area and the surrounding gingival area were designated equally. Trueness was calculated by overlapping all the data of each group with the model design reference data, and precision was calculated by overlapping the data in each group in a pairwise manner. Surface deviation data were calculated using root-mean-square estimation (RMSE) to perform overall volume comparisons [32]. The RMSE was calculated using the following Equation (1):

$$\text{RMSE} = \frac{1}{\sqrt{n}} \cdot \sqrt{\sum_{i=1}^{n} (x_{1,i} - x_{2,i})^2} \quad (1)$$

All scan data were analyzed statistically to compare the trueness and precision values between groups, and the mean discrepancy obtained from the comparisons of two data sets was used for statistical analysis. A 3D comparative analysis was used to determine the accuracy of the model output; that is, the accuracy of the scanner comprised a combination of trueness (measure of the differences from the reference model) and precision (measure of the similarity between measurements).

Statistical analyses of the results in each group were performed using standard statistical software (SPSS version 25.0, SPSS, IBM SPSS Statistics, Armonk, USA). All of the acquired data were subjected to Levene's test to evaluate homoscedasticity, and the Shapiro–Wilk normality test was used to test for the presence of normality. Differences between the groups according to the presence or absence of a cross-arch plate and the internal structure were analyzed using the two-way ANOVA test, with the one-way ANOVA test used to verify the difference in accuracy according to the internal structure in each of Groups P and U. The Bonferroni test was used as a posttest. The student's *t*-test was used to compare differences between with and without a cross-arch plate in groups with the same internal structure. The significance cutoff in all tests was $\alpha = 0.05$.

3. Results

Figure 4 shows the results of two-way ANOVAs of trueness according to the presence or absence of a cross-arch plate and differences in the internal structure. The deviation was 91.0 ± 7.8 μm (mean ± SD) in Group P and 139.1 ± 25.4 μm in Group U, and the accuracy was significantly higher when a cross-arch plate was present ($F = 376.5$, $p < 0.001$). The internal structure also significantly affected the accuracy ($F = 23.4$, $p < 0.001$). The accuracy was low in the 1.5 mm and 4 mm-thick shell models with a hollow internal structure, and high in the models in which the internal structure was not hollowed out (e.g., fully filled model). The interaction between the two factors ($F = 15.5$, $p < 0.001$) was also found to have a significant effect on trueness.

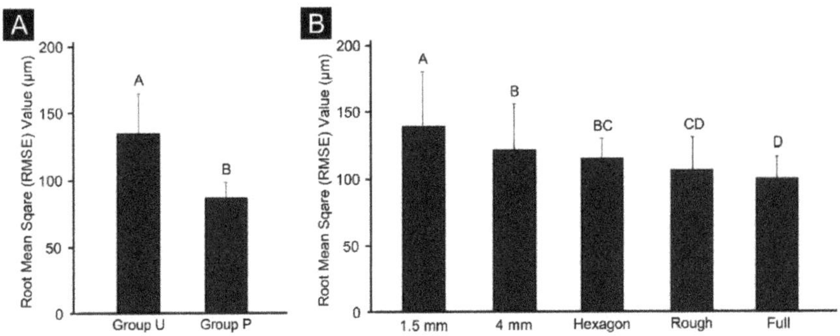

Figure 4. Results of the two-way ANOVAs of trueness (**A**) between Groups U and P, and (**B**) between the groups with different internal structures. Uppercase letters indicate significant differences. Data are the mean and SD values.

In Group U, the overall RMSE value was high, and it differed markedly depending on the internal structure, being the highest in the 1.5 mm thick model, followed by the 4 mm thick model. In the 1.5 mm thick model, the accuracy was higher in the group filled with the hexagon shape, and highest in the fully filled model. In Group P, the internal structure had lower effects than in Group U, with the accuracy being significantly higher in the roughly filled and fully filled groups (Figure 5).

Figure 6 shows the results of the two-way ANOVA of precision according to the presence or absence of a cross-arch plate and differences in internal structure. The deviation was 62.97 ± 9.8 μm in Group P and 71.6 ± 16.81 μm in Group U, and the accuracy was significantly higher in the presence of a cross-arch plate ($F = 31.1$, $p < 0.001$). The internal structure also significantly affected the accuracy ($F = 7.5$, $p < 0.001$). The output stability was low for the model with a hollow internal structure (e.g., the 4 mm-thick shell model), and high in the hexagon-filled model. The interaction between the two factors was also found to have a significant effect on precision ($F = 3.618$, $p = 0.006$).

The precision did not differ significantly with the internal structure in Group P, while in Group U, there were significant differences in the 1.5 mm hollow model, the roughly filled model, and the fully filled model, and in the 4 mm hollow model and the hexagon-filled model. In Group P, the precision was lowest in the 4 mm hollow model and highest in the roughly filled and fully filled models. In Group U, the precision was the highest in the hexagon-filled model and lowest in the 4 mm hollow model (Figure 7).

3D color maps were used to visualize the characteristic elements of each group (Figure 8). In Group U, the contraction of the arch around the left and right posterior teeth occurred in the lingual direction. In contrast, Group P with a cross-arch plate structure had relatively stable output results.

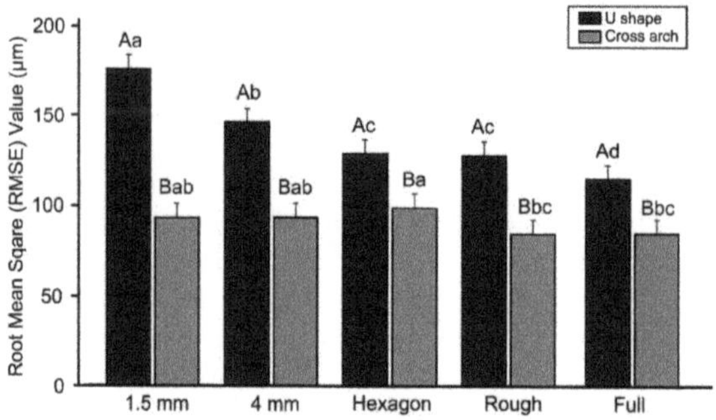

Figure 5. Results of the trueness analysis between Groups P and U. Lowercase letters indicate significant differences between internal structures within the Groups U or P each, and uppercase letters indicate significant differences between Groups P and U within the same internal-structure.

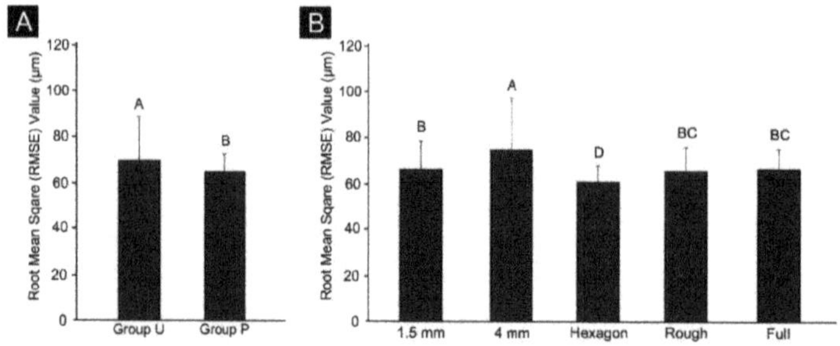

Figure 6. Results of the two-way ANOVA of precision (**A**) between Groups P and U and (**B**) between each internal-structure group. Uppercase letters indicate significant differences. Data are the mean and SD values.

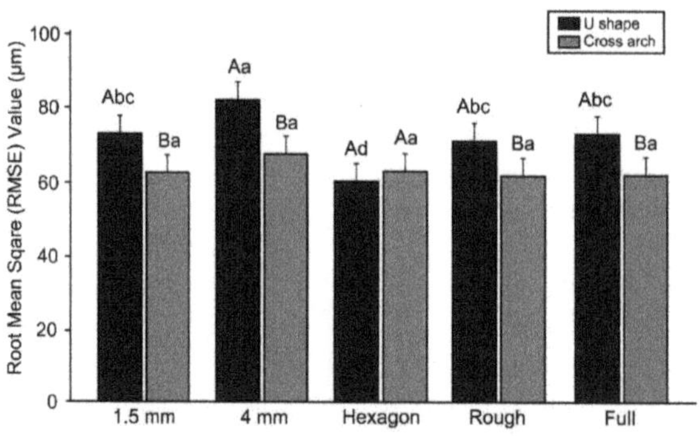

Figure 7. Precision comparison between Groups P and U. Lowercase letters indicate significant differences between internal structures within the Groups U or P each, and uppercase letters indicate significant differences between Groups P and U within the same internal-structure.

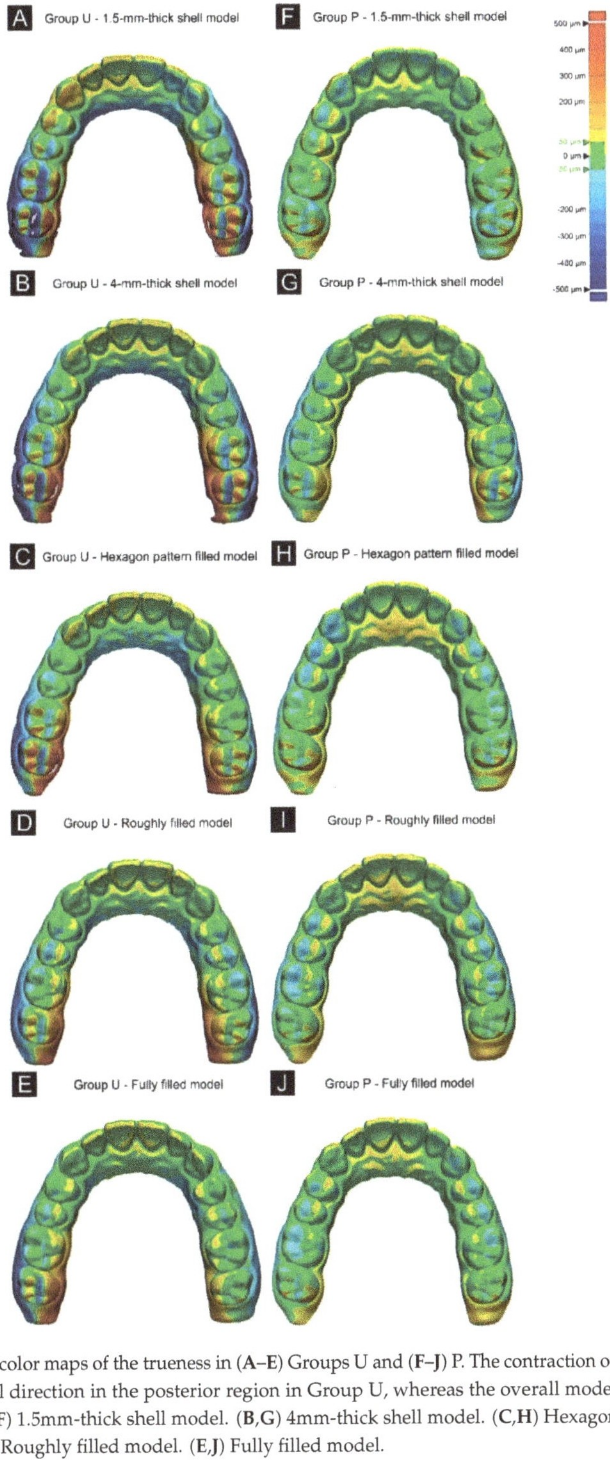

Figure 8. 3D color maps of the trueness in (**A–E**) Groups U and (**F–J**) P. The contraction occurred mainly in the lingual direction in the posterior region in Group U, whereas the overall model was stable in Group P. (**A**,**F**) 1.5mm-thick shell model. (**B**,**G**) 4mm-thick shell model. (**C**,**H**) Hexagon pattern filled model. (**D**,**I**) Roughly filled model. (**E**,**J**) Fully filled model.

4. Discussion

This study confirmed that the presence or absence of a cross-arch plate and differences in the internal structure resulted in significant variations in the characteristics of 3D printed models produced using the DLP method. In the trueness analysis of Groups U and P, the overall error was large for Group U, whereas the output result was stable for Group P. The color-map analysis of model overlap revealed that the error in Group U manifested in the model contraction on both lingual sides in the posterior region. Group P, with a cross-arch support plate, was found to be stable. It seems that the shrinkage in the polymerization process is caused by differences in the overall volume in Group U [33,34]. Therefore, the first null hypothesis was rejected. Both 3D printing and post-curing are processes involving the polymerization of a photopolymer resin, and it has been reported that shrinkage during this process affects the dimensional accuracy of produced objects [35–37]. In Group U, only the support structure for 3D printing could resist shrinkage, whereas in Group P, the presence of a cross-arch stabilization structure is thought to have resulted in the overall volume stability during each curing process. Thus, the second null hypothesis was also rejected. Camardella et al. [36] also concluded that there are differences in output stability according to various types of base shapes. Among the U-shaped models that those authors investigated, the average interdental distance differed by −0.7 mm when compared with the model group with a general base, and the model group that included a cross bar was arranged in a U shape, and there was no significant difference from the group with the general base. These findings are similar to the present study confirming that the stability of 3D printing increased when there was a cross-arch stabilization structure, and accordingly it shows the necessity for a cross-arch stabilization structure in the 3D printing process of the model.

Park et al. [38] performed a linear analysis of U-shaped models printed using two types of resin with the same DLP printer, and for both models the minimum deviation occurred in the front of the model and with contraction in the molar region. The median trueness values did not differ significantly between the two DLP groups, but the distribution of the values in the lower 50% relative to the median value has varied markedly with the resin type, which means that the trueness differed with the resin type. This reflects the contraction of the posterior teeth according to the resin type, and can be interpreted as the stability of 3D printing increasing when a cross-arch stabilization structure is present, accounting the results obtained in the present study.

In this study, the accuracy was low for the printed models, with a 1.5 mm or 4 mm-thick shell and a hollow interior. These models require less photopolymer resin than the fully filled model in the 3D printing process, with the 1.5 mm hollow model consuming only 54.9–62.7% of resin required to produce the fully filled model; however, that model had the lowest accuracy. The presence or absence of the cross-arch plate also affected the accuracy, and it was thought that hollowing the model reduced the overall volume stability during the printing and post-curing processes [39]. Rungrojwittayakul et al. [31] compared the trueness and precision between the U-shaped models with hollow and solid internal structures and a shell thickness of 2 mm. An error of 45 μm was found for the model with a shell thickness of 2 mm produced by continuous liquid interface production (CLIP), while the error was 35 μm for the solid model. For models with a shell thickness of 2 mm printed using a DLP 3D printer the error was 77 μm, with the same error found for the solid model. This meant that there was no significant difference in the printing accuracy between the solid and hollow models produced using either a CLIP or DLP printer. That study showed a similar trend to our study, but since cross-arch bars were applied to all of the models in that study, there was a similarity between the results with the hollow and fully filled groups of Group P in which a cross-arch plate was applied. On the other hand, the absence of a cross-arch plate in the design with a U shape resulted in the same difference between our studies.

In this study, 3D printing was performed using a selective pixel application method in the roughly filled model. This technique utilizes a microscopic mirror during DLP printing, which is controlled at the software level so that the UV light does not cause excessive curing. When printing a model using a DLP 3D printer, large curing areas can be associated with UV-light leak on the edges of the cured

3D printed layer and the masking surface of the LCD screen, possibly resulting in overcuring, which increases the volume of the product [40–42]. In the present study, the interiors of the fully filled and roughly filled models were designed to be solid, and the range of the applied light source was wider than for the 1.5 and 4 mm hollow models. Therefore, if the selective pixel application method was not utilized, model deformation may have occurred during printing, and so this method was included in the study design. However, this study found very little difference in accuracy between the roughly filled and fully filled models, and the amounts of photopolymer resin consumed were almost the same.

Moreover, the application of the optimal curing time per layer in 3D printing during the preparation process can explain why there was no difference in the overcuring accuracy between the selective pixel application model and the fully filled model in this study. The application of an appropriate design using the slicing software and the output equipment stage (e.g., for the curing times of the various layers) will optimize the accuracy of the model output. The trueness of the hexagon-filled model was not better than those for the fully filled and roughly filled models. However, the hexagon-filled model in Group U showed the best precision. Since the internal structure was reinforced with a hexagon structure and the density of the internal structure was lower, the most stable output environment was achieved during printing due to the appropriate UV exposure being applied. Yang and Huang [43], similarly, found very high stability for a model having an internal honeycomb structure, and another previous study found that an object containing an internal structure with appropriate porosity can produce accurate printing results and superior mechanical properties such as stability and strength [44]. The hexagon-filled model has the advantage of reducing resin consumption, but the design of this internal structure requires a complicated modeling process and did not show higher accuracy in the trueness evaluation, and so it seems that there are not many advantages in using this model.

This study found that the cross-arch stabilization plate structure plays a very important role in producing a high-accuracy dental model, and modeling in a solid form is superior to hollow modeling despite requiring the use of more resin. 3D printed models can be used in the dental clinical environment not only for consultation and diagnosis, but also for prosthesis production, and an appropriate production method needs to be determined depending on the intended purpose. The most cost-effective approach would be to reduce resin consumption by making a U-shaped 1.5 mm hollow model for consultations. However, for fabricating an accurate prosthesis, the use of a cross-arch plate and the fully filled model design that involves completely filling the interior appears to be the best approach.

Further studies are needed for applications that were not covered in this study. Since this study focused on the modeling conditions, analyses were conducted with one type of 3D printer, and various types of photopolymer resin were not used. Future investigations of the 3D printing process using various printing methods and types of resin with various components would provide wider insights. It is also worth studying the effects of using various types of equipment with various light sources, wavelengths, and temperatures in the post-curing stage after the 3D printing process, including changes in the volume of the final products.

5. Conclusions

The trueness error was larger in the U-shaped group than in the cross-arch plate group in this study, and was the largest in the 1.5 mm group, while it was smallest for the roughly filled and fully filled models in the cross-arch plate group. This precision was not stable in the U-shaped group, whereas it was stable in the cross-arch plate group. Meanwhile, the output stability was highest for the hexagon-filled model in the U-shaped group, and the lowest for the 4 mm model in the cross-arch plate group.

Author Contributions: Conceptualization, J.-E.K. and S.-H.S.; data curation, S.-H.S.; formal analysis, S.-H.S., Y.-J.K., J.-H.L. and J.-E.K.; methodology, S.-H.S., Y.-J.K. and J.-H.K.; project administration, J.-E.K., and J.-S.S.; resources, J.-E.K., and J.-S.S.; software, S.-H.S. and Y.-J.K.; supervision, J.-E.K.; validation, J.-E.K. and J.-S.S.; visualization, S.-H.S. and J.-E.K.; writing—original draft, S.-H.S., J.-H.L. and J.-E.K.; writing—review and editing, S.-H.S., J.-H.L.,Y.-J.K., J.-H.K., J.-E.K. and J.-S.S. All authors have read and agreed to the published version of the manuscript.

Funding: This study was supported by the Advanced Technology Center(ATC) Program funded by the Ministry of Trade, Industry and Energy (MOTIE, Korea) (10077361, Integrated System for Dental Diagnosis, Treatment Simulation & PSI (Patient Specific Instrument) Design).

Conflicts of Interest: The authors declare no conflict of interest.

References

1. Ender, A.; Attin, T.; Mehl, A. In vivo precision of conventional and digital methods of obtaining complete-arch dental impressions. *J. Prosthet. Dent.* **2016**, *115*, 313–320. [CrossRef] [PubMed]
2. McGuinness, N.J.; Stephens, C.D. Storage of Orthodontic Study Models in Hospital Units in the U.K. *Br. J. Orthod.* **1992**, *19*, 227–232. [CrossRef] [PubMed]
3. Attaran, M. The rise of 3-D printing: The advantages of additive manufacturing over traditional manufacturing. *Bus. Horizons* **2017**, *60*, 677–688. [CrossRef]
4. Jeong, I.-D.; Lee, J.-J.; Jeon, J.-H.; Kim, J.-H.; Kim, H.-Y.; Kim, W.-C. Accuracy of complete-arch model using an intraoral video scanner: An in vitro study. *J. Prosthet. Dent.* **2016**, *115*, 755–759. [CrossRef] [PubMed]
5. Martorelli, M.; Gloria, A.; Bignardi, C.; Calì, M.; Maietta, S. Design of Additively Manufactured Lattice Structures for Biomedical Applications. *J. Heal. Eng.* **2020**, *2020*, 2707560. [CrossRef]
6. Giudice, A.L.; Ronsivalle, V.; Grippaudo, C.; Lucchese, A.; Muraglie, S.; Lagravère, M.O.; Isola, G. One Step before 3D Printing—Evaluation of Imaging Software Accuracy for 3-Dimensional Analysis of the Mandible: A Comparative Study Using a Surface-to-Surface Matching Technique. *Materials* **2020**, *13*, 2798. [CrossRef]
7. Farronato, G.; Giannini, L.; Galbiati, G.; Pisani, L.; Mortellaro, C.; Maspero, C. Verification of the Reliability of the Three-dimensional Virtual Presurgical Orthodontic Diagnostic Protocol. *J. Craniofacial Surg.* **2014**, *25*, 2013–2016. [CrossRef]
8. Unkovskiy, A.; Bui, P.H.-B.; Schille, C.; Geis-Gerstorfer, J.; Huettig, F.; Spintzyk, S. Objects build orientation, positioning, and curing influence dimensional accuracy and flexural properties of stereolithographically printed resin. *Dent. Mater.* **2018**, *34*, e324–e333. [CrossRef]
9. Paris, H.; Mokhtarian, H.; Coatanéa, E.; Museau, M.; Ituarte, I.F. Comparative environmental impacts of additive and subtractive manufacturing technologies. *CIRP Ann.* **2016**, *65*, 29–32. [CrossRef]
10. Gaspar, M.; Weichert, F. Integrated construction and simulation of tool paths for milling dental crowns and bridges. *Comput. Des.* **2013**, *45*, 1170–1181. [CrossRef]
11. Khaledi, A.-A.; Farzin, M.; Akhlaghian, M.; Pardis, S.; Mir, N. Evaluation of the marginal fit of metal copings fabricated by using 3 different CAD-CAM techniques: Milling, stereolithography, and 3D wax printer. *J. Prosthet. Dent.* **2019**, *124*, 81–86. [CrossRef]
12. Baumers, M.; Dickens, P.; Tuck, C.; Hague, R. The cost of additive manufacturing: Machine productivity, economies of scale and technology-push. *Technol. Forecast. Soc. Chang.* **2016**, *102*, 193–201. [CrossRef]
13. Javaid, M.; Haleem, A. Current status and applications of additive manufacturing in dentistry: A literature-based review. *J. Oral Biol. Craniofacial Res.* **2019**, *9*, 179–185. [CrossRef] [PubMed]
14. Wang, W.; Chao, H.; Tong, J.; Yang, Z.; Tong, X.; Li, H.; Liu, X.; Liu, L. Saliency-Preserving Slicing Optimization for Effective 3D Printing. *Comput. Graph. Forum* **2015**, *34*, 148–160. [CrossRef]
15. Jeong, Y.-G.; Lee, W.-S.; Lee, K.-B. Accuracy evaluation of dental models manufactured by CAD/CAM milling method and 3D printing method. *J. Adv. Prosthodont.* **2018**, *10*, 245–251. [CrossRef] [PubMed]
16. Park, M.-E.; Shin, S.-Y. Three-dimensional comparative study on the accuracy and reproducibility of dental casts fabricated by 3D printers. *J. Prosthet. Dent.* **2018**, *119*, 861.e1–861.e7. [CrossRef] [PubMed]
17. Choi, J.-W.; Ahn, J.-J.; Son, K.; Huh, J.-B. Three-Dimensional Evaluation on Accuracy of Conventional and Milled Gypsum Models and 3D Printed Photopolymer Models. *Materials* **2019**, *12*, 3499. [CrossRef]
18. Nugrahani, F.; Jazaldi, F.; A I Noerhadi, N. Comparison of conventional study model measurements and 3D digital study model measurements from laser scanned dental impressions. *J. Phys. Conf. Ser.* **2017**, *884*, 012060. [CrossRef]

19. Osman, R.B.; Van Der Veen, A.J.; Huiberts, D.; Wismeijer, D.; Alharbi, N. 3D-printing zirconia implants; a dream or a reality? An in-vitro study evaluating the dimensional accuracy, surface topography and mechanical properties of printed zirconia implant and discs. *J. Mech. Behav. Biomed. Mater.* **2017**, *75*, 521–528. [CrossRef]
20. Nestler, N.; Wesemann, C.; Spies, B.C.; Beuer, F.; Bumann, A. Dimensional accuracy of extrusion- and photopolymerization-based 3D printers: In vitro study comparing printed casts. *J. Prosthet. Dent.* **2020**. [CrossRef]
21. Alharbi, N.; Osman, R.B.; Wismeijer, D. Factors Influencing the Dimensional Accuracy of 3D-Printed Full-Coverage Dental Restorations Using Stereolithography Technology. *Int. J. Prosthodont.* **2016**, *29*, 503–510. [CrossRef] [PubMed]
22. Jin, M.-C.; Yoon, H.-I.; Yeo, I.-S.L.; Kim, S.-H.; Han, J.-S. The effect of build angle on the tissue surface adaptation of maxillary and mandibular complete denture bases manufactured by digital light processing. *J. Prosthet. Dent.* **2020**, *123*, 473–482. [CrossRef] [PubMed]
23. Osman, R.B.; Alharbi, N.; Wismeijer, D. Build Angle: Does It Influence the Accuracy of 3D-Printed Dental Restorations Using Digital Light-Processing Technology? *Int. J. Prosthodont.* **2017**, *30*, 182–188. [CrossRef]
24. Zhang, Z.-C.; Li, P.-L.; Chu, F.-T.; Shen, G. Influence of the three-dimensional printing technique and printing layer thickness on model accuracy. *Fortschritte der Kieferorthopädie* **2019**, *80*, 194–204. [CrossRef] [PubMed]
25. Loflin, W.A.; English, J.D.; Borders, C.; Harris, L.M.; Moon, A.; Holland, J.N.; Kasper, F.K. Effect of print layer height on the assessment of 3D-printed models. *Am. J. Orthod. Dentofac. Orthop.* **2019**, *156*, 283–289. [CrossRef]
26. Jongsma, L.A.; Kleverlaan, C.J. Influence of temperature on volumetric shrinkage and contraction stress of dental composites. *Dent. Mater.* **2015**, *31*, 721–725. [CrossRef]
27. Dikova, T.; Dzhendov, D.; Ivanov, D.; Bliznakova, K. Dimensional accuracy and surface roughness of polymeric dental bridges produced by different 3D printing processes. *Arch. Mater. Sci. Eng.* **2018**, *2*, 65–75. [CrossRef]
28. Abudayyeh, I.; Gordon, B.; Ansari, M.M.; Jutzy, K.; Stoletniy, L.; Hilliard, A.A. A practical guide to cardiovascular 3D printing in clinical practice: Overview and examples. *J. Interv. Cardiol.* **2017**, *31*, 375–383. [CrossRef]
29. Ye, N.; Wu, T.; Dong, T.; Yuan, L.; Fang, B.; Xia, L. Precision of 3D-printed splints with different dental model offsets. *Am. J. Orthod. Dentofac. Orthop.* **2019**, *155*, 733–738. [CrossRef]
30. Prasad, S.; Kader, N.A.; Sujatha, G.; Raj, A.T.; Patil, S. 3D printing in dentistry. *J. 3D Print. Med.* **2018**, *2*, 89–91. [CrossRef]
31. Rungrojwittayakul, O.; Kan, J.Y.; Shiozaki, K.; Swamidass, R.S.; Goodacre, B.J.; Goodacre, C.J.; Lozada, J.L. Accuracy of 3D Printed Models Created by Two Technologies of Printers with Different Designs of Model Base. *J. Prosthodont.* **2019**, *29*, 124–128. [CrossRef] [PubMed]
32. Ozsoy, U. Comparison of Different Calculation Methods Used to Analyze Facial Soft Tissue Asymmetry: Global and Partial 3-Dimensional Quantitative Evaluation of Healthy Subjects. *J. Oral Maxillofac. Surg.* **2016**, *74*, 1847.e1–1847.e9. [CrossRef] [PubMed]
33. Cui, K.; Shang, X.; Luo, C.; Shen, Z.; Gao, H.; Xiong, G. A Kind of Accuracy Improving Method Based on Error Analysis and Feedback for DLP 3D Printing. In Proceedings of the 2019 IEEE International Conference on Service Operations and Logistics, and Informatics (SOLI), Zhengzhou, China, 6–8 November 2019; pp. 5–9.
34. Barker, T.M.; Earwaker, W.J.S.; A Lisle, D. Accuracy of stereolithographic models of human anatomy. *Australas. Radiol.* **1994**, *38*, 106–111. [CrossRef]
35. Choi, J.-Y.; Kim, N.-K.; Kim, Y.; Lee, J.-K.; Kim, M.-K. Analysis of errors in medical rapid prototyping models. *Int. J. Oral Maxillofac. Surg.* **2002**, *31*, 23–32. [CrossRef] [PubMed]
36. Camardella, L.T.; Vilella, O.D.V.; Breuning, H. Accuracy of printed dental models made with 2 prototype technologies and different designs of model bases. *Am. J. Orthod. Dentofac. Orthop.* **2017**, *151*, 1178–1187. [CrossRef]
37. Hazeveld, A.; Slater, J.J.R.H.; Ren, Y. Accuracy and reproducibility of dental replica models reconstructed by different rapid prototyping techniques. *Am. J. Orthod. Dentofac. Orthop.* **2014**, *145*, 108–115. [CrossRef]
38. Park, J.-M.; Jeon, J.; Koak, J.-Y.; Kim, S.-K.; Heo, S.-J. Dimensional accuracy and surface characteristics of 3D-printed dental casts. *J. Prosthet. Dent.* **2020**. [CrossRef]

39. Wu, D.; Zhao, Z.; Zhang, Q.; Qi, H.J.; Fang, D. Mechanics of shape distortion of DLP 3D printed structures during UV post-curing. *Soft Matter* **2019**, *15*, 6151–6159. [CrossRef]
40. Mitteramskogler, G.; Gmeiner, R.; Felzmann, R.; Gruber, S.; Hofstetter, C.; Stampfl, J.; Ebert, J.; Wachter, W.; Laubersheimer, J. Light curing strategies for lithography-based additive manufacturing of customized ceramics. *Addit. Manuf.* **2014**, 110–118. [CrossRef]
41. Kang, H.-W.; Park, J.H.; Cho, D.-W. A pixel based solidification model for projection based stereolithography technology. *Sens. Actuators A: Phys.* **2012**, *178*, 223–229. [CrossRef]
42. Borlaf, M.; Serra-Capdevila, A.; Colominas, C.; Graule, T. Development of UV-curable ZrO2 slurries for additive manufacturing (LCM-DLP) technology. *J. Eur. Ceram. Soc.* **2019**, *39*, 3797–3803. [CrossRef]
43. Yang, M.-Y.; Huang, J.-S. Numerical analysis of the stiffness and strength of regular hexagonal honeycombs with plateau borders. *Compos. Struct.* **2004**, *64*, 107–114. [CrossRef]
44. Melchels, F.P.; Bertoldi, K.; Gabbrielli, R.; Velders, A.H.; Feijen, J.; Grijpma, D.W. Mathematically defined tissue engineering scaffold architectures prepared by stereolithography. *Biomaterials* **2010**, *31*, 6909–6916. [CrossRef] [PubMed]

materials

Article

Realization of a Dental Framework by 3D Printing in Material Cobalt-Chromium with Superior Precision and Fitting Accuracy

André Edelmann *, Lisa Riedel and Ralf Hellmann

Applied Laser and Photonics Group, University of Applied Sciences Aschaffenburg, 63743 Aschaffenburg, Germany; s7040@h-ab.de (L.R.); ralf.hellmann@th-ab.de (R.H.)
* Correspondence: andre.edelmann@th-ab.de; Tel.: +49-(0)6022-81-3698

Received: 02 October 2020; Accepted: 25 November 2020; Published: 27 November 2020

Abstract: We report on the generation of a cobalt-chromium dental framework with superior precision and fitting accuracy using selective laser melting. The objective of this study is the reduction of surface roughness and the possibility to manufacture a dental framework with high precision for passive fit with attachments, in particular a round tack. After selective laser melting, the dental framework is thermally post processed at 750 °C, shot-blasted with glass and highly polished. Nominal to actual 3D form deviation is analyzed by stripe light projection, revealing deviations being less than 250 μm, i.e., warpage is as low as to permit dental application and accurate passive fit. In particular, the critical area of the dental framework, the fixture to the implant (overdenture) shows negligible deviations. This superior fitting accuracy is confirmed by joining the bar with a testing stylus.

Keywords: additive manufacturing; dental application; superior accuracy

1. Introduction

Dental implant therapy is since more than 30 years a common practice in the contemporary restorative and surgical dentistry of partially and fully edentulous patients [1–6]. Different polymers and metals were qualified in terms of biocompatibility, with respect to their soft tissue responses and good clinical performance over long periods [7–9]. Among a variety of implant component shapes, one of the most distinguished representatives is the dental implant bar [10,11]. With reference to selective laser melting (SLM), as a beneficial additive manufacturing method for dental technology, titanium and cobalt-chrome alloys are the most prominent and approved metals for dental implant therapy [12–15].

For full anatomical restorations, the dental bar is designed to support partial dentures. Bars are typically employed in a variety of advanced designs with different, complex attachments and retentions (Figure 1 exemplifies details of such a bar), to take into account complex clinical situations and provide maximum comfort for the patient. Dental bars are manufactured in various geometries, such as, e.g., Preci-Horax bars, Dolder bars with joints, abutments and attachments, as well as freely designable bar shapes [10,16]. For a long time, cast bars with welded or soldered prefabricated attachments were the standard in implant-supported restoration of the maxilla and mandible [17,18]. However, these conventional restorations may shrink, expand or have unwanted inclusions as a result of the casting and joining processes [19,20]. During the last decade, precision milling evolved as current the state-of-the-art manufacturing technology to meet the increasing expectations in accuracy and stress-free fit as well as design flexibility [19,21,22].

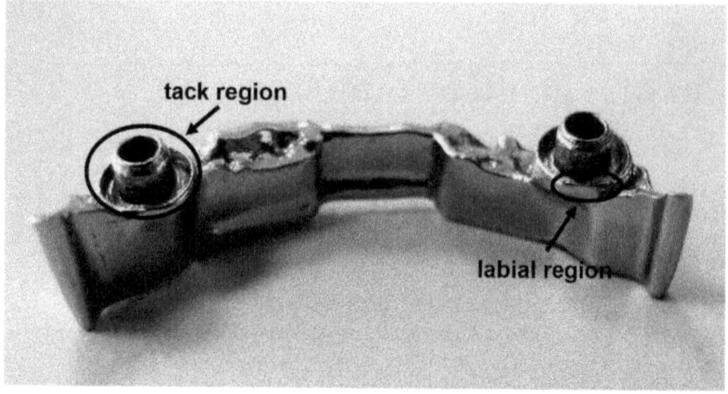

Figure 1. SLM fabricated dental framework.

Proper angulation and positioning of dental implants and the superstructure are essential to achieve acceptable prosthetic outcomes and long term success of implants and implant-supported prostheses, in turn striving superior demands on the fitting accuracy of bars with respect to shape divergence and surface roughness, e.g., in the labial region of the bar as indicated in Figure 1. In addition, surface properties should promote the integration of soft tissue while minimizing plaque and bacterial retention [23].

Therefore, different corrective techniques such as abrasive blasting, precision grinding or electrical discharge machining are employed to improve the surface and accuracy of dental bars. Though a clear definition of acceptable deviations in precision is not yet available [11], it was shown by Romero et al. and others that gaps in the range between 10 μm and 200 μm will be sufficient in meeting the criteria of passive fit between a cast bar superstructure and its interface with an implant abutment [24–27]. This prevents stress in the prosthesis-abutment-screw-implant complex, and, as a consequence, technical complications such as, e.g., fracture of the abutment, prosthesis or implant or biological complications including discomfort or pain to the patient or even bone fracture, respectively [9,28]. In fact, CNC-milled implant superstructures outperform the accuracy of fit that can be achieved with cast metal frameworks [29–31].

As a novel method in prosthodontics and orthodontics, additive manufacturing (AM) combines the advantages of high design flexibility, short manufacturing cycles enabling individual and small series production, high precision and a balanced selection of qualified polymer materials and metals. AM thus has the potential and is indeed already in use, beyond pure rapid prototyping, to replace conventional technologies, shorten process chains and improve dental implant technology [32–34]. Nonetheless, the demanding requirements in terms of precision and passive fit, as well as surface quality still challenge AM.

Against this background, we highlight the potential of SLM by exemplifying a complex shaped bar made of CoCrW. To facilitate the details of the complex design, in particular a thin walled hollow cylinder attachment as part of a full dental framework, which has not been previously reported by SLM, and to improve the surface roughness achievable with SLM, powders with different particle size distributions have been comparatively studied. The reduction of surface roughness is associated with reducing the necessary efforts in post processing, in turn enabling rapid, individualized manufacturing [11]. In addition and detail, achievable density and surface roughness have been optimized by investigating the influence of the applied laser fluence. Smallest shape deviations and high passive fit of highly polished bars lead to good passive fit as demonstrated by a testing stylus, typically used by dental laboratory technicians. In particular, the area of support of the tack that facilitates the connection to the implant is sensitive to roughness and shape deviations hampering precise passive fit.

2. Materials and Methods

2.1. Selective Laser Melting Conditions

For SLM, we employed a Realizer SLM 50 (Realizer GmbH, Bielefeld, Germany) equipped with a $P_L = 100$ W yttrium fiber laser (IPG, YLM-100). Spot size of the laser is set to $d_{spot} = 20$ µm at focus position. The machine processes under argon atmosphere with a 0.1% oxygen level. The build platform was kept at $\vartheta_{plate} = 200$ °C to maintain the machined part at an elevated temperature as to avoid deformation by curling due to residual stress. The input energy density E_d is varied in the range of 52 J/mm^3 to 92 J/mm^3 by varying the hatch distance y_{hatch} and keeping the laser power at $P_L = 55$ W, the exposure time at $t_{exp} = 20$ µm and the point distance at $x_{point} = 6$ µm, and layer thickness $z_{layer} = 50$ µm constant, respectively. The thus resulting energy density is calculated by Equation (1) [13,35].

$$E_d = \frac{P_L \, t_{exp}}{x_{point} \, y_{hatch} \, z_{layer}} \tag{1}$$

2.2. Powder Characterization

In this study, we analyze and process commercially available CoCrW metal powder (Eisenbacher GmbH, Wörth am Main, Germany). The chemical composition of this powder is as listed in Table 1.

Table 1. Chemical composition of CoCrW powder.

wt%	Cobalt	Chromium	Tungsten	Silicon	Manganous	Iron	Others
Powder	62.44	27.50	8.09	1.52	0.2	0.11	<0.1

Important fabrication material parameters for processing metallic powder in AM systems are the flowability and the powder density. If the flowability is too low, a homogenous covering of powder over the build plate in the SLM machine cannot be ensured and, in addition, a low powder density can lead to a higher porosity of the fabricated components [36]. For a more detailed investigation of the build quality regarding the powder characteristics, we divide the powder by sieving into the fraction A32 and A45. The notation refers to the d90 value of the grain size distribution. The fraction in A32 contains powder where 90% of the grain sizes are below $d_g < 32$ µm, whereas 90% of grain sizes in fraction A45 are below $d_g < 45$ µm. For each of these two powder batches we measure the flow time and the powder density. The results are shown in Table 2. The flowability, which influences the coating of the powder bed, is determined by measuring the flow rate using a Hall-Flowmeter according DIN EN ISO 4490. The powder density, influencing the homogeneity and density of the powder bed and thus the accessible relative density of the SLM built part, is measured according DIN ISO 697.

Table 2. Flowability and powder density of powder A32 and A45.

	A 32	A45
flow time (s)	19.1 ± 0.1	14.5 ± 0.3
powder density (g/cm^3)	3.6 ± 0.1	3.1 ± 0.1

Comparing powder sections A32 with A45, a higher flow time is found for A32. For this sieved particle size, the averaged grain sizes are smaller and, as a result, a higher probability of agglomeration by intermolecular interactions such as Van-der-Waals forces and higher contact surfaces of smaller particles come predominantly into play. As a result, higher stiction appears and the flowability is reduced [37,38]. In addition, the lowest powder density is found for A45, as for the A32 powder fraction an increase of finer grain sizes gets relevant and larger particles cannot fill the free spaces [39,40].

The moisture of the powder, which reduces the flow rate and thus the coating of the powder bed and which may also lead to higher gas porosity, is determined by weighting in combination with a drying chamber (PCE-MA 110, PCE Germany GmbH). We determine the moisture of both powder batches being under 0.01% and, therefore, exclude any influence of moisture to the flowability and powder density.

Figure 2 depicts the morphology of the powder and the particle size distribution of the different powder batches A32 and A45. In the powder samples, a spherical characteristic with minor satellites is observed which are free of porosity. The particle size distribution of the powder was analyzed by a Camsizer X2 based on dynamic digital image analysis methods according to ISO 13322-2 (Retsch Technology GmbH). This particle size distribution and morphology allows good flowability and packing density, as was demonstrated in a flowability test conducted using the Hall flowmeter funnel.

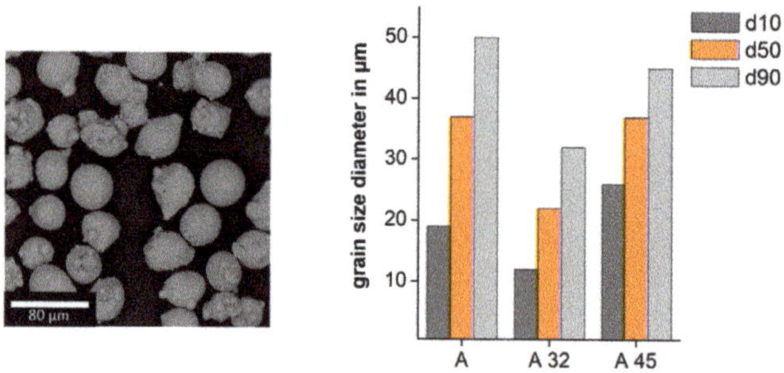

Figure 2. SEM images of Powder A (**left**) and particle size distribution of powder batch A, A32 and A45 (**right**).

2.3. Mechanical Properties

We evaluate the mechanical properties of SLM specimens based on powder batch A and comparing the results with the product specifications of CoCrW-powder (Eisenbacher Dentalwaren, Wörth am Main, Germany) [41]. By using tensile test specimens we measure the tensile strength with $\sigma_m = 365$ MPa, Young's modulus with $E = 170$ GPa, elongation with $\epsilon_b = 18\%$ and yield strength with $\sigma_{ys} = 567$ MPa (AG-Xplus, Shimadzu, Kyoto, Japan). The Vickers hardness HV10/30 on the top surface of test cubes (edge length $a = 10$ mm) results to $h_{vickers} = 365$ HV (Falcon 5000, Innovatest, Maastricht, The Netherlands). For the thermal expansion coefficient we obtain $\Delta l = 14.5 \times 10^{-6}\,\mathrm{K}^{-1}$ (DIL 402 Expedis, Netzsch, Selb, Germany) by using cylindrical specimens with a diameter of $d = 6$ mm and a length of $l = 50$ mm and applying a heating rate of $r_{heat} = 5$ K/s up to $\vartheta_{max} = 300$ °C. The mechanical properties are combined in Tables 3 and 4.

Table 3. Tensile strength, Young's modulus, elongation and yield strength of SLM fabricated CoCrW specimens.

	Tensile Strength	Young's Modulus	Elongation	Yield Strength
SLM	969 MPa	170 GPa	18%	567 MPa
reference [41]	1021 MPa	196 GPa	8%	642 MPa

Table 4. Vickers hardness and thermal expansion coefficient of SLM fabricated CoCrW specimens.

	Hardness	Thermal Expansion
SLM	365 HV	14.5×10^{-6} K^{-1}
reference [41]	356 HV	14.25×10^{-6} K^{-1}

Additionally we have taken polished cut images of test specimens in combination with SEM and EDX analysis. We have found, in gerneral, homogeneous microstructure with grain boundaries, at which we observe segregations of Wolfram. In Figure 3 the images of the mircostructure is shown.

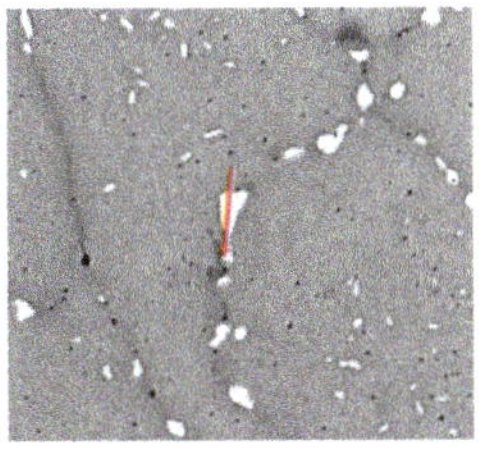

Figure 3. SEM image of CoCrW microstructure.

2.4. Experimental Flow Chart

The flow chart of the experimental tasks carried out in this report is shown in Figure 4. Beside the metallurgical and physical examination of powders and test specimen, the generation of the dental framework is conducted as follows. Beginning from digital data, obtained by anonymized patient data and prepared in .stl-data format, we have additively built both specimen for testing and the dental bar by SLM (implant fabrication). Here we focus particularly on the surface roughness by optimizing the particle size distribution of the metal powder. After post processing by thermal treatment and polishing, the dental framework is characterized with particular focus on 3D form deviation and fitting accuracy.

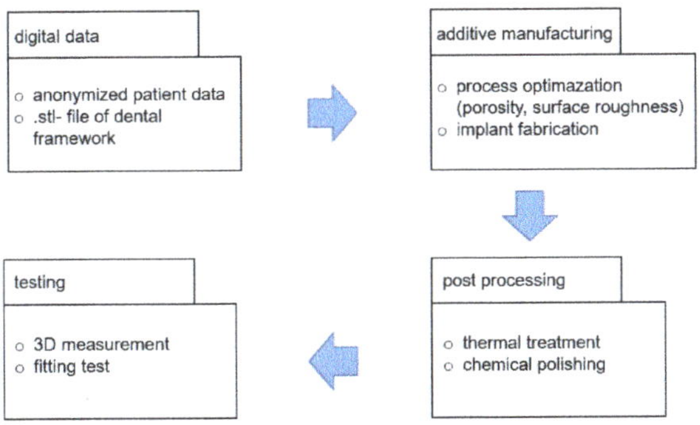

Figure 4. Experimental work flow carried out to fabricate the dental framework.

3. Results and Discussion

3.1. Optimization of Density and Roughness

In medical application and in particular in dental restoration, a high quality of the additive manufactured parts is needed. An important quality factor refers to the remaining porosity in the SLM part. By using well defined process parameters, the porosity of SLM parts is, in general accessible, below one percent. As previous, comprehensive studies on selective laser melting have shown, the porosity in the material sensitively depends on the energy density [42–46]. If the energy density is too high, gas porosity appears and if, in contrast, the input of the energy is to low, lack-of-fusion porosity appears [47].

In the following, we compare the processing of the fine powder section A32 and the coarse powder A45, as to evaluate the remaining porosity in the volume of the SLM part. We process both powder batches with the same process parameters, yet varying the applied energy density from $E_d = 52\ \mathrm{J/mm^3}$ to $E_d = 92\ \mathrm{J/mm^3}$. While we keep the laser power P_L, the point distance x_{point}, the exposure time t_{exp} and the layer thickness with z_{layer} constant, respectively, we vary the hatch distance y_{hatch} to accomplish different energy densities (as shown in Section 2.1). For each parameter set we built four cuboids with the dimensions of $V = 4 \times 4 \times 3$ mm^3 and measure the porosity by applying Archimedes method. The results for powder A32 and powder A45 are summarized in Figure 5.

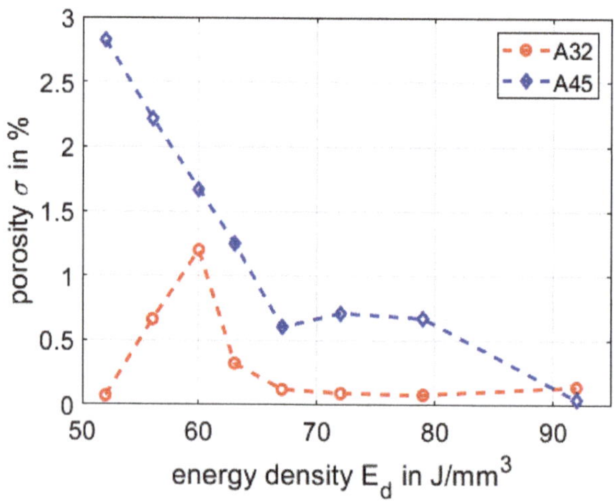

Figure 5. Comparison of the porosity of A32 and A45 in dependency of the energy density.

By processing powder A45 and increasing the energy density, the porosity drops from $\sigma = 2.8\%$ to $\sigma = 0.04\%$. We attribute this decrease to larger particle sizes, leading to lack-of-fusion porosities by lower energy inputs. In contrast, applying the finer powder A32, we find a peak value of the porosity with $\sigma = 1.2\%$ at an energy density of $E_d = 60$ J/mm^3, whereas for energy densities between $E_d = 67$ J/mm^3 and $E_d = 92$ J/mm^3, respectively, we have measured a rather low and stable porosity between $\sigma = 0.1\%$ and $\sigma = 0.2\%$. Here we assume the optimum between the lack-of-fusion and gas porosity. Considering both powder fraction A32 and A45, we find porosities of below one percent at higher energy densities of $E_d = 67$ J/mm^3. Therefore we define the process window for both powder fractions between $E_d = 67$ J/mm^3 and $E_d = 92$ J/mm^3. In this range the porosity is below one percent for both powder fractions, indicating an appropriate build quality.

One of the further limiting factors in the fabrication of high accuracy additive manufactured parts refers to the surface roughness, which we quantify by the common roughness parameter R_z. Deviations in the surface roughness lead to deviations in the accuracy of the part geometry and increase the necessary post processing efforts. Therefore, we discuss the two considered powder batches regarding the accessible surface roughness in dependence of the applied energy input during SLM. Surface roughness was analyzed using a laser scanning microscope (LSM VK-X200, Keyence).

The surface roughness of SLM parts, in general, depends on the grain size distribution of processed powder and used process parameters [48–50]. Furthermore, the surface roughness appears different on top and side surfaces, with respect to the build direction. In Figure 6 the surface roughness R_z is shown for the top and side surfaces for the powder A32 and powder A45 as function of the applied energy density. A suitable process window regarding the porosity is already defined by the porosity between the energy density of $E_d = 63$ J/mm^3 and $E_d = 92$ J/mm^3.

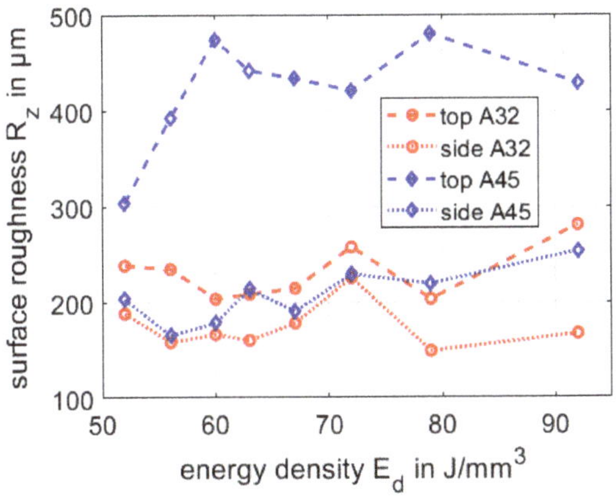

Figure 6. Comparison of surface roughness of the top and side surfaces.

Comparing the surface roughness as given in Figure 6, R_Z of the top surface of powder A45 is highest with $R_Z > 400$ µm, whereas the corresponding values of A32 (top), A32 (side) and A45 (side), respectively, are below $R_Z < 300$ µm. The roughness of the top surfaces of specimen made of A32 and A45 can jointly be explained by the particle size distribution. By processing coarser powder particles a rough surface appears due to sintering of particles on the top surface. The cavities between coarser powder particles cannot be filled with finer powder particles. In contrast, the side surfaces roughness of powder A45 and A32 is rather similar to each other, i.e., the influence of particle size distribution is less pronounced. Here smaller particles of both powder batches are sintered at the side surfaces and the quality of the SLM side surfaces depends mainly on the energy input [50]. As an interim conclusion, best surface roughness for the top and side surfaces is found for powder batch A32 with $R_Z < 300$ µm for the top and $R_Z < 200$ µm for the side. For dental application a low value of the surface roughness is needed allowing the fabrication of geometries with high accuracy and lowest effort in surface finishing of the respective components.

3.2. Fabrication of Dental Framework

To highlight the potential of of CoCrW for dental applications, we exemplify the SLM fabrication by generating a sophisticated dental framework (dental bar with attachements). In Figure 7 the finished dental framework is shown, after post processing with a thermal treatment of up to 750 °C, glass spheres blasting of the surface (grain size of 90–150 µm) and chemical polishing (the polishing step is done by a dental laboratory). Thermal treatment was carried out in a standard oven (Nabertherm) at a temperature of 750 °C (heating phase 45 min), temperature hold for 55 min and natural cooling. The resulting fitting accuracy is tested by a dental testing gauge (stylus) without significant deviation.

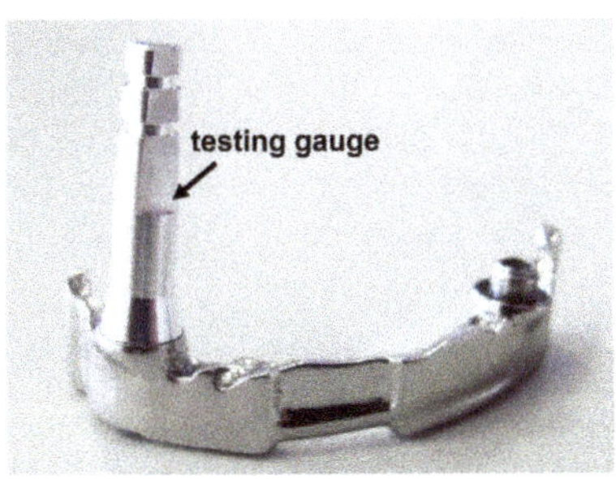

Figure 7. Dental framework with testing gauge.

Verification of the geometrical accuracy of the dental framework is done by 3D inspection (3D scanning) and comparison of the actual values with the nominal values. Shape deviations and shape variance analysis as compared to the original CAD data is provided by stripe line projection using Atos Core and ATOS Professional V8-SR1 software (GOM, Brunswick, Germany). The results are shown in Figure 8 in different orientations. The maximum deviation for the whole dental framework is less than $d_x \leq 0.25$ mm. This fabrication accuracy excludes thermal warpage of the structure and well-defined energy input during the build process. In particular the critical area around the fixture of the dental implant shows very good precision with deviations to the nominal value of less than $d_x \leq 15$ µm.

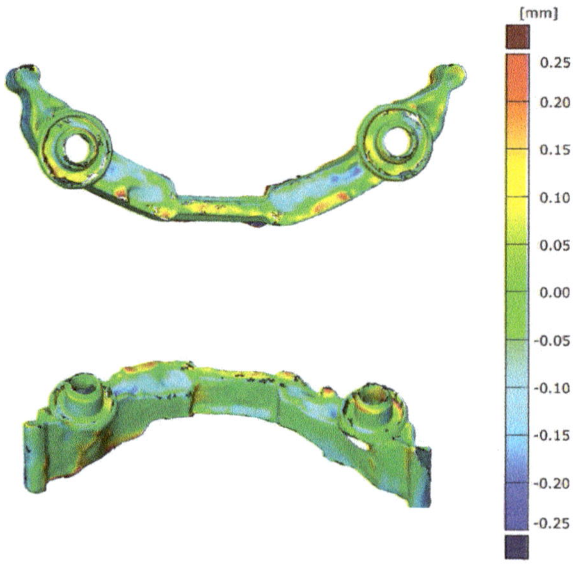

Figure 8. Nominal/actual value comparison of the dental framework—top view (above) and side view (below).

4. Conclusions

We demonstrated additive manufacturing of a dental framework (dental bar) with superior precision and fitting accuracy. In particular, using a fine sized particle distribution leads to significant improvement of the surface roughness fulfilling the recommendations for dental applications. A proper setting of the SLM laser and scanning parameters, in particular the applied laser energy density, leads to a minimized shape deviation and warping of the fabricated dental implant. As a result and to exemplify and highlight the potential of selective laser melting, a CoCrW dental implant components, a dental bar with attachments on the contact area and small sized round tack with thin walls and sufficient roughness, is demonstrated, which is commonly difficult to process with conventional processes.

Author Contributions: Conceptualization, A.E. and R.H.; methodology, A.E.; validation, A.E. and L.R.; formal analysis, A.E. and L.R.; investigation, A.E. and L.R.; data curation, A.E. and L.R.; writing—original draft preparation, A.E. and R.H.; writing—review and editing, A.E. and R.H.; visualization, A.E.; supervision, R.H.; project administration, R.H.; funding acquisition, R.H. All authors have read and agreed to the published version of the manuscript.

Funding: This research received no external funding.

Conflicts of Interest: The authors declare no conflict of interest.

Abbreviations

The following abbreviations are used in this manuscript:

SLM	selective laser melting
AM	additive manufacturing

References

1. Jemt, T. Failures and complications in 391 consecutively inserted fixed prostheses supported by Brånemark implants in edentulous jaws: A study of treatment from the time of prosthesis placement to the first annual checkup. *Int. J. Oral Maxillofac. Implants* **1991**, *6*, 270–276.
2. Wee, A.G.; Aquilino, S.A.; Schneider, R.L. Strategies to achieve fit in implant prosthodontics: A review of the literature. *Int. J. Prosthodont.* **1999**, *12*, 167–178. [PubMed]
3. Kalpana, D.; Sanjana, J.R.; Kumara Raju Kurapati, S.; Joel Koshy, J. Comparative evaluation of one piece and two piece dental implants—A review. *Int. J. Sci. Res.* **2017**, *6*, 49–50.
4. Pjetursson, B.E.; Asgeirsson, A.G.; Zwahlen, M.; Sailer, I. Improvements in implant dentistry over the last decade: Comparison of survival and complication rates in older and newer publications. *Int. J. Oral Maxillofac. Implants* **2014**, *29*, 308–324. [CrossRef] [PubMed]
5. Devaraju, K.; Rao, S.J.; Joseph, J.K.; Kurapati, S.K. Comparison of biomechanical properties of different implant-abutment connections. *Indian J. Dent. Sci.* **2018**, *10*, 180–183.
6. Thalji, G.; McGraw, K.; Cooper, L.F. Maxillary Complete Denture Outcomes: A Systematic Review of Patient-Based Outcomes. *Int. J. Oral Maxillofac. Implants* **2016**, *31*, 169–181. [CrossRef]
7. Örtorp, A.; Jemt, T. CNC-milled titanium frameworks supported by implants in the edentulous jaw: A 10-year comparative clinical study. *Clin. Implant Dent. Relat. Res.* **2012**, *14*, 88–99. [CrossRef]
8. Lowe, L.G.; Shcherbukhin, V.M. An implant-supported, cobalt-chromium milled bar and nonflanged attachment-retained overdenture to rehabilitate the edentulous mandible. *J. Prosthet. Dent.* **2009**, *102*, 46–51. [CrossRef]
9. Kioleoglou, I.; Pissiotis, A.; Konstantinos, M. Accuracy of fit of implant-supported bars favricated on definitive casts made of different dental stones. *J. Clin. Exp. Dent.* **2018**, *10*, 252–263.
10. Rinke, S.; Rasing, H.; Gersdorff, N.; Buergers, R.; Roediger, M. Implant supported over dentures with different bar designs: A retrospective evaluation after 5–19 years of clinical function. *J. Adv. Prosthodont.* **2015**, *7*, 338–343. [CrossRef]
11. Gehrke, P.; Dinkel, J.; Fischer, C.; Schmenger, K.; Sader, R. Surface roughness and necessity of manual refinishing requirements of CAD/CAM-manufatured titanium and cobalt-chrome bars—A pilot study. *Open Dent. J.* **2019**, *13*, 316–326. [CrossRef]
12. Chen, G.; Zeng, X.; Wang, Z.; Guan, K.; Peng, C. Fabrication of removable partial denture framework by selective laser melting. *Adv. Mater. Res.* **2011**, *317–319*, 174–178. [CrossRef]
13. Hong, M.-H.; Ki Min, B.; Kwon, T.-Y. The influence of process parameters on the surface roughness of a 3D-printed CoCr Dental alloy produced via selective laser melting. *Appl. Sci.* **2016**, *6*, 401–411. [CrossRef]
14. Kanazawa, M.; Iwaki, M.; Shunsuke, M.; Naoyuki, N. Fabrication of titanium alloy framework for complete dentures by selective laser melting. *J. Prosthet. Dent.* **2014**, *112*, 1441–1447. [CrossRef] [PubMed]
15. Konieczny, B.; Szczesio-Wlodarczyk, A.; Sokolowski, J.; Bociong, K. Challenges of Co–Cr Alloy Additive Manufacturing Methods in Dentistry—The Current State of Knowledge (Systematic Review). *Materials* **2020**, *13*, 3524. [CrossRef]
16. Weinländer, M.; Piehslinger, E.; Krennmair, G. Removable implant prosthodontic rehabilitation of the edentulous mandible: Five-year results of different prosthetic anchorage concepts. *Int. J. Oral Maxillofac. Implants* **2010**, *25*, 589–597.
17. Mericske-Stern, R. Prosthetic considerations. *Aust. Dent. J.* **2008**, *53*, 49–59. [CrossRef]
18. Waddell, J.N.; Payne, A.G.; Swain, M.V.; Kieser, J.A. Scanning electron microscopy observations of failures of implant overdenture bars: A case series report. *Clin. Implant Dent. Relat. Res.* **2010**, *12*, 26–38. [CrossRef]

19. Abduo, J.; Lyons, K.; Bennani, V.; Waddell, N.; Swain, M. Fit of screwretained fixed implant frameworks fabricated by different methods: A systematic review. *Int. J. Prosthodont.* **2011**, *24*, 207–220.
20. Paniz, G.; Stellini, E.; Meneghello, R.; Cerardi, A.; Gobbato, E.A.; Bressan, E. The precision of fit of cast and milled full-arch implant-supported restorations. *Int. J. Oral Maxillofac. Implants* **2013**, *28*, 687–693. [CrossRef]
21. Katsoulis, J.; Mericske-Stern, R.; Yates, D.M.; Izutani, N.; Enkling, N.; Blatz, M.B. In vitro precision of fit of computer-aided design and computeraided manufacturing titanium and zirconium dioxide bars. *Dent. Mater.* **2013**, *29*, 945–953. [CrossRef] [PubMed]
22. Miyazaki, T.; Hotta, Y.; Kunii, J.; Kuriyama, S.; Tamaki, Y. A review of dental CAD/CAM: Current status and future perspectives from 20 years of experience. *Dent. Mater. J.* **2009**, *28*, 44–56. [CrossRef] [PubMed]
23. Bollen, C.M.; Lambrechts, P.; Quirynen, M. Comparison of surface roughness of oral hard materials to the threshold surface roughness for bacterial plaque retention: A review of the literature. *Dent. Mater.* **1997**, *13*, 258–269. [CrossRef]
24. Romero, G.G.; Engelmeier, R.; Powers, J.M.; Canterbury, A. Accuracy of three corrective techniques for implant bar fabrication. *J. Prosthet. Dent.* **2000**, *84*, 602–607. [CrossRef] [PubMed]
25. Abduo, J.A.; Lyons, K.L. Effect of vertical misfit on strain within screw-retained implant titanium and zirconia frameworks. *J. Prosthodont Res.* **2012**, *56*, 102–109. [CrossRef]
26. Karl, M.; Winter, W.; Taylor, T.D.; Heckmann, S.M. In vitro study on passive fit in implant-supported 5-unit fixed partial dentures. *Int. J. Oral Maxillofac. Implants* **2004**, *19*, 30–37.
27. Hanif, A.; Qureshi, S.; Sheikh, Z.; Rashid, H. Complications in implant dentistry. *Eur. J. Dent.* **2017**, *11*, 135–140. [CrossRef]
28. Clelland, N.L.; Papazoglou, E.; Carr, A.B.; Gilat, A. Comparison of strains transferred to a bone sumulant among implant overdenture bars with various levels of misfir. *J. Prosthodont.* **1995**, *4*, 243–250. [CrossRef]
29. Torsello, F.; di Torresanto, V.M.; Ercoli, C.; Cordaro, L. Evaluation of the marginal precision of one-piece complete arch titanium frameworks fabricated using five different methods for implant-supported restorations. *Clin. Oral Implant. Res.* **2008**, *19*, 772–779. [CrossRef]
30. Takahashi, T.; Gunne, J. Fit of implant frameworks: An in vitro comparison between two fabrication techniques. *J. Prosthet. Dent.* **2003**, *89*, 256–260. [CrossRef]
31. Buzayan, M.M.; Yunus, N.B. Passive fit in screw retained multi-unit implant prosthesis understanding and achieving: A review of the literature. *J. Indian Prosthodont. Soc.* **2014**, *14*, 16–23. [CrossRef] [PubMed]
32. Di Giacomo, A.P.; Cury, P.R.; Airton, D.; DaSilva, M.; DaSilva, V.L.; Sergio, D.; Ajzen, A. A selective laser sintering prototype guide used to fabricate immediate interim fixed complete arch prostheses in flapless dental implant surgery: Technique description and clinical results. *J. Prosthet. Dent.* **2016**, *116*, 874–879. [CrossRef] [PubMed]
33. Jamshidinia, M.; Wang, L.; Tong, W.; Ajlouni, R.; Kovacevic, R. Fatigue properties of a dental implant produced by electron beam melting. *J. Mater. Process. Technol.* **2015**, *226*, 255–263. [CrossRef]
34. Lima, J.; Anami, L.; Araujo, R.; Pavanelli, C. Removable Partial Dentures: Use of Rapid Prototyping. *J. Prosthodont.* **2014**, *23*, 588. [CrossRef]
35. Cherry, J.; Davies, H.; Mehmood, S.; Lavery, N.; Brown, S.; Sienz, J. Investigation into the effect of process parameters on microstructural and physical properties of 316L stainless steel parts by selective laser melting. *Int. J. Adv. Manuf. Technol.* **2015**, *76*, 869–879. [CrossRef]
36. Spierings, A.B.; Levy, G. Comparision of density of stainless steel parts produced with selective laser melting using different powder grades. In Proceedings of the Annual International Solid Freeform Fabrication Symposium, Austin, TX, USA, 3–5 August 2009.
37. Nguyen, Q.B.; Nai, M.L.S.; Zhu, Z.; Sun, C.N.; Wei, J.; Zhou, W. Characteristics of Inconel Powders for Powder-Bed Additive Manufacturing. *Engineering* **2017**, *3*, 695–700. [CrossRef]
38. Clayton, J. Optimising metal powders for additive manufacturing. *Met. Powder Rep.* **2014**, *69*, 14–17. [CrossRef]
39. Lee, Y.S.; Zhang, W. Mesoscopic simulation of heat transfer and fluid flow in laser powder bed additive manufacturing. In Proceedings of the International Solid Free Form Fabrication Symposium, Austin, TX, USA, 12 August 2015.
40. Karapatis, N.P.; Egger, G.; Gygax, P.E.; Glardon, R. Optimization of powder layer density in selective laser sintering. In Proceedings of the 1999 International Solid Freeform Fabrication Symposium, Austin, TX, USA, 25 April 1999.

41. Eisenbacher Dentalwaren ED GmbH. *Product Specification of Kera S-Powder*; Eisenbacher Dentalwaren ED GmbH: Wörth am Main, Germany, 2015
42. Maamoun, A.H.; Xue, Y.F.; Elbestawi, M.A.; Veldhuis, S.C. Effect of Selective Laser Melting Process Parameters on the Quality of Al Alloy Parts: Powder Characterization, Density, Surface Roughness, and Dimensional Accuracy. *Materials* **2018**, *11*, 2343. [CrossRef]
43. Prashanth, K.G.; Scudino, S.; Maity, T.; Das, J.; Eckert, J. Is the energy density a reliable parameter for materials synthesis by selective laser melting? *Mater. Res. Lett.* **2017**, *5*, 386–390. [CrossRef]
44. Aboulkhaira, N.T.; Everitt, N.M.; Ashcroft, I.; Tuck, C. Reducing porosity in AlSi10Mg parts processed by selective laser melting. *Addit. Manuf.* **2014**, *1–4*, 77–86. [CrossRef]
45. Zhang, L.-C.; Attar, H. Selective Laser Melting of Titanium Alloys and Titanium Matrix Composites for Biomedical Applications: A Review. *Adv. Eng. Mater.* **2016**, *18*, 463–475. [CrossRef]
46. Kempen, K.; Thijs, L.; Van Humbeeck, J.; Kruth, J.-P. Mechanical properties of AlSi10Mg produced by Selective Laser Melting. *Phys. Procedia* **2012**, *39*, 439–446. [CrossRef]
47. Pleass, C.; Jothi, S. Influence of powder characteristics and additive manufacturing process parameters on the microstructure and mechanical behaviour of Inconel 625 fabricated by Selective Laser Melting. *Addit. Manuf.* **2018**, *24*, 419–431. [CrossRef]
48. Dadbakhsh, S.; Hao, L.; Jerrard, P.G.E.; Zhang, D.Z. Experimental investigation on selective laser melting behaviour and processing windows of in situ reacted Al/Fe2O3 powder mixture. *Powder Technol.* **2012**, *231*, 112–121. [CrossRef]
49. Calignano, F.; Manfredi, D.; Ambrosio, E.P.; Iuliano, L.; Fino, P. Influence of process parameters on surface roughness of aluminum parts produced by DMLS. *Int. J. Adv. Manuf. Technol.* **2013**, *67*, 2743–2751. [CrossRef]
50. Yang, T.; Liu, T.; Liao, W.; MacDonald, E.; Wei, H.; Chen, X.; Jiang, L. The influence of process parameters on vertical surface roughness of the AlSi10Mg parts fabricated by selective laser melting. *J. Mater. Process. Technol.* **2019**, *266*, 26–36. [CrossRef]

materials

MDPI

Article

A Clinical Trial to Evaluate the Efficacy and Safety of 3D Printed Bioceramic Implants for the Reconstruction of Zygomatic Bone Defects

Ui-Lyong Lee [1,2,*], Jun-Young Lim [3], Sung-Nam Park [3], Byoung-Hun Choi [3], Hyun Kang [4] and Won-Cheul Choi [2,5,*]

1 Department of Oral and Maxillofacial Surgery, Chung-Ang University Hospital, Soeul 06973, Korea
2 Chung-Ang 3D Craniofacial Research Society, Chun-Ang University, Seoul 06974, Korea
3 CGbio 3D Innovation Center, Seongnam-si 13211, Korea; jylim77@cgbio.co.kr (J.-Y.L.); snsimin@daewoong.co.kr (S.-N.P.); byounghunchoi@daewoong.co.kr (B.-H.C.)
4 Department of Anesthesiology and Pain Medicine, Chung-Ang University College of Medicine, Seoul 06974, Korea; roman00@naver.com
5 Department of Orthodontics, Chung-Ang University Hospital, Seoul 06974, Korea
* Correspondence: davidjoy@caumc.or.kr (U.-L.L.); abbalove70@gmail.com (W.-C.C.)

Received: 16 September 2020; Accepted: 9 October 2020; Published: 12 October 2020

Abstract: The purpose of this study was to evaluate the clinical efficacy and safety of patient-specific additive-manufactured $CaOSiO_2$-P_2O_5-B_2O_3 glass-ceramic (BGS-7) implants for reconstructing zygomatic bone defects at a 6-month follow-up. A prospective, single-arm, single-center, clinical trial was performed on patients with obvious zygoma defects who needed and wanted reconstruction. The primary outcome variable was a bone fusion between the implant and the bone evaluated by computed tomography (CT) at 6 months post surgery. Secondary outcomes, including implant immobilization, satisfaction assessment, osteolysis, subsidence of the BGS-7 implant, and safety, were assessed. A total of eight patients were enrolled in the study. Two patients underwent simultaneous reconstruction of the left and right malar defects using a BGS-7 3D printed implant. Cone beam CT analysis showed that bone fusion at 6 months after surgery was 100%. We observed that the average fusion rate was 76.97%. Osteolysis around 3D printed BGS-7 implants was not observed. The mean distance displacement of all 10 implants was 0.4149 mm. Our study showed no adverse event in any of the cases. The visual analog scale score for satisfaction was 9. All patients who enrolled in this trial were aesthetically and functionally satisfied with the surgical results. In conclusion, this study demonstrates the safety and promising value of patient-specific 3D printed BGS-7 implants as a novel facial bone reconstruction method.

Keywords: bioceramic; patient-specific; 3D printing; additive manufacturing; clinical trial

1. Introduction

Tumor resection, trauma, osteoradionecrosis, and various other causes may result in maxillofacial bone defects. The ultimate goal of reconstruction of maxillofacial bone defects is to restore bone defects and facial shape to their original form, minimize malocclusion, and restore masticatory function. In addition, the morbidity of the donor and recipient should be minimized and reconstruction should be done with a minimum number of operations [1]. There are many options for the reconstruction of maxillofacial bone defects. Grafting with allograft bone has been documented to be a useful tool in reconstructing jawbone defects [2,3]. Among them, microvascular bone transfer has become the gold standard for reconstruction. However, donor site morbidity, prolonged hospitalization time, and a lengthy recovery period with delayed functional rehabilitation are frequently noted [4]. Hence, there is an increasing need for an alternative option to microvascular free osteocutaneous flaps [5]. Ready-made implants made of various materials are also used to reconstruct maxillofacial defects. However, ready-made implants are inconvenient because they require secondary processing before implantation in accordance with the anatomical structure of the patient. In order to overcome this, patient-specific implants using 3D printing technology have recently been developed. Since the implants developed by 3D printing technology are customized, secondary processing is not necessary, and the implants can be transplanted quickly.

The development of CAD–CAM (computer aided design/computer aided manufacturing) technology and additive manufacturing with adequate strength and biocompatibility makes the foundation for the application of patient-specific three-dimensional printed titanium implants in the field of maxillofacial bone reconstruction [6–8]. A multicenter study using patient-specific CAD/CAM reconstruction plates for mandibular reconstruction has been performed, showing good outcomes [9], while a case was reported about the successful reconstruction of facial bone defects using a 3D printed titanium mesh [5]. Recent success in the manufacture of patient-specific 3D printed metal devices by additive manufacturing has been demonstrated [1,5,10].

However, titanium implants can eventually bring about subsidence because of the stress shielding effect and the differences in the modulus of elasticity [11]. Moreover, metallic artifacts due to the titanium pose difficulty in the evaluation of bone–implant fusion and detection of possible pathology in the maxillofacial area. To overcome these limitations, bioactive glass-ceramics with improved mechanical strength have been developed for bone grafting and repair. These bioactive glass-ceramics form apatite layers in the physiological condition of the bone and chemically bind to bone directly, resulting in improved bone-bonding strength [12,13].

Among the many types of bioactive glass-ceramics, $CaOSiO_2$-P_2O_5-B_2O_3 glass-ceramics (BGS-7) have been reported to induce osteoblastic differentiation of human mesenchymal stem cells, which results in an improved bone–implant contact ratio [14–16]. Furthermore, the intravenous administration of BGS-7 in rats did not show any toxicity for 90 days [17]. A 4-year follow-up study demonstrated similar fusion rates and clinical outcomes in both BGS-7 spine cage and autologous bone with a titanium cage in one-level posterior lumbar interbody fusion [11]. Besides, technology has been developed to make BGS-7 into a patient-specific implant through a fused deposition manufacturing method.

This clinical trial was designed to evaluate the safety and effectiveness of the patient-specific implant, manufactured by 3D printing process technology with BGS-7 for zygoma reconstruction.

2. Materials and Methods

2.1. Study Design

The Investigational New Drug application (IND) was approved by the Korean Food and Drug Administration (761) for this clinical trial. IND means that the clinician who intends to conduct clinical trials using the drug or medical device to collect safety efficacy data for the human body applies for approval from the Korean Ministry of Food and Drug Safety. The study protocol was approved by the Ethics Committee of Chung-Ang University Hospital (IRB no.3DB-1701) and registered at cris.nih.go.kr (KTC0002655). This study was performed according to the principles of the Declaration of Helsinki, 2000 [18]. In addition, written informed consent was obtained from all participants before participating in the trial. The study has been registered in the Korean Trial Register (NTR1289). The primary outcome variable was the fusion between the implant and the bone evaluated by computed tomography (CT) at 6 months after surgery. Secondary variables, including immobilization of the implant by CT, a visual analog scale (VAS) for satisfaction, osteolysis, subsidence of the BGS-7 implant, and safety, were assessed. A 4-year follow-up study evaluating fusion rates and clinical outcomes using BGS-7 spine cage in 1-level posterior lumbar interbody fusion has been performed [9]. Since the spine study used the BGS-7 spine cage, which is the same material used in this study, the primary outcome and secondary outcomes used in that study were also evaluated in this study.

The inclusion criteria and exclusion criteria of this study were as follows (Table 1).

Table 1. The inclusion criteria and exclusion criteria of this study.

Inclusion Criteria	Exclusion Criteria
1. Adults aged 19 to under 75 who have completed craniofacial growth 2. Those with obvious zygoma defects, who need and want reconstruction 3. In the case of women of childbearing potential, those who consent to contraceptive use during the clinical trial participation period (more than 6 months after surgery) 4. Those who voluntarily agreed to participate in clinical trials and were willing to comply with the study protocol.	1. People with uncontrolled metabolic diseases (e.g., diabetes, osteomalacia, thyroid disease) 2. People who are taking or are planning to take drugs that can affect bone metabolism (Bisphosphonate, Recombinant human parathyroid hormone, Denosumab, etc.) 3.Those with uncontrolled gingivitis, periodontitis, and dental caries 4. People with severe heart disease or severe liver dysfunction 5. Persons with infectious diseases with a risk of recurrence 6. People with blood diseases (leukemia, hemophilia, sepsis, etc.) 7. People who cannot stop taking steroids, anti-thrombotics, or anticoagulants before surgery 8. People who cannot stop systemic corticosteroids or anabolic steroids for 3 months after surgery 9. People with osteomalacia and Paget's disease 10. People who have experienced radiation therapy at the surgical site 11. People who are allergic to implant materials 12. Patients with syphilis and severe epilepsy 13. Drug abuse or alcoholics 14. Smokers 15. People who are pregnant or have a pregnancy plan during the clinical trial period 16. In case the investigator judges that participation in the clinical trial is inappropriate because other ethical or clinical trial results may be affected.

2.2. *Computer-Aided Virtual Surgery, Design, and Fabrication of Patient-Specific Devices*

Cone beam computed tomography (CBCT, 3D eXam, Kavo Dental GmbH, Biberach, Germany) of the patients was taken while patients were in an upright position. The CBCT data of the maxillofacial regions were obtained with a 0.4 mm voxel size and 512 × 512 matrices using 120 kVp, 11 mA, 17.8 s of scan time, and a 12-inch detector field (Figure 1A). Patient data were stored in the Digital Imaging and Communications in Medicine (DICOM) format and reconstructed into 3D bone images using the Mimics program (Materialise Co, Leuven, Belgium). By using the thresholding function of the program, we perform the process of mask-drawing the bone part for each slice cut, and 3D rendering by connecting each mask through the 3D calculation function. Following the completion of the 3D bone image-rendering, zygoma implants were designed using 3 Matics software (Materialise Co, Leuven, Belgium). The zygomatic bone defect is to be reconstructed accurately and matched to the original defect of the patient. The defect part is designed to be smoothly connected based on the normal bone, but the shape may be designed slightly differently depending on the surgical method or the fixing method selected by the surgeon. The basic contour of the reconstruction implant was taken from the other side of the non-defect zygomatic bone. The design can be modified according to the request of the surgeon.

After loading the stereolithography (STL) file of the implant with the confirmed design, we set 3D printing conditions such as printing position, printing direction, resolution, nozzle size, and support configuration. During 3D printing, the stacking direction is set parallel to the force direction that the implant will receive when the implant is later inserted into the body. In consideration of the occurrence of shrinkage during the sintering process, ceramics must be built up to a larger size than the final sample. BGS 7 powder was mixed with the binder according to the mixing ratio using a mixer to make the paste. This paste was filled in a stainless-steel syringe barrel and installed on the printer. After installation, printing conditions such as speed and discharge amount were appropriately set, and additive manufacturing was performed using the fused deposition modeling method (video). Additive-manufactured products were dried overnight.

The dried additive-manufactured products were placed in a furnace, and then, a sintering process was performed. As the heating process proceeded, the strength of the product increased, and shrinkage occurred. After the sintering was completed, the product was washed and dried using an ultrasonic cleaner. Cleansing was performed to remove any foreign substances or residues that may remain after removal of the support. After cleansing and drying, the product was put in a wrapping paper, and the packaging paper was hot-sealed, and then, gamma-ray sterilization was performed at a dose of 15–25 kGy.

2.3. Surgical Procedure

All cases were reconstructed with a bioceramic 3D printed zygoma implant (EASYMADE, CG Bio Co, Seoul, Korea), and implants were fixed using a mini-plate or wire via a transoral approach. Intraoperatively, the fibrous tissue filled the gap of nonunion. The soft tissue interposed between the non-united bones has to be removed completely. After removing all the fibrous tissue and exposing the bony margin of both sides, the 3D printed implant was applied and fixed with a mini-plate and or wire (Figure 1C). The method of fixing a screw hole through the implant itself was considered. However, since there was a possibility that the implant could break during the screw tightening process, the plate was fixed by pressing the implant downward (Figure 1D). Therefore, depression was designed to be placed on the implant (Figure 1B). Alternatively, we drilled a small hole in the implant and fixed it using a wire through the hole. In some cases, plates and wires were used together to fix them. All patients received the same anesthetic protocol. Anesthesia was induced with intravenous administration of 2 mg/kg propofol and 0.6 mg/kg rocuronium. Using 2–3% sevoflurane in 1.5 L/min N_2O and 1.5 L/min O_2, anesthesia was maintained. Noninvasive arterial blood pressure (NIBP), electrocardiography, and pulse oximetry were monitored continuously during the operation. Lactated Ringer's solution (3–6 mL/kg/h) and 6% hydroxyethyl starch were infused throughout surgery. A total of 30 mg ketorolac was administered just before the end of surgery for pain control and 5 mL of dexamethasone was administered intravenously after surgery.

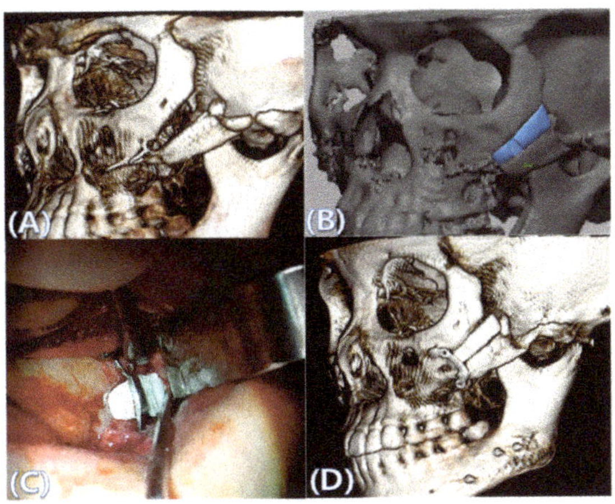

Figure 1. (**A**) The malar complex is dislocated inferiorly and rotated externally, which leads to facial asymmetry, bony gap, and facial drooping. (**B**) The implant for reconstructing the defected part is basically designed to be smoothly connected based on the normal bone. (**C**) After removing all the intervening soft tissue and exposing the bony margin of both sides, a 3D printed implant was applied and fixed with a mini-plate. (**D**) CT taken at 6 months after surgery shows that the bony defect is well reconstructed.

2.4. Evaluation

The primary outcome variable was the fusion between the implant and the bone evaluated by computed tomography (CT) at 6 months after surgery. The other variables assessed included immobilization of the implant by CT, a visual analog scale (VAS) for satisfaction, osteolysis, subsidence of the BGS-7 implant, and safety.

The VAS is a 10 cm long horizontal line. The patient expressed his or her satisfaction by pointing a vertical mark on the 10 cm long line. The measurement in centimeters was changed to the same number of points, ranging from 0 to 10 points. The question was, "Are you satisfied with your zygoma implant?"

The evaluation of CT used for bone fusion was performed by an independent and experienced oral and maxillofacial surgeon who did not participate in the clinical trial. Surgical variables such as operating time, blood loss, length of hospital stay in addition to adverse events, and post operative complications were also documented.

2.5. Cone Beam CT and 3D Comparison

CBCT was performed immediately after surgery and 6 months after surgery to evaluate bone fusion, the fusion area, and the immobilization of implants. A CT Digital Imaging and Communications in Medicine (DICOM) file, taken 6 months after surgery, was loaded into the in vivo 5 software (Anatomage, San Jose, CA, USA). The multi-planar plane was re-oriented so that the longest axis of the implant was perpendicular to the reference plane, and the minor axis was horizontal to the reference plane (Figure 2B–D). A cross-section was created based on the newly reorientated plane (Figure 2A).

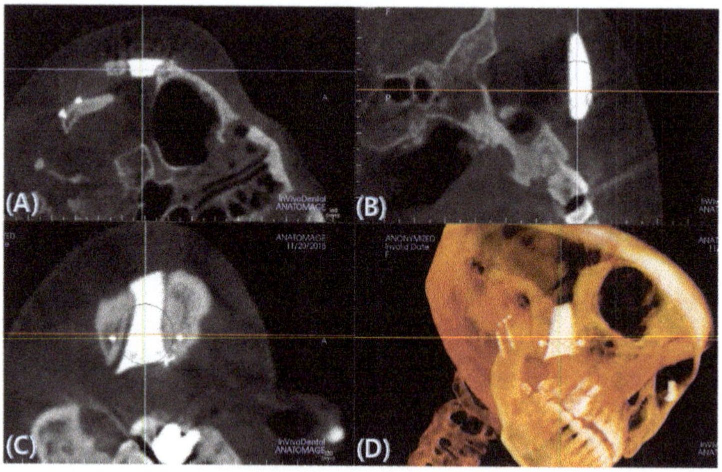

Figure 2. (**A**) A cross-section is created based on the newly reorientated plane. (**B–D**) The multi-planar plane is re-oriented so that the longest axis of the implant is perpendicular to the reference plane and the minor axis is horizontal to the reference plane.

To assess bone fusion, the newly formed axial planes (Figure 2A) were evaluated one by one at 0.4 mm intervals. "Fusion" is defined as the case where complete bone contact occurs in more than 50% of the total area of the interface where the implant meets the bone. Each section was checked, and the total number of sections was counted. For each case, we calculated the ratio of the number of fused cross-sections to the total number of cross-sections. Osteolysis around the BGS-7 implants and subsidence to the surrounding bone were both measured using axial, sagittal, and coronal cuts. An oral and maxillofacial surgeon independently reviewed and scored them as "fusion", if the calculated fusion rate was over 50%.

CT data taken immediately post surgery (reference data) and 6 months after surgery (measured data) were converted to stereolithography (STL) files and imported into Geomagic Control X software (3D systems, Rock Hill, SC, USA), and initial alignment was applied to superimpose the measured data onto the reference data (Figure 3A). A best-fit algorithm was implemented to overlay the measured data taken to the reference data, and the 3D Compare tool was utilized to measure deviation at 10 evenly spaced points on the implant surface (Figure 3B).

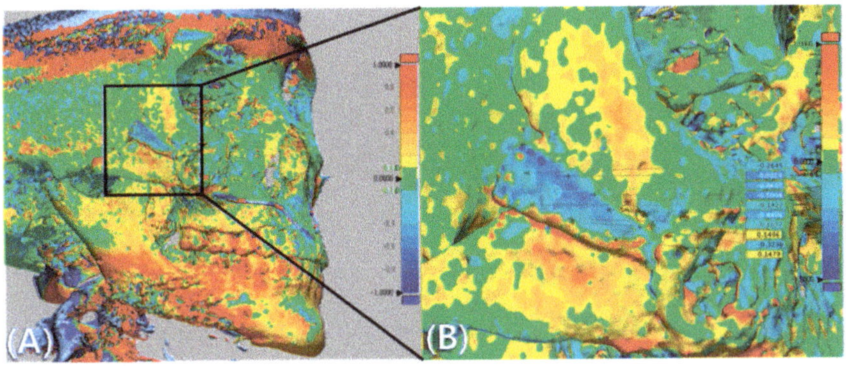

Figure 3. (**A**) CT data were converted into stereolithography (STL) files and imported into Geomagic Control X, and superimposition of CT data taken immediate post surgery (reference data) and CT data taken at 6 months after surgery (measured data) was performed using the Geomagic Control X software. The images were positioned using both the Initial Alignment and Best-Fit Alignment tools. The colors show overlays of 2 CT scan data. (**B**) Deviations between reference data and measured data were measured at ten evenly spaced points on the implants. The specific values of deviation on the implants are demonstrated. The value of deviation across the entire scan is color-graded from 1 mm (blue) to +1 mm (red).

2.6. Sample Size Determination

This study was a prospective, single-arm, single-center, clinical trial aimed at collecting initial safety and efficacy information for medical devices, designing follow-up clinical trials, providing criteria for evaluation items, and evaluation methods. Because it is an exploratory clinical trial, it does not statistically calculate the number of subjects.

2.7. Statistical Analysis

All data were analyzed using SPSS (Statistical Package for the Social Sciences) (IBM, Chicago, IL, USA) ($\alpha = 0.05$). Between-case differences for distances between random points were analyzed with a linear mixed-effects model (LMEM), which was made with cases as independent fixed factors, and each distance as a random effect. The number of cuts was analyzed with an LMEM, which was made with cases and fusion status as independent fixed factors, and each cut as a random effect.

3. Results

3.1. Baseline Characteristics

Between April 2017 and January 2019, a total of eight patients were enrolled in the study. Two patients underwent simultaneous reconstruction of the left and right malar defects using a BGS-7 3D printed implant (Cases 4, 5, 9, and 10). One patient (Case 3) refused to continue in the study 3 months after surgery. Consequently, the study was performed with Case 3's CBCT taken at 3 months after reconstruction. Of the 10 cases, one case was a male (10%). The mean age was 34.8 years, and none of the patients were smokers. All patients presented with various sizes of zygomatic bone defects in various areas due to previous malarplasty. Baseline characteristics are shown in Table 2.

Table 2. Summary of demographic characteristics, zygoma defect configuration, and virtual design of a patient-specific implants.

Screening Number	Gender/Age	Cause of Defect	Defect	Defect Area (mm)	Virtual Planning	Fixation Method
1S-01	F/29	Zygoma plasty	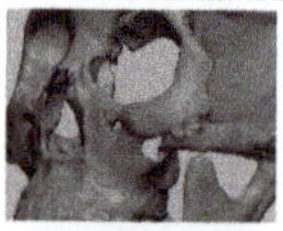	X = 16.4 Y = 9.8 Z = 3.8	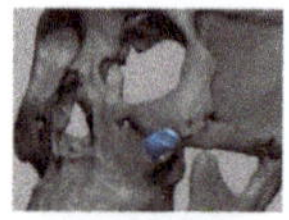	Plate
1S-02	F/24	Zygoma plasty	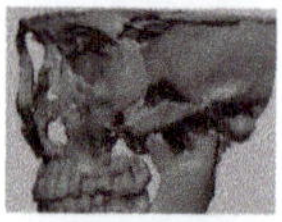	X = 32.4 Y = 12 Z = 4.8	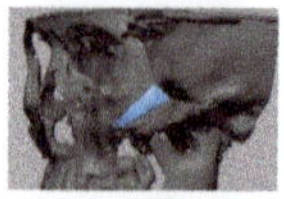	Plate
1S-03	M/25	Zygoma plasty	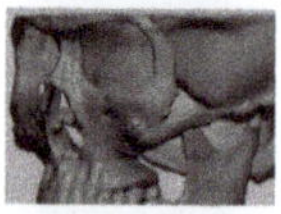	X = 17.3 Y = 13.3 Z = 5	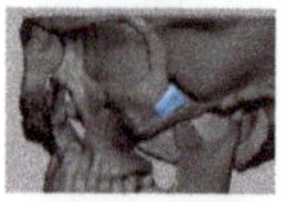	Plate
1S-04	F/28	Zygoma plasty	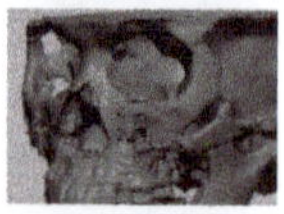	X = 28.4 Y = 10.9 Z = 5	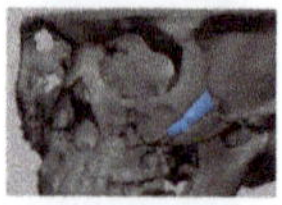	Plate
1S-05	F/28	Zygoma plasty	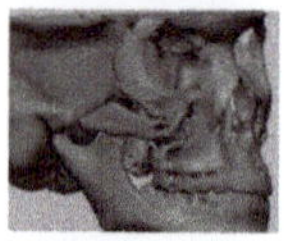	X = 26 Y = 8.2 Z = 4.4	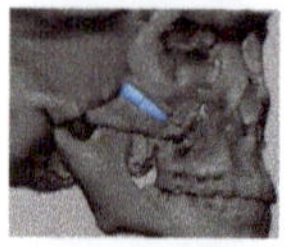	Plate
1S-06	F/41	Zygoma plasty	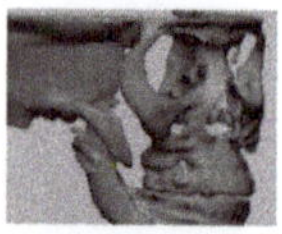	X = 29 Y = 19.2 Z = 5	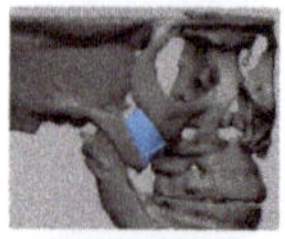	Plate and wire
1S-07	F/26	Zygoma plasty	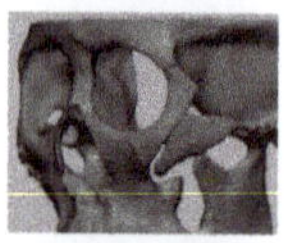	X = 18.1 Y = 7 Z = 4.1	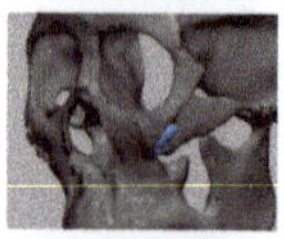	Plate
1S-08	F/53	Zygoma plasty	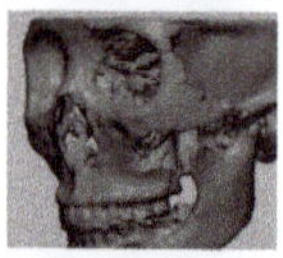	X = 37 Y = 21.5 Z = 5	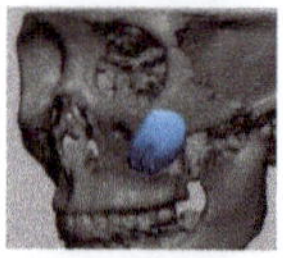	Plate and wire
1S-09	F/53	Zygoma plasty	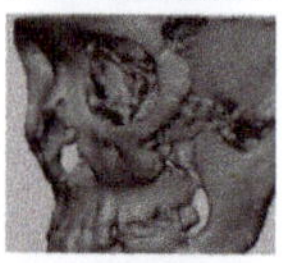	X = 21.8 Y = 13.3 Z = 5	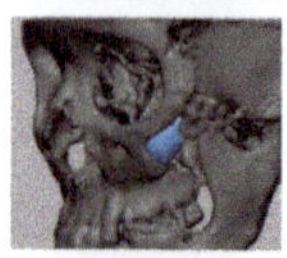	Wire
1S-10	F/53	Zygoma plasty	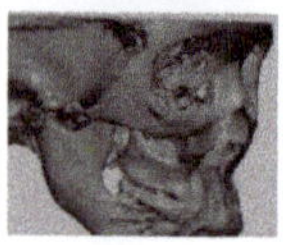	X = 16.8 Y = 13 Z = 4	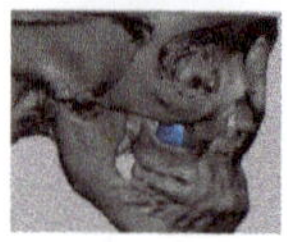	Wire

3.2. *Fusion Rate Analysis Using 3D CT*

Cone beam CT analysis showed that all patients exhibited bone fusion at 6 months after surgery (10/10). According to the results of analyzing the fusion rate using CBCT, we observed that the average fusion rate was 76.97%, and the standard deviation was 11.36. In all cases, the fusion rate exceeded 50%. The minimum was 58.33%, and the maximum was 88.24% (Figure 4). The LMEM showed no evidence of significant differences in average fusion rate between each cases ($F(9, 9) = 0.900$, $p = 0.561$), but significant differences for fusion status were observed ($F(1, 9) = 40.438$, $p < 0.001$) (Figure 4). In this study, osteolysis around the 3D printed BGS-7 implants was not observed.

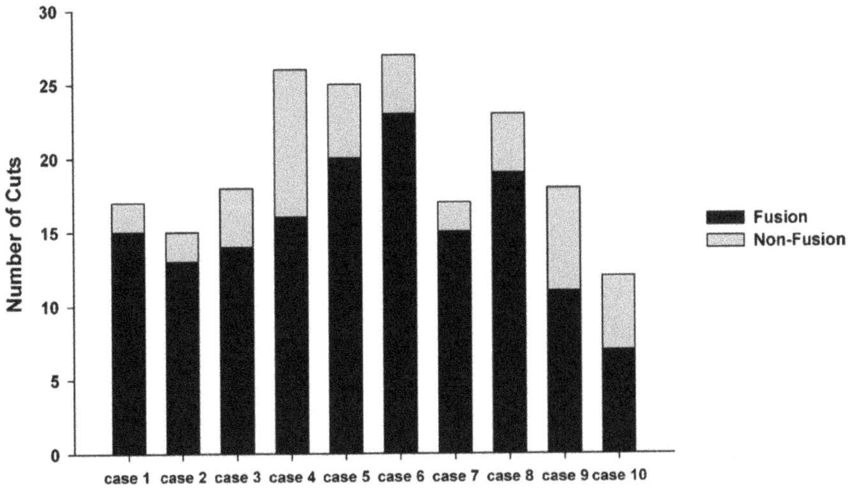

Figure 4. Linear mixed-effects model (LMEM) showed no evidence of significant difference between each cases ($F(9, 9) = 0.900$, $p = 0.561$), but significant differences for fusion status ($F(1, 9) = 40.438$, $p < 0.001$).

3.3. *3D Comparison between Immediate Post Operative and 6 Months Post Operative*

Table 3. shows the distance displacement of the measurements at 10 randomly distributed points on the 3D printed BGS-7 implants. There were statistically significant differences in the distance displacement of the 10 BGS-7 implants ($p < 0.001$). LMEM also showed a significant difference between cases ($F(9, 16.76) = 6.095$, $p = 0.001$) (Figure 5). The maximum and minimum mean distance displacements were 0.889 and 0.1156 mm, respectively, while the mean deviation distance displacement of all 10 implants was 0.4149 mm.

Table 3. The displacement of the measurements at 10 randomly distributed points on the 3D printed BGS-7 implants.

	Point 1	2	3	4	5	6	7	8	9	10	Aver.	SD
Case 1	0.3853	0.3461	0.5375	0.3455	0.4526	0.233	0.1499	0.1982	0.0476	0.0812	0.2776	0.1616
2	0.1469	0.3044	0.0014	0.2874	0.0191	0.1403	0.0927	0.0263	0.0695	0.0675	0.1155	0.1064
3	0.0979	0.0137	0.1259	0.0966	0.0821	0.1918	0.2396	0.3076	0.2452	0.3689	0.1741	0.1170
4	0.3342	0.0045	0.0888	0.2472	0.6319	0.6853	0.6889	0.6646	0.871	0.9915	0.5207	0.3327
5	0.1479	0.3236	0.1486	0.1077	0.4406	0.1422	0.5004	0.4437	0.5019	0.2645	0.3021	0.1602
6	0.4378	0.3892	0.337	0.3052	0.8668	0.7413	1.2819	1.4485	1.4251	1.6551	0.8887	0.5231
7	0.4298	0.2216	0.3879	0.2224	0.2695	0.2097	0.4689	0.3944	0.1436	0.456	0.3203	0.1192
8	0.4187	0.3392	0.5911	0.8404	0.5219	0.7681	0.7887	0.2335	0.1735	0.011	0.4686	0.2826
9	0.3199	0.1057	0.2524	0.1483	0.2272	0.3322	0.1833	0.4457	0.0755	0.045	0.2135	0.1270
10	0.3489	0.2618	0.9525	0.4041	0.288	1.3645	1.1981	0.6722	1.8174	1.3628	0.8670	0.5513

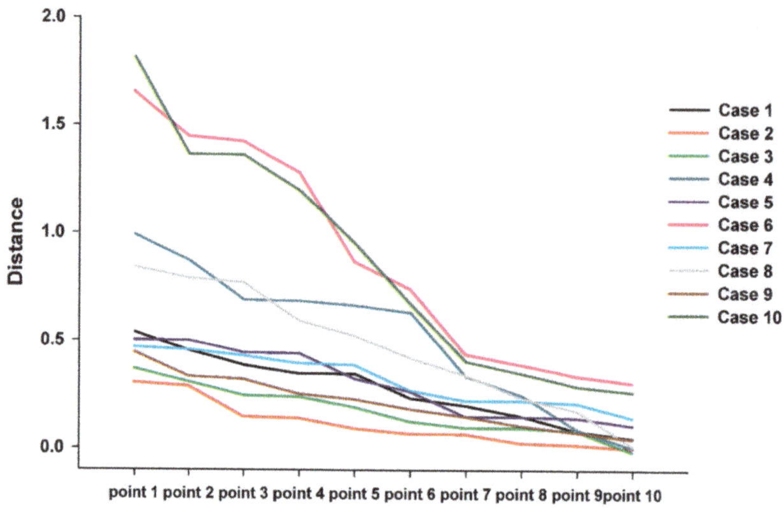

Figure 5. Linear mixed-effects model (LMEM) also showed significant differences between cases ($F(9, 16.76) = 6.095, p = 0.001$).

In the color map using the 3D inspection program, the displacement was the same as the measured displacement (Figure 6). In Figure 6, if the outer surface is blue, it means that the CT taken at 6 months after surgery is lower than the CT taken immediately after surgery. Most implants were displaced downward 6 months after surgery when compared to CT taken immediately after surgery. This result shows that the implant is attached closer to the surrounding bone under the downward pressure of the skin.

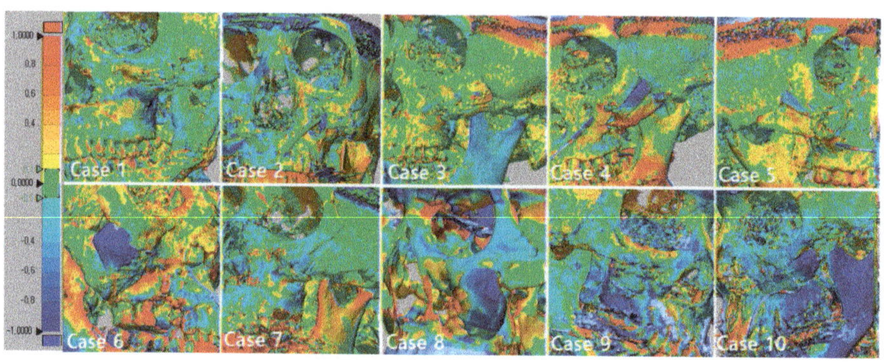

Figure 6. 3D comparison between immediately after surgery and after 6 months. This figure shows that the implant was attached closer to the surrounding bone. The specific values of deviation on the implants are demonstrated. The value of deviation across the entire scan is color-graded from 1 mm (blue) to +1 mm (red).

3.4. Results of Satisfactory Scale and Adverse Events

The VAS (Visual Analogue Scale) score for satisfaction was 9 at 6 months after surgery. All patients who performed the survey were aesthetically and functionally satisfied with the results of the operation. In case 3, we were unable to measure VAS because of loss to follow-up 3 months after surgery. In this follow-up study, there were no post operative complications, and no adverse events were reported in any of the patients.

4. Discussion

Reduction malarplasty is frequently utilized to contour the facial bone in Asia by repositioning the prominent malar bone. Improper fixation can result in nonunion or malunion of the malar complex due to the pulling force of the masseter muscle [19]. Consequently, the malar complex is displaced inferiorly and rotated externally, which leads to facial deformity, cheek drooping, or jaw movement restriction [20].

Instead of repositioning the displaced malar complex, which is due to malunion or nonunion after zygoma plasty, reconstruction of the bony gap in the zygomatic bone with a prosthesis can be a good alternative. Reconstruction surgery using a prosthesis is much simpler and less time consuming than repositioning the displaced malar complex and can be performed using a transoral approach. Most patients complain of the depression that occurred on the skin covering the gaps in the zygoma. They wanted to reduce this depression. After reconstruction surgery, all patients were satisfied with the aesthetics because the dents on their faces disappeared.

The development of implant materials has evolved rapidly over the years. In addition, the development of CAD–CAM technology and titanium 3D printing with adequate strength and biocompatibility has led to the application of patient-specific titanium implants in maxillofacial bone reconstruction [6–8]. However, titanium implants can eventually lead to subsidence due to the difference in the stress shielding effect and elastic modulus [11]. In addition, titanium metal artifacts can make bone assessments, such as fusion with implants and detection of possible pathologies in the maxillofacial region, difficult. To overcome these limitations, patient-specific additive-manufactured implants made of BG (BGS-7) were tested through this clinical trial. Among the many types of bioactive glass-ceramics, $CaOSiO_2$-P_2O_5-B_2O_3 glass-ceramics (BGS-7) have been reported to induce osteoblastic differentiation of human mesenchymal stem cells, which results in an improved bone–implant contact ratio [14–16]. Previous in vitro and in vivo studies have demonstrated that the BGS-7 cage for implantation in posterior lumbar interbody fusion has high bioactivity and chemical bonding ability [11,14–16]. The BGS-7 interbody fusion cages used for spinal surgery are not patient-specific and ready-made. The shape of the spine cage is not complicated and has a large contact area with the bone.

In contrast, implants for reconstructing zygoma defects vary in shape and size, and the contact area with zygomatic bone is not wide. However, since it is not a site under a large load, we conducted a clinical trial on malar defects for the first time to evaluate the efficacy and stability of the 3D printed bioceramic implant. As far as we know, this is the first clinical trial to reconstruct a facial bone using a patient-specific bioceramic implant.

Due to the lack of clinical data on facial bone reconstruction using additive-manufactured bioceramic implants, this trial was designed to evaluate clinical and radiological outcomes of reconstruction with bioceramic 3D printed implants. This clinical trial on patients receiving additive-manufactured bioceramic implants has shown that the implants are safe and result in clinical and radiological improvement. The lack of a control group is a weakness of this study. However, there was no standard treatment for the bony gap on the zygoma that occurred after the zygoma plasty, and the number of patients undergoing zygoma reconstruction surgery was small, so it was almost impossible to make a control group.

The authors evaluated the fusion rates of implants with bone using CBCT. A common method for assessing bone—implant ° integration is to measure bone–implant contact area. In the case of a dental implant, since the dental implant is drilled on a compact bone and the implant is placed, it is theoretically possible for the entire implant surface to make contact with the bone. However, in the case of a zygoma implant, the implant is placed by placing it on the bone. As this implant is designed to reconstruct the gap, there are many areas where the implant and bone do not make contact. Therefore, for these implants, a new standard for measuring the fusion rate is needed. In this study, the fusion rate was calculated by calculating the ratio of the area in contact with the bone to the area designed to contact the bone during implant design. The average fusion rate was 76.97%, and the standard deviation was 11.36. In all cases, the fusion rate exceeded 50%, with the minimum being 58.33%, and the maximum being 88.24%. In this study, osteolysis around 3D printed BGS-7 implants was not observed. Statistical analysis showed no evidence of a significant difference between cases ($F(9, 9) = 0.900$, $p = 0.561$), but significant differences for fusion status were observed ($F(1, 9) = 40.438$, $p < 0.001$) (Figure 4).

The mean removal torque of BGS-7 implants installed in rabbit ileum was significantly higher than that of titanium and PEEK (Polyether ether ketone) at 2 and 4 weeks, and the other three implant types at 8 weeks [15]. In vitro study results showed sufficient hydroxycarbonate apatite layer formation on $CaOSiO_2$-P_2O_5-B_2O_3 glass-ceramics (BGS-7) after soaking in simulated body fluid [21]. In addition, CaO-SiO_2-P_2O_5-B_2O_3 glass-ceramics are known to be used as a coating material to enhance osseointegration between bones and implants [14,22]. Titanium implants coated with hydroxyapatite have been shown to accelerate bone healing and prompt an enhancement in initial implant osseointegration [23–30]. The method used to fix the implant in this clinical trial is to fix it by pressing the implant using the mini-plate and a wire. Initial stability is important for proper osseointegration in dental implants [19–21].

Consequently, it was especially important to evaluate whether the BGS-7 implant was immobilized at the planned position until fusion with the bone. We analyzed the immobilization of the delivered implants using 3D comparison. A best-fit algorithm superimposed CT data taken immediately after surgery and 6 months after surgery, and deviation at 10 evenly spaced locations on the implant surface was measured (Figure 6). The maximum and minimum mean displacements were 0.889 and 0.1155 mm, respectively, while the mean distance displacement of all 10 implants was 0.415 mm. Most implants were displaced downward 6 months after surgery when compared to immediately after surgery. It can be seen that the implant was attached closer to the surrounding bone. Our study showed no adverse events in any of the cases. Therefore, this clinical trial shows that excellent osseointegration of the BGS-7 implants promotes effective bone fusion around the zygomatic bone. The BGS-7 implants can be successfully fixed using a mini-plate or wire. When performing zygoma reconstruction surgery using a patient-specific BGS-7 implant, most of the surgery took less than an hour because there was no need to harvest bones elsewhere in the body. Patients were discharged the day after surgery because there was no donor site morbidity and it took less time for surgery. As hospitalization period was shortened, overall medical expenses also decreased (data not shown).

5. Conclusions

The 6 months follow-up showed a high fusion rate and clinical results for reconstructing malar defects using patient-specific 3D printed BGS-7 implants. Furthermore, all patients who enrolled in this trial were aesthetically and functionally satisfied with the results of the operation with BGS-7 implants. Therefore, this study demonstrates the safety and promising value of patient-specific 3D printed BGS-7 implants for new facial bone reconstruction.

Author Contributions: Conceptualization, U.-L.L. and J.-Y.L.; methodology, U.-L.L.; software, B.-H.C.; validation, W.-C.C.; investigation, S.-N.P.; resources, S.-N.P.; writing—original draft preparation, U.-L.L. and H.K.; writing—review and editing, W.-C.C.; visualization, B.-H.C.; supervision, U.-L.L.; project administration, U.-L.L. and J.-Y.L.; funding acquisition, U.-L.L. All authors have read and agreed to the published version of the manuscript.

Funding: This research was funded by a research grant for clinical studies from CGBio Inc. and, this research was supported by the KIAT (Korea Institute for Advancement of Technology) grant funded by the Korea Government (MOTIE: Ministry of Trade Industry and Energy) (N0008804, 2019).

Conflicts of Interest: The authors declare no conflict of interest.

Table 3. Root mean square error (RMSE) values of trueness.

Trueness	0°	45°	90°	*p* Value
RMSE (mm)	0.129 ± 0.006 [a]	0.086 ± 0.004 [b]	0.109 ± 0.005 [c]	0.001 *

Data are presented as mean ± SD. * One-way ANOVA among three groups yielded $p < 0.05$. [abc] Different superscript letters indicate statistically significant differences based on Tukey's highly significant difference (HSD) test for the post hoc comparison test at $p < 0.05$.

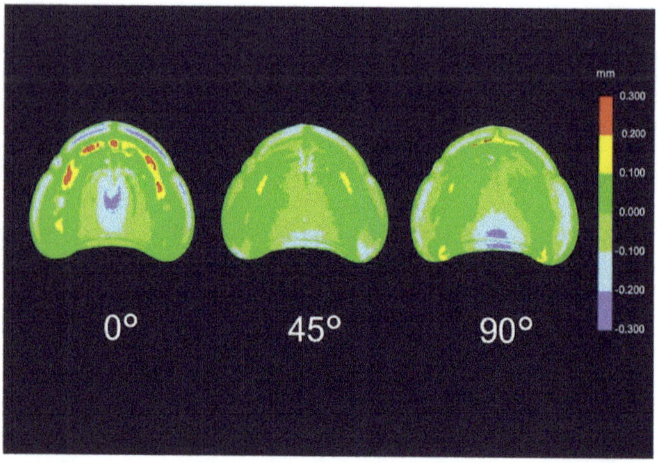

Figure 4. Deviation analysis of trueness. Color map deviation patterns of the denture mucosal surface with different printing directions. The trueness indicates the average deviation between the experimental data and the master data as follows: positive deviation, yellow to red; negative deviation, light blue to blue; and acceptable deviation, light green to green.

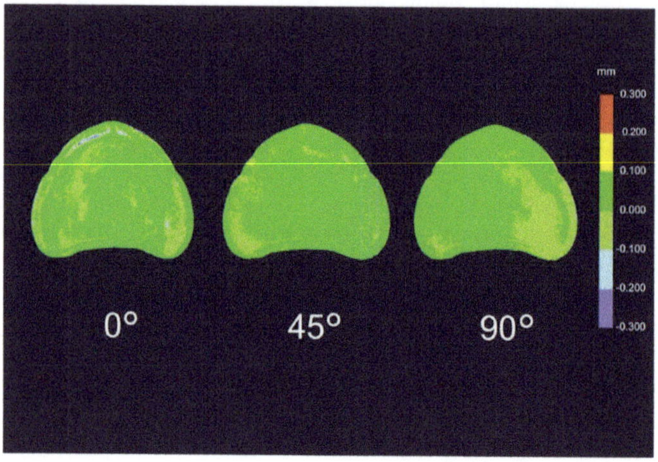

Figure 5. Deviation analysis of precision. Color map deviation patterns of the denture mucosal surface with different printing directions. The precision indicates the average deviation among the experimental data as follows: positive deviation, yellow to red; negative deviation, light blue to blue; and acceptable deviation, light green to green.

References

1. Lee, U.-L.; Kwon, J.-S.; Woo, S.-H.; Choi, Y.-J. Simultaneous Bimaxillary Surgery and Mandibular Reconstruction With a 3-Dimensional Printed Titanium Implant Fabricated by Electron Beam Melting: A Preliminary Mechanical Testing of the Printed Mandible. *J. Oral Maxillofac. Surg.* **2016**, *74*, 1501.e1–1501.e15. [CrossRef] [PubMed]
2. Barone, A.; Covani, U. Maxillary Alveolar Ridge Reconstruction With Nonvascularized Autogenous Block Bone: Clinical Results. *J. Oral Maxillofac. Surg.* **2007**, *65*, 2039–2046. [CrossRef] [PubMed]
3. Grassi, F.R.; Grassi, R.; Vivarelli, L.; Dallari, D.; Govoni, M.; Nardi, G.M.; Kalemaj, Z.; Ballini, A. Design Techniques to Optimize the Scaffold Performance: Freeze-dried Bone Custom-made Allografts for Maxillary Alveolar Horizontal Ridge Augmentation. *Materials* **2020**, *13*, 1393. [CrossRef] [PubMed]
4. Ettl, T.; Driemel, O.; Dresp, B.V.; Reichert, T.E.; Reuther, J.; Pistner, H. Feasibility of alloplastic mandibular reconstruction in patients following removal of oral squamous cell carcinoma. *J. Cranio-Maxillofac. Surg.* **2010**, *38*, 350–354. [CrossRef] [PubMed]
5. Shan, X.-F.; Chen, H.-M.; Liang, J.; Huang, J.-W.; Cai, Z.-G. Surgical Reconstruction of Maxillary and Mandibular Defects Using a Printed Titanium Mesh. *J. Oral Maxillofac. Surg.* **2015**, *73*, 1437.e1–1437.e9. [CrossRef] [PubMed]
6. Bertollo, N.; Da Assunção, R.; Hancock, N.J.; Lau, A.; Walsh, W.R. Influence of Electron Beam Melting Manufactured Implants on Ingrowth and Shear Strength in an Ovine Model. *J. Arthroplast.* **2012**, *27*, 1429–1436. [CrossRef]
7. Hrabe, N.W.; Heinl, P.; Flinn, B.; Körner, C.; Bordia, R.K. Compression-compression fatigue of selective electron beam melted cellular titanium (Ti-6Al-4V). *J. Biomed. Mater. Res. Part B Appl. Biomater.* **2011**, *99*, 313–320. [CrossRef]
8. Joshi, G.V.; Duan, Y.; Neidigh, J.; Koike, M.; Chahine, G.; Kovacevic, R.; Okabe, T.; Griggs, J.A. Fatigue testing of electron beam-melted Ti-6Al-4V ELI alloy for dental implants. *J. Biomed. Mater. Res. Part B Appl. Biomater.* **2012**, *101*, 124–130. [CrossRef]
9. Wilde, F.; Hanken, H.; Probst, F.; Schramm, A.; Heiland, M.; Cornelius, C.-P. Multicenter study on the use of patient-specific CAD/CAM reconstruction plates for mandibular reconstruction. *Int. J. Comput. Assist. Radiol. Surg.* **2015**, *10*, 2035–2051. [CrossRef]
10. Watson, J.; Hatamleh, M.; Alwahadni, A.; Srinivasan, D. Correction of Facial and Mandibular Asymmetry Using a Computer Aided Design/Computer Aided Manufacturing Prefabricated Titanium Implant. *J. Craniofacial Surg.* **2014**, *25*, 1099–1101. [CrossRef]
11. Lee, J.H.; Kim, S.K.; Kang, S.S.; Han, S.J.; Lee, C.-K.; Chang, B.-S. A Long-Term Follow-up, Multicenter, Comparative Study of the Radiologic, and Clinical Results Between a $CaO\text{-}SiO_2\text{-}P_2O_5\text{-}B_2O_3$ Bioactive Glass Ceramics (BGS-7) Intervertebral Spacer and Titanium Cage in 1-Level Posterior Lumbar Interbody Fusion. *Clin. Spine Surg.* **2020**. [CrossRef] [PubMed]
12. Kokubo, T.; Ito, S.; Huang, Z.T.; Hayashi, T.; Sakka, S.; Kitsugi, T.; Yamamuro, T. Ca, P-rich layer formed on high-strength bioactive glass-ceramic A-W. *J. Biomed. Mater. Res.* **1990**, *24*, 331–343. [CrossRef] [PubMed]
13. Ohtsuki, C.; Kamitakahara, M.; Miyazaki, T. Bioactive ceramic-based materials with designed reactivity for bone tissue regeneration. *J. R. Soc. Interface* **2009**, *6*, S349–S360. [CrossRef] [PubMed]
14. Lee, J.H.; Nam, H.; Chang, B.-S.; Lee, C.-K.; Ryu, H.-S.; Seo, J.-H. Bioactive ceramic coating of cancellous screws improves the osseointegration in the cancellous bone. *J. Orthop. Sci.* **2011**, *16*, 291–297. [CrossRef]
15. Lee, J.H.; Hong, K.S.; Baek, H.-R.; Seo, J.-H.; Lee, K.M.; Ryu, H.-S.; Lee, H.-K. In Vivo Evaluation of $CaO\text{-}SiO_2\text{-}P_2O_5\text{-}B_2O_3$ Glass-Ceramics Coating on Steinman Pins. *Artif. Organs* **2013**, *37*, 656–662. [CrossRef]
16. Lee, J.H.; Seo, J.-H.; Lee, K.M.; Ryu, H.-S.; Baek, H.-R. Fabrication and Evaluation of Osteoblastic Differentiation of Human Mesenchymal Stem Cells on Novel $CaO\text{-}SiO_2\text{-}P_2O_5\text{-}B_2O_3$ Glass-Ceramics. *Artif. Organs* **2013**, *37*, 637–647. [CrossRef]
17. Lee, J.H.; Ryu, H.-S.; Seo, J.-H.; Chang, B.-S.; Lee, C.-K. A 90-day intravenous administration toxicity study of $CaO\text{-}SiO_2\text{-}P_2O_5\text{-}B_2O_3$ glass-ceramics (BGS-7) in rat. *Drug Chem. Toxicol.* **2009**, *33*, 38–47. [CrossRef]
18. World Medical Association General Assembly World Medical Association Declaration of Helsinki: Ethical Principles for Medical Research Involving Human Subjects Revised October 7, 2000. *HIV Clin. Trials* **2001**, *2*, 92–95. [CrossRef]

19. Cho, J.; Kwon, J.-S.; Lee, U.-L. Occlusion-Fit Three-Dimensional–Printed Zygoma Repositioner. *J. Craniofacial Surg.* **2018**, *29*, 731–732. [CrossRef]
20. Baek, R.-M.; Kim, J.; Lee, S.W. Revision reduction malarplasty with coronal approach. *J. Plast. Reconstr. Aesthetic Surg.* **2010**, *63*, 2018–2024. [CrossRef]
21. Lee, J.H.; Ryu, H.-S.; Seo, J.-H.; Lee, D.-Y.; Chang, B.-S.; Lee, C.-K. Negative Effect of Rapidly Resorbing Properties of Bioactive Glass-Ceramics as Bone Graft Substitute in a Rabbit Lumbar Fusion Model. *Clin. Orthop. Surg.* **2014**, *6*, 87–95. [CrossRef] [PubMed]
22. Lee, J.H.; Ryu, H.-S.; Lee, D.-S.; Hong, K.S.; Chang, B.-S.; Lee, C.-K. Biomechanical and histomorphometric study on the bone–screw interface of bioactive ceramic-coated titanium screws. *Biomaterials* **2005**, *26*, 3249–3257. [CrossRef] [PubMed]
23. LeGeros, R. Calcium Phosphate Materials in Restorative Dentistry: A Review. *Adv. Dent. Res.* **1988**, *2*, 164–180. [CrossRef] [PubMed]
24. Jarcho, M. Retrospective analysis of hydroxyapatite development for oral implant applications. *Dent. Clin. North Am.* **1992**, *36*, 19–26. [PubMed]
25. Piattelli, A.; Cordioli, G.P.; Trisi, P.; Passi, P.; A Favero, G.; Meffert, R.M. Light and confocal laser scanning microscopic evaluation of hydroxyapatite resorption patterns in medullary and cortical bone. *Int. J. Oral Maxillofac. Implant.* **1993**, *8*, 309–315.
26. Ozawa, S. Evaluation of implant materials (hydroxyapatite, glass-ceramics, titanium) in rat bone marrow stromal cell culture. *Biomaterials* **1996**, *17*, 23–29. [CrossRef]
27. Zablotsky, M. The surgical management of osseous defects associated with endosteal hydroxyapatite-coated and titanium dental implants. *Dent. Clin. North Am.* **1992**, *36*, 117.
28. De Lange, G.; Donath, K. Interface between bone tissue and implants of solid hydroxyapatite or hydroxyapatite-coated titanium implants. *Biomaterials* **1989**, *10*, 121–125. [CrossRef]
29. Rocca, M.; Fini, M.; Giavaresi, G.; Aldini, N.N.; Giardino, R. Osteointegration of hydroxyapatite-coated and uncoated titanium screws in long-term ovariectomized sheep. *Biomaterials* **2002**, *23*, 1017–1023. [CrossRef]
30. Cook, S.D.; Kay, J.F.; A Thomas, K.; Jarcho, M. Interface mechanics and histology of titanium and hydroxylapatite-coated titanium for dental implant applications. *Int. J. Oral Maxillofac. Implant.* **1987**, *2*, 15–22.

materials

MDPI

Article

Effect of Printing Direction on the Accuracy of 3D-Printed Dentures Using Stereolithography Technology

Tamaki Hada [1], Manabu Kanazawa [1,*], Maiko Iwaki [2], Toshio Arakida [1], Yumika Soeda [1], Awutsadaporn Katheng [1], Ryosuke Otake [1] and Shunsuke Minakuchi [1]

1 Gerodontology and Oral Rehabilitation, Graduate School of Medical and Dental Sciences, Tokyo Medical and Dental University, Yushima, Bunkyo, Tokyo 113-8549, Japan; t.hada.gerd@tmd.ac.jp (T.H.); aragerd@tmd.ac.jp (T.A.); y.soeda.gerd@tmd.ac.jp (Y.S.); katheng.gerd@tmd.ac.jp (A.K.); r.otake.gerd@tmd.ac.jp (R.O.); s.minakuchi.gerd@tmd.ac.jp (S.M.)

2 General Dentistry, Graduate School of Medical and Dental Sciences, Tokyo Medical and Dental University, Yushima, Bunkyo, Tokyo 113-8549, Japan; m.iwaki.gerd@tmd.ac.jp

* Correspondence: m.kanazawa.gerd@tmd.ac.jp; Tel.: +81-3-5803-4645

Received: 6 July 2020; Accepted: 30 July 2020; Published: 2 August 2020

Abstract: This study evaluated the effects of the differences in the printing directions of stereolithography (SLA) three-dimensional (3D)-printed dentures on accuracy (trueness and precision). The maxillary denture was designed using computer-aided design (CAD) software with an STL file (master data) as the output. Three different printing directions (0°, 45°, and 90°) were used. Photopolymer resin was 3D-printed (n = 6/group). After scanning all dentures, the scanning data were saved/output as STL files (experimental data). For trueness, the experimental data were superimposed on the master data sets. For precision, the experimental data were selected from six dentures with three different printing directions and superimposed. The root mean square error (RMSE) and color map data were obtained using a deviation analysis. The averages of the RMSE values of trueness and precision at 0°, 45°, and 90° were statistically compared. The RMSE of trueness and precision were lowest at 45°, followed by 90°; the highest occurred at 0°. The RMSE of trueness and precision were significantly different among all printing directions ($p < 0.05$). The highest trueness and precision and the most favorable surface adaptation occurred when the printing direction was 45°; therefore, this may be the most effective direction for manufacturing SLA 3D-printed dentures.

Keywords: accuracy verification; complete denture; precision; printing; stereolithography; three-dimensional trueness

1. Introduction

With the recent and rapid advances in digital technology, new digital tools called computer-aided design (CAD) and computer-aided manufacturing (CAM) have become popular in the field of dentistry [1,2]. The designing and manufacturing of prosthetic devices using such digital tools have helped to reduce the burden on dentists and dental technicians [3]. There are two main processing methods for CAD-CAM systems: subtractive manufacturing (SM) and additive manufacturing (AM).

SM has been used for the production of dental prostheses such as crown bridges and implants, and its effectiveness has been confirmed. Additionally, SM has been actively applied to removable dentures [4–8]. The most common method involves designing the complete denture using CAD software, milling the denture base using a denture base resin disc, and bonding the existing artificial teeth [5,6]. This method of milling a ready-made disk can be processed with high accuracy because there is no polymerization shrinkage of the material itself, although it depends on the size and number of milling burs [9,10]. However, since only one denture base can be machined per denture base resin disc, the disc has many surplus parts after milling. Furthermore, milling burs are prone to becoming extremely worn out because the time required for milling one denture base can be long, which is not economical.

AM is a method of manufacturing a dental prosthesis by laminating and molding photopolymer resin and metal powder. Recently, a method of printing artificial teeth and a denture base separately using a three-dimensional (3D) printer and bonding the two with a photopolymer resin has been practically used [11,12]. The cost of 3D printers is low, and the printing time is short and economical; therefore, we have greater opportunities to use 3D printing in dental laboratories and dental clinics [13]. Typical examples of modeling methods for 3D printers are selective laser melting (SLM) for powder bed fusion [14,15], fused deposition modeling (FDM) for material jetting [16] and material extrusion [17], and stereolithography (SLA) and digital light processing (DLP) for vat photopolymerization. These methods are classified into seven types according to the ISO standard (ISO17296-2:2015 AM Part 2: Overview of process categories and feedstock). SLA is a method involving laser beam raster scanning of the surface of a liquid tank filled with a methacrylate-based photocurable resin to create a model [18]. The advantage of this method is that it is possible to produce transparent objects and create large, high-resolution models. Furthermore, by setting detailed parameters such as the print pitch, it is possible to form complex shapes with undercuts that are difficult to shear, and further applications in the dental field are expected [19].

Benefits to using 3D printing to create complete dentures are the quicker manufacturing time and less expensive cost compared to those of conventional methods [20]. In general, the number of models that can be planted on a platform depends on the shape and printing direction; vertical printing can produce more models than horizontal printing. There have been many studies of SLA 3D printers because their accuracy in creating printed objects differs on the basis of the printing direction, parameter settings, and the type of material used. Unkovskiy et al. [21] examined the precision of bar-shaped test specimens based on the printing direction used. Tahayeri et al. [22] examined the precision when changing the printing direction and parameters such as light intensity, exposure time, and slice thickness during the manufacturing of bar-shaped test specimens using various 3D printer materials. These studies demonstrated that several factors, such as the parameters and printing directions of the SLA 3D printer, affect precision. However, most specimens have simple shapes such as a bar [21,22], crown [23,24], and prism [25]. No studies have evaluated the effects of the differences in the printing directions (0°, 45°, and 90°) (Figure 1) on the accuracy (trueness and precision) of clinical dentures. Therefore, this study aimed to evaluate the effects of differences in the printing directions (0°, 45°, and 90°) on the accuracy (trueness and precision) of SLA 3D printing when creating dentures. The null hypothesis was that the three different printing directions would not show any differences in accuracy (trueness and precision).

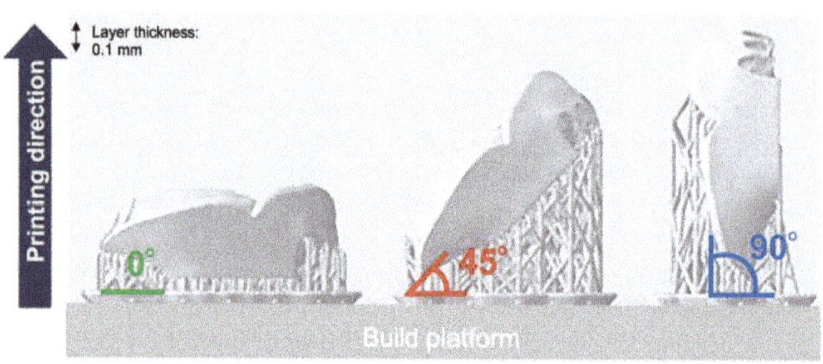

Figure 1. Schematic of three different print directions (0°, 45°, and 90°).

2. Materials and Methods

The flow chart of the SLA 3D printing accuracy verification protocol for dentures is shown in Figure 2. The surface of the maxillary edentulous model (G2-402U; Nissin Dental Products, Kyoto, Japan) and the artificial teeth (Velasia SA Antieria A3 ST5; Shofu, Kyoto, Japan) were coated with scanning powder (high-resolution scanning spray; 3M, St. Paul, MN, USA) and scanned with a 3D optical scanner (NeWay; Open Technologies, Rezzato, Italy) to obtain surface image data. A maxillary denture was designed by CAD software (Geomagic Freeform; 3D Systems, Rock Hill, SC, USA). The artificial teeth data were deleted from the denture data using Boolean logic operations, and a socket part for inserting the artificial teeth into the denture base was prepared. Then, the denture base was saved as a standard tessellation language (STL) file (master data) and sent to the 3D printing software (PreForm Software; Formlabs, Somerville, MA, USA). Three groups of dentures were assigned according to three different printing directions (Figure 3): 0°, print layer vertical to the z-axis direction (n = 6); 45°, print layer 45° to the z-axis direction (n = 6); and 90°, print layer horizontal to the z-axis direction (n = 6). A commercially available methacrylate-based photopolymer resin (Clear; Formlabs) was printed using a desktop SLA 3D printer (Form 2; Formlabs). Eighteen dentures with a thickness layer of 100 µm (z resolution) were fabricated (n = 6 per group). Tables 1 and 2 show the composition and processing parameters of this photopolymer resin. The dentures were washed with isopropyl alcohol (99.9 %) for 15 min (Form Wash; Formlabs) to remove excess resin. Once they were completely dry, polymerization was performed at 60 °C for 10 min in a 350- to 500-nm wavelength light-emitting diode oven (Form Cure; Formlabs) according to the manufacturer's instructions. Up to 24 h before the start of measurements, the denture base was stored in a lightproof container at a constant temperature of 23 °C.

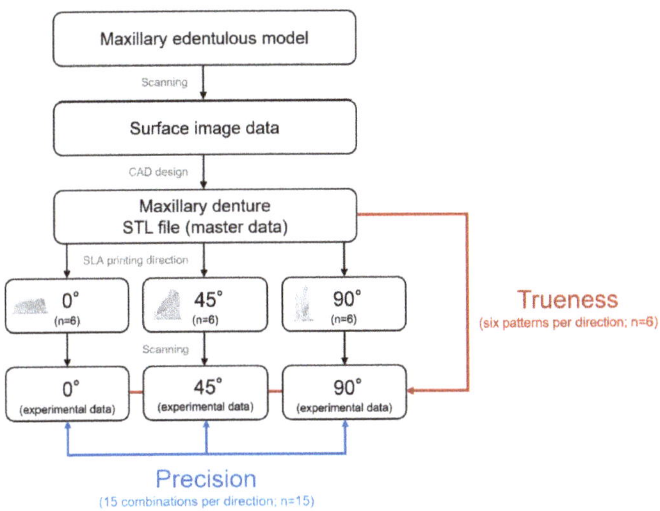

Figure 2. Flow chart of the stereolithography (SLA) 3D printing accuracy verification protocol for dentures.

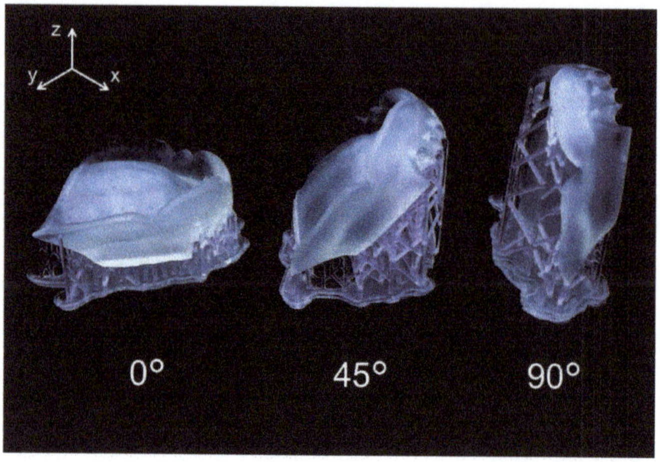

Figure 3. Dentures created using 3D printing with three different printing directions.

Table 1. Composition of transparent photopolymer resin.

Composition	Value (%)
Methacrylated oligomer	≥75–≤90
Methacrylated monomer	≥25–≤50
Diphenyl (2,4,6-trimethylbenzoyl) phosphine oxide	<1

Table 2. Print parameters and settings.

Printing Parameters	Settings
x-y resolution	150 μm
z resolution (layer thickness)	100 μm
Laser specifications	405 nm
Printing direction	0°, 45°, 90°

2.1. Accuracy Verification

In this study, materials and measuring equipment were calibrated according to the manufacturer's recommendations to precisely analyze the accuracy of the denture and eliminate bias in measurement methods. After 3D printing, the supporting materials were removed, and a 3.5-magnification optical loupe was used to visually inspect the denture surface for defects. The mucosal surface of the denture base was coated with scanning powder (high-resolution scanning spray; 3M) with an average particle size of 3.0 μm. All dentures were scanned with a 3D optical scanner (NeWay; Open Technologies). Scanning data were saved/output as STL files (experimental data). The International Standards Organization defined both trueness (closeness of measured values to the true value) and precision (closeness of measured values during repeated measurements) as accuracy (ISO 5725-1) [26]. During accuracy research of 3D printing, it was observed that the trueness value increased when the printed object and the CAD-designed object were dimensionally close, and that the precision value increased when the printed objects were dimensionally close. During the trueness test, experimental data were superimposed on master data (six patterns per direction). During the precision test, two sets of experimental data were selected from six dentures created using three different printing directions and superimposed on each other (15 combinations per direction). Superposition was performed automatically using the iterative tangent point algorithm after manually aligning the data along the flange of the internal surface to create the same coordinate system. A deviation analysis was performed using 3D analysis software (CATIA V5; Dassault Systèmes, Vélizy-Villacoublay, France). The distance between each set of data obtained by the deviation analysis was calculated and output as a text file. The root mean square error (RMSE) value (mm) was used to quantify the trueness and precision and was calculated using the following formula:

$$\text{RMSE} = \frac{1}{\sqrt{n}} \cdot \sqrt{\sum_{i=1}^{n} (x_{1,i} - x_{2,i})^2} \tag{1}$$

where $x_{1,i}$ refers to the measurement point $_i$ in the master data, $x_{2,i}$ refers to the measurement point of $_i$ in the experimental data, and n refers to the total number of points. The average of the RMSE values calculated for each denture was considered the representative value. Subsequently, a color map was created for qualitative expression. The nominal deviation was set to ±100 µm, and the maximum critical deviation was set to ±300 µm. The color map shows the average deviation between experimental data and master data for trueness and the average deviation among experimental data for precision as follows: positive deviation, yellow to red (area where the experimental data were larger than the master data and exceed the limit of the allowable range [100 µm]); negative deviation, light blue to blue (area where the experimental data were smaller than the master data and exceed the lower limit of the allowable range [−100 µm]); and acceptable deviation, light green to green.

2.2. Statistical Analyses

Statistical analyses were performed using statistical analysis software (IBM SPSS statistics 22.0; IBM Corp., Armonk, NY, USA). The Shapiro-Wilk test found normality in the data distribution, and the homogeneity of variance was satisfied according to Levene's test. Therefore, for trueness and precision, the averages of the RMSE values at 0°, 45°, and 90° were statistically compared using one-way analyses of variance (ANOVA) and Turkey's test for multiple comparisons with a significance level of $\alpha = 0.05$.

3. Results

The RMSE values of trueness were the lowest for dentures printed at 45° (0.086 ± 0.004 mm; $p = 0.001$), followed by those for dentures printed at 90° (0.109 ± 0.005 mm; $p = 0.001$) and at 0° (0.129 ± 0.006 mm; $p = 0.001$) (Table 3). The RMSE values for trueness were the highest at 0°. There was a significant difference in the RMSE values for trueness among all printing directions ($p < 0.05$). The color map shows that deviations existed in both positive and negative directions (Figure 4). The palate showed a light green color under all conditions, and the part equivalent to the ridge showed a green color (acceptable deviation). At 0°, yellow and red colors (positive deviation) were observed from near the incisive papilla to the left and right, and a light blue-to-blue color (negative deviation) appeared prominently at the central palate and denture border. At 45°, a yellow color (positive deviation) was observed near the linguogingival residual, and a light blue color (negative deviation) was observed near the palate folds and labial denture border. At 90°, a yellow color (positive deviation) was noticeable at the part equivalent to the incisive papilla and pterygomandibular fold, and a light blue-to-blue color (negative deviation) appeared near the palatine foveola. The RMSE values of precision were lowest for dentures printed at 45° (0.050 ± 0.003 mm; $p = 0.001$), followed by those printed at 90° (0.069 ± 0.002 mm; $p = 0.001$) and at 0° (0.072 ± 0.004 mm; $p = 0.001$) (Table 4). The RMSE values of trueness were the highest at 0°, and there was a significant difference between the RMSE values for precision using all printing directions ($p < 0.05$). The color map showed colors from light green-to-green (acceptable deviation) for most of the printing directions (Figure 5). Almost uniform color appeared at 45°. While observing the part where the deviation appeared in the color map, a staircase effect [27–35] of the print layer that could be confirmed with the naked eye occurred frequently (Figure 6). Positive deviations had a concave staircase effect, and negative deviations had a convex staircase effect (Figure 7).

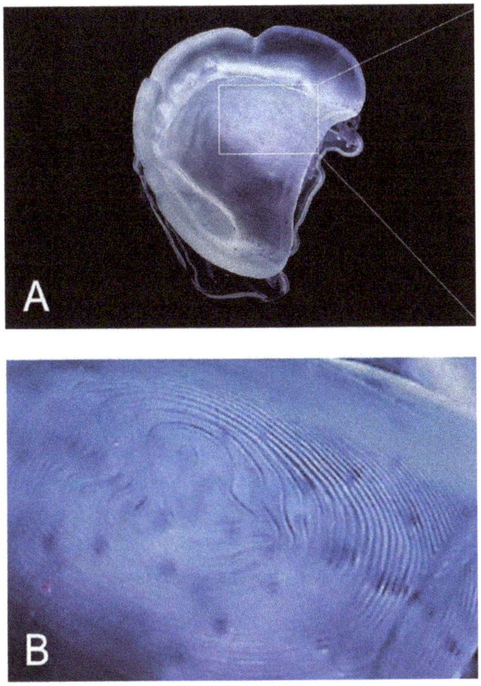

Figure 6. Staircase effects of the print layers on the surface of the denture mucosa. Many appeared when the printing direction was 0° and were clearly visible to the naked eye. (**A**) Total image. (**B**) Enlarged image of the staircase effects.

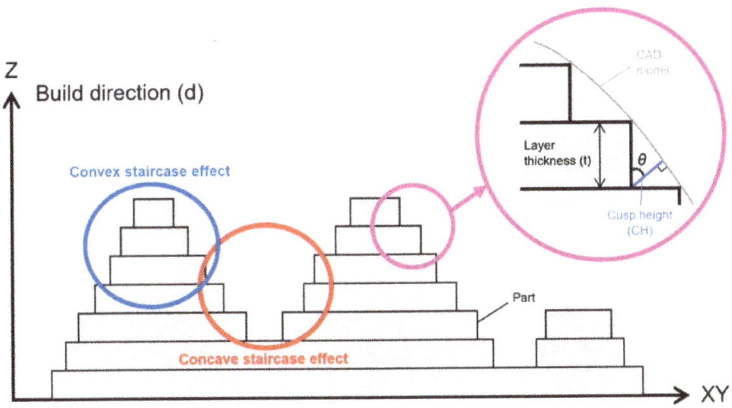

Figure 7. Concave staircase effects (positive deviation: red) and convex staircase effects (negative deviation: blue) in the trueness color map. The maximum deviation between the surface of the print layer and the CAD model surface caused by the staircase effect was called the cusp height (CH) [29–31]. The CH depends on the printing direction (d), the angle (θ) formed by the normal CAD model surface, and the thickness (t) of the printed layer. A thick print layer and/or a large cos (θ) value generated a large CH and reduced the surface accuracy.

Table 4. RMSE values of precision.

Precision	0°	45°	90°	*p* Value
RMSE (mm)	0.072 ± 0.004 ^{a}	0.050 ± 0.003 ^{b}	0.069 ± 0.002 ^{c}	0.001 *

Data are presented as mean ± SD. * One-way ANOVA among the three groups yielded $p < 0.05$. ^{abc} Different superscript letters indicate statistically significant difference based on Tukey's highly significant difference (HSD) test for the post hoc comparison test at $p < 0.05$.

Experimental data were superimposed on the master data, and the distance between each data point was obtained by the deviation analysis of six patterns (n = 6) for each direction. The root mean square error (RMSE) in mm was subsequently calculated.

Two sets of experimental data were selected from six dentures in the three different printing directions and superimposed on each other. The distance between each data point was obtained by a deviation analysis of 15 combinations for each direction (n = 15). The root mean square error (RMSE) in mm was subsequently calculated.

4. Discussion

During this in vitro study, we investigated the differences in the three printing directions when creating dentures with a 3D printer and found that the accuracy (trueness and precision) was significantly different with each direction. Therefore, the null hypothesis that three different printing directions used for SLA 3D printing dentures do not affect accuracy (trueness and precision) was rejected.

In terms of trueness, the mean deviation of the RMSE values in this study was 0.086–0.129 mm; however, the mean deviation of the RMSE values in a previous in vitro study [32] that evaluated the trueness of 3D printing full-arch models was 0.085 mm. The trueness of our study was similar to that reported in that previous study [32].

In this study, the RMSE values of trueness were largest when printing was performed at 0° in the z-axis direction (the print layer vertical to the z-axis direction). In other words, the fit of the denture printed at 0° was the least clinically favorable among the three printing directions. According to the color map of the deviation in the trueness of the mucosal surface of the denture (Figure 4), at 0°, a positive deviation was noticeable from near the incisive papilla to the left and right, and a negative deviation was prominent in the central palate and denture border. Positive deviations indicate a gap between the experimental data and the master data, suggesting that poor matching between the denture and mucosa may lower the stability and maintenance force of the denture. Negative deviations indicate that the master data are smaller than the experimental data, suggesting that denture adjustment may be necessary because of the strong contact between the denture and mucosa. According to a previous study [27], the surface accuracy of a printed object depends on the surface roughness. Furthermore, the staircase effect was caused by the thickness of the printed layer and the gradient of the surface of the object [27,29,30]. The maximum deviation between the surface of the printed layer and the CAD model surface caused by the staircase effect was expressed as the cusp height (CH) [29–31]. The CH depends on the printing direction (d), the angle (θ) formed by the normal CAD model surface, and the thickness (t) of the printed layer [$CH = t \cos(\theta)$]. A thick print layer and/or large cos (θ) value generated large CH and reduced the surface accuracy [33,34]. Therefore, Dolenc et al. [35] concluded that it was necessary to reduce the staircase effect to improve the surface quality of the object. In this study, when a denture printed at 0° with a constant print layer thickness (100 μm), a large cos (θ) value was generated at the part equivalent to the ridge crest, palate, and denture border. As a result, it was suggested that a remarkable staircase effect appeared in these three parts, and that positive and negative deviations were observed.

In our study, the RMSE values of trueness were minimal when printed at 45° in the z-axis direction (Table 3). In other words, dentures printed at 45° showed the best clinical fit among the three printing directions. A previous study [31] reported that printing an object at an angle reduced the surface area of each printed layer, thereby minimizing the ability to remove the object from the resin tank and greatly increasing the success rate of printing; the conclusion of that study [31] was consistent with that of our study, which indicated that printing at 45° showed the best accuracy. The color map of the deviation (Figure 4) showed a positive deviation near the linguogingival residual, suggesting the possibility of lowering the retention of the denture. No staircase effect was found when observing the part where the deviation appeared. Therefore, when observing the polished surface side, many support structures were denser than those created using the other two printing directions (0° and 90°). This was consistent with a previous study [24] that found positive deviations in the area with more support structures and the opposite side. When the part had many support structures, the part shrunk to the side of the support structure because it was damaged by more ultraviolet exposure than the less dense areas of the support structure. Therefore, it was suggested that the positive deviation that appeared near the linguogingival residual affected the support structures densely planted on the opposite side of the mucosal surface. However, negative deviations appeared near the palate folds and the labial denture border. Observation of this part showed a slight convex staircase effect. When dentures were printed at 45°, a large cos (θ) occurred near the palate folds and the labial denture border. As a result, a notable staircase effect appeared in these two places, suggesting a negative deviation.

The RMSE values of the trueness of the dentures printed at 90° were smaller than the RMSE values when dentures were printed at 0° and larger than the RMSE values when dentures were printed at 45° (Table 3). In other words, the fit of dentures printed at 90° was better than that of those printed at 0° and worse than that of those printed at 45°. A previous study [30] found that if the printing direction exceeded 45°, then overhang areas (a shape that cannot be supported without a support material) occurred, and it was necessary to add support structures to the surface of the object, which could adversely affect the surface accuracy of the object. Furthermore, in this study, the support structures were added not only to the polished surface side of the dentures printed at 90° but also to a part of the mucosal surface side to avoid displaying the printing error (overhang area) of the 3D printing software (PreForm Software; Formlabs). This suggested that the RMSE values of the trueness of the denture printed at 90° were larger than the values of those printed at 45°. In the color map of the deviation that occurred when printing was performed at 90° (Figure 4), the positive deviations were prominent at the part equivalent to the incisive papilla and the pterygomandibular fold, and a negative deviation was prominent near the palatine foveola. Observation of this area revealed the concave staircase effects (positive deviations) in the area corresponding to the part equivalent to the incisive papilla. When dentures were printed at 90°, a large cos (θ) occurred at the part equivalent to the incisive papilla. As a result, staircase effects appeared, suggesting a significant positive deviation. However, there were no staircase effects near the pterygomandibular fold and the palatine foveola where the positive and negative deviations appeared. Observation of this area revealed many additional support structures. Therefore, positive and negative deviations were suggested to be technical errors due to removing extra support structures to avoid overhang areas.

Regarding precision, the average deviations of the RMSE values in this study were 0.050–0.072 mm; however, in a previous in vitro study [23] that evaluated the precision of the crown fabricated by the SLA 3D printer using RMSE values, the maximum RMSE value was 0.042 mm. The difference was approximately 0.03 mm, which is clinically acceptable. Therefore, the precision of the SLA 3D printer used this time was relatively good. The RMSE value for precision was the least when dentures were printed at 45° in the z-axis direction, and it was the highest when dentures were printed at 0° in the z-axis direction (print layer vertical to the load direction). This suggested a tendency similar to the RMSE values for trueness. A comparison of the differences between the RMSE values for precision and the RMSE values for trueness showed that the RMSE values for precision were lower than the RMSE values for trueness by approximately 55–58%. It was suggested that the reason why the RMSE values for precision became small was that the dentures were printed near the center with high accuracy, thus avoiding the edge [21] of the platform where the accuracy was poor when printing the dentures. The color map of the deviation in precision (Figure 5) showed a green color in most areas in each of the printing directions. This was because the trueness of the experiment data was superimposed on the master data using CAD software, and the precision of the experiment was due to the superimposition of experimental data and other experimental data combined. Therefore, it was suggested that the precision of the printed objects showed the same tendency.

A post hoc power analysis was performed using the analysis software (G*Power 3.1.9.4 software; Kiel University, Kiel, Germany). Because the significance level was $\alpha = 0.05$ in this study, the power of 1-β was 0.8 or more; therefore, the sample size in this study was appropriate. To verify accuracy, the RMSE values were used to numerically evaluate the trueness and precision [36]. The RMSE value is widely used to quantitatively evaluate dimensional accuracy by calculating the phase difference between each point of the denture data of the three-dimensional space [37].

Reproducing the denture morphology designed by CAD with the highest accuracy is important for accurately fitting the denture in the patient's mouth and enabling long-term use [9]. The findings suggested that investigating differences in printing directions was essential to determining the overall clinical performance of 3D printing dentures. In this in vitro study, we selected the SLA 3D printer, which is widely used in various fields, and a corresponding photopolymer resin. The denture base after polymerization was stored in a lightproof container to prevent deformation due to ultraviolet rays [21,23].

The results of this study indicated that printing at 45° was recommended to minimize the effects on the accuracy of 3D printing dentures using SLA technology. If the denture printing direction deviates from this range, the denture will still be usable; however, to improve the accuracy of the denture, the printing direction must be at least 45°–90°.

The main limitation of this study was its in vitro nature. In this study, we used one type of SLA 3D printer and photopolymer resin corresponding to the model. The parameters of this model were fixed and could not be freely adjusted. Therefore, the same tendency was not always observed when using other types of SLA 3D printers. Clear photopolymer resin was chosen for this study because it was an in vitro study. We also conducted material property tests of the same materials and designs [38]. Therefore, we believe it is important to verify the accuracy using standardized materials and designs. However, there are various types of photopolymer resins other than those used in this study, and some resins could be used in open mode in printers made by other companies. Therefore, it is necessary to investigate the method that can produce the most accurate denture with various types of 3D printers, photopolymer resins, or a combination of these. The creation of dentures with 3D printers is simple, quick, and inexpensive compared to other conventional methods; therefore, it is expected that 3D printing will become more popular in the future to reduce the burden on dentists and dental technicians. Further studies investigating the effects of different 3D printing directions on accuracy in vivo are required.

5. Conclusions

The accuracy (trueness and precision) of dentures printed using an SLA 3D printer depends on the denture printing direction. The 45° printing direction showed the highest accuracy compared to the 0° and 90° printing directions.

Author Contributions: Conceptualization, T.H.; formal analysis, T.H.; investigation, T.A., Y.S., A.K., and R.O.; methodology, T.H.; resources, T.H.; software, T.H.; supervision, S.M. and M.K.; writing—original draft, T.H.; writing—review and editing, M.K. and M.I. All authors have read and agreed to the published version of the manuscript.

Funding: This research received no external funding.

Acknowledgments: The authors thank the CAD-CAM team for providing support for this study.

Conflicts of Interest: The authors declare no conflict of interest.

References

1. Miyazaki, T.; Hotta, Y.; Kunii, J.; Kuriyama, S.; Tamaki, Y. A review of dental CAD/CAM: Current status and future perspectives from 20 years of experience. *Dent. Mater. J.* **2009**, *28*, 44–56. [CrossRef] [PubMed]
2. Bidra, A.S.; Taylor, T.D.; Agar, J.R. Computer-aided technology for fabricating complete dentures: Systematic review of historical background, current status, and future perspectives. *J. Prosthet. Dent.* **2013**, *109*, 361–366. [CrossRef]
3. Kattadiyil, M.T.; Goodacre, C.J.; Baba, N.Z. CAD/CAM complete dentures: A review of two commercial fabrication systems. *J. Calif. Dent. Assoc.* **2013**, *41*, 407–416. [PubMed]
4. Kawahata, N.; Ono, H.; Nishi, Y.; Hamano, T.; Nagaoka, E. Trial of duplication procedure for complete dentures by CAD/CAM. *J. Oral Rehabil.* **1997**, *24*, 540–548. [CrossRef]
5. Kanazawa, M.; Inokoshi, M.; Minakuchi, S.; Ohbayashi, N. Trial of a CAD/CAM system for fabricating complete dentures. *Dent. Mater. J.* **2011**, *30*, 93–96. [CrossRef]
6. Katase, H.; Kanazawa, M.; Inokoshi, M.; Minakuchi, S. Face simulation system for complete dentures by applying rapid prototyping. *J. Prosthet. Dent.* **2013**, *109*, 353–360. [CrossRef]
7. Zhang, Y.D.; Jiang, J.G.; Liang, T.; Hu, W.P. Kinematics modeling and experimentation of the multi-manipulator tooth-arrangement robot for full denture manufacturing. *J. Med. Syst.* **2011**, *35*, 1421–1429. [CrossRef]
8. Goodacre, C.J.; Garbacea, A.; Naylor, W.P.; Daher, T.; Marchack, C.B.; Lowry, J. CAD/CAM fabricated complete dentures: Concepts and clinical methods of obtaining required morphological data. *J. Prosthet. Dent.* **2012**, *107*, 34–46. [CrossRef]
9. Goodacre, B.J.; Goodacre, C.J.; Baba, N.Z.; Kattadiyil, M.T. Comparison of denture base adaptation between CAD-CAM and conventional fabrication techniques. *J. Prosthet. Dent.* **2016**, *116*, 249–256. [CrossRef]
10. Srinivasan, M.; Cantin, Y.; Mehl, A.; Gjengedal, H.; Müller, F.; Schimmel, M. CAD/CAM milled removable complete dentures: An in vitro evaluation of trueness. *Clin. Oral Investig.* **2017**, *21*, 2007–2019. [CrossRef]
11. Dentsply Sirona Inc., Charlotte. Dentsply Sirona Support: Introducing Lucitone Digital Dentures. 2019. Available online: https://lp.dentsplysirona.com/en-us/lucitone-digital-print.html (accessed on 7 January 2020).
12. Formlabs Inc., Somerville. Formlabs Support: 3D Printed Digital Dentures. 2019. Available online: https://formlabs.com/uk/dental/digital-dentures/ (accessed on 7 January 2020).
13. Fullerton, J.N.; Frodsham, G.C.M.; Day, R.M. 3D printing for the many, not the few. *Nat. Biotechnol.* **2014**, *32*, 1086–1087. [CrossRef] [PubMed]
14. Revilla-León, M.; Meyer, M.J.; Özcan, M. Metal additive manufacturing technologies: Literature review of current status and prosthodontic applications. *Int. J. Comput. Dent.* **2019**, *22*, 55–67. [PubMed]
15. Janeczek, M.; Szymczyk, P.; Dobrzynski, M.; Parulska, O.; Szymonowicz, M.; Kuropka, P.; Rybak, Z.; Zywicka, B.; Ziolkowski, G.; Marycz, K.; et al. Influence of surface modifications of a nanostructured implant on osseointegration capacity- preliminary in vivo study. *RSC Adv.* **2018**, *8*, 15533–15546. [CrossRef]
16. Liang, X.; Liao, W.; Cai, H.; Jiang, S.; Chen, S. 3D-printed artificial teeth: Accuracy and application in root canal therapy. *J. Biomed. Nanotechnol.* **2018**, *14*, 1477–1485. [CrossRef]
17. Zhou, Z.; Buchanan, F.; Mitchell, C.; Dunne, N. Printability of calcium phosphate: Calcium sulfate powders for the application of tissue engineered bone scaffolds using the 3D printing technique. *Mater. Sci. Eng. C Mater. Biol. Appl.* **2014**, *38*, 1–10. [CrossRef]
18. Gibson, I.; Rosen, D.W.; Stucker, B. *Additive Manufacturing Technologies*, 2nd ed.; Springer: Boston, MA, USA, 2015; pp. 63–106.
19. Takeda, Y.; Lau, J.; Nouh, H.; Hirayama, H. A 3D printing replication technique for fabricating digital dentures. *J. Prosthet. Dent.* 2019. [CrossRef]
20. Berman, B. 3-D printing: The new industrial revolution. *Bus. Horiz.* **2012**, *55*, 155–162. [CrossRef]
21. Unkovskiy, A.; Bui, P.H.; Schille, C.; Geis-Gerstorfer, J.; Huettig, F.; Spintzyk, S. Objects build orientation, positioning, and curing influence dimensional accuracy and flexural properties of stereolithographically printed resin. *Dent. Mater.* **2018**, *34*, e324–e333. [CrossRef]
22. Tahayeri, A.; Morgan, M.; Fugolin, A.P.; Bompolaki, D.; Athirasala, A.; Pfeifer, C.S.; Ferracane, J.L.; Bertassoni, L.E. 3D printed versus conventionally cured provisional crown and bridge dental materials. *Dent. Mater.* **2018**, *34*, 192–200. [CrossRef]

23. Alharbi, N.; Osman, R.B.; Wismeijer, D. Factors influencing the dimensional accuracy of 3D-printed full-coverage dental restorations using stereolithography technology. *Int. J. Prosthodont.* **2016**, *29*, 503–510. [CrossRef]
24. Osman, R.B.; Alharbi, N.; Wismeijer, D. Build Angle: Does it influence the accuracy of 3D-printed dental restorations using digital light-processing technology? *Int. J. Prosthodont.* **2017**, *30*, 182–188. [CrossRef] [PubMed]
25. Ide, Y.; Nayar, S.; Logan, H.; Gallagher, B.; Wolfaardt, J. The effect of the angle of acuteness of additive manufactured models and the direction of printing on the dimensional fidelity: Clinical implications. *Odontology* **2017**, *105*, 108–115. [CrossRef] [PubMed]
26. International Organization of Standardization, Geneva. ISO 5725-1:1998. Accuracy (Trueness and Precision) of Measurement Methods and Results–Part 1: General Principles and Definitions. 1998. Available online: https://www.iso.org/obp/ui/#iso:std:iso:5725:-1:ed-1:v1:en (accessed on 9 January 2020).
27. Arnold, C.; Monsees, D.; Hey, J.; Schweyen, R. Surface quality of 3D-printed models as a function of various printing parameters. *Materials* **2019**, *12*, 1970. [CrossRef] [PubMed]
28. Formlabs Inc., Somerville. Formlabs Support: What Does Resolution Mean in 3D Printing? Pt. 2. 2016. Available online: https://formlabs.com/blog/horizontal-resolution-meaning-3d-printing/ (accessed on 26 November 2019).
29. Jaiswal, P.; Patel, J.; Rai, R. Build orientation optimization for additive manufacturing of functionally graded material objects. *Int. J. Adv. Manuf. Technol.* **2018**, *96*, 223–235. [CrossRef]
30. Pandey, P.M.; Reddy, N.V.; Dhande, S.G. Slicing procedures in layered manufacturing: A review. *Rapid Prototyp. J.* **2003**, *9*, 274–288. [CrossRef]
31. Cheng, W.; Fuh, J.Y.H.; Nee, A.Y.C.; Wong, Y.S.; Loh, H.T.; Miyazawa, T. Multi-objective optimization of part-building orientation in stereolithography. *Rapid Prototyp. J.* **1995**, *1*, 12–23. [CrossRef]
32. Choi, J.W.; Ahn, J.J.; Son, K.; Huh, J.B. Three-dimensional evaluation on accuracy of conventional and milled gypsum models and 3D printed photopolymer models. *Materials* **2019**, *12*, 3499. [CrossRef]
33. Alexander, P.; Allen, S.; Dutta, D. Part orientation and build cost determination in layered manufacturing. *Comput. Aided Des.* **1998**, *30*, 343–356. [CrossRef]
34. Matos, M.A.; Rocha, A.M.A.C.; Pereira, A.I. Improving additive manufacturing performance by build orientation optimization. *Int. J. Adv. Manuf. Technol.* **2020**, *107*, 1993–2005. [CrossRef]
35. Dolenc, A.; Mäkelä, I. Slicing procedures for layered manufacturing techniques. *Comput. Aided Des.* **1994**, *26*, 119–126. [CrossRef]
36. Oh, K.C.; Lee, B.; Park, Y.B.; Moon, H.S. Accuracy of three digitization methods for the dental arch with various tooth preparation designs: An in vitro study. *J. Prosthodont.* **2019**, *28*, 195–201. [CrossRef] [PubMed]
37. Congalton, R.G. *Assessing the Accuracy of Remotely Sensed Data: Principles and Practices*, 3rd ed.; CRC: Boca Raton, FL, USA, 2008; pp. 49–61.
38. Hada, T.; Kanazawa, M.; Iwaki, M.; Arakida, T.; Minakuchi, S. Effect of printing direction on stress distortion of three-dimensional printed dentures using stereolithography technology. *J. Mech. Behav. Biomed. Mater.* **2020**, *10*. [CrossRef]

materials

MDPI

Article

In Vitro Mechanical and Biological Properties of 3D Printed Polymer Composite and β-Tricalcium Phosphate Scaffold on Human Dental Pulp Stem Cells

Shuaishuai Cao [1,2], Jonghyeuk Han [3], Neha Sharma [1,2], Bilal Msallem [1,2], Wonwoo Jeong [3], Jeonghyun Son [3], Christoph Kunz [1], Hyun-Wook Kang [3,*] and Florian M. Thieringer [1,2,*]

1. Department of Oral and Cranio-Maxillofacial Surgery, University Hospital Basel, Spitalstrasse 21, 4031 Basel, Switzerland; shuaishuai.cao@unibas.ch (S.C.); neha.sharma@usb.ch (N.S.); bilal.msallem@usb.ch (B.M.); christoph.kunz@usb.ch (C.K.)
2. Medical Additive Manufacturing Research Group, Department of Biomedical Engineering, University of Basel, Gewerbestrasse 16, 4123 Allschwil, Switzerland
3. Biomedical Engineering, School of Life Sciences, Ulsan National Institute of Science and Technology (UNIST), 50, UNIST-gil, Ulsan 44919, Korea; g14619@unist.ac.kr (J.H.); wwjeong@unist.ac.kr (W.J.); mgm4336@unist.ac.kr (J.S.)

* Correspondence: hkang@unist.ac.kr (H.-W.K.); florian.thieringer@usb.ch (F.M.T.)

Received: 18 May 2020; Accepted: 6 July 2020; Published: 8 July 2020

Abstract: 3D printed biomaterials have been extensively investigated and developed in the field of bone regeneration related to clinical issues. However, specific applications of 3D printed biomaterials in different dental areas have seldom been reported. In this study, we aimed to and successfully fabricated 3D poly (lactic-co-glycolic acid)/β-tricalcium phosphate (3D-PLGA/TCP) and 3D β-tricalcium phosphate (3D-TCP) scaffolds using two relatively distinct 3D printing (3DP) technologies. Conjunctively, we compared and investigated mechanical and biological responses on human dental pulp stem cells (hDPSCs). Physicochemical properties of the scaffolds, including pore structure, chemical elements, and compression modulus, were characterized. hDPSCs were cultured on scaffolds for subsequent investigations of biocompatibility and osteoconductivity. Our findings indicate that 3D printed PLGA/TCP and β-tricalcium phosphate (β-TCP) scaffolds possessed a highly interconnected and porous structure. 3D-TCP scaffolds exhibited better compressive strength than 3D-PLGA/TCP scaffolds, while the 3D-PLGA/TCP scaffolds revealed a flexible mechanical performance. The introduction of 3D structure and β-TCP components increased the adhesion and proliferation of hDPSCs and promoted osteogenic differentiation. In conclusion, 3D-PLGA/TCP and 3D-TCP scaffolds, with the incorporation of hDPSCs as a personalized restoration approach, has a prospective potential to repair minor and critical bone defects in oral and maxillofacial surgery, respectively.

Keywords: 3D printing; dental biomaterials; polymer printing; ceramic printing; human dental pulp stem cell; in vitro research; bone regeneration

1. Introduction

Oral and maxillofacial bone defects caused by trauma, tumors, and malformations are common clinical scenarios causing physiological and psychological afflictions to the patients. With complex bone defect architectures and unique functions, reconstructive possibilities in this field are still a challenge for the current states of available clinical treatments. Ultimately, the goal of oral and maxillofacial bone reconstruction is to imitate and reconstruct the original anatomical features to provide desirable long-term functional and esthetical results [1].

In the past decade, many techniques, such as forming, subtractive manufacturing, electrospinning, or combinations of these processes have been applied to fabricate artificial bone substitutes [2–4]. However, these methods have several limitations, for example, low controllability of internal pore design (i.e., pore size, pore-interconnectivity, and tortuosity, etc.) and limitations in creating specific three-dimensional (3D) shapes [1,5]. To overcome the limitations of these methods, 3D printing (3DP) has been applied. 3DP technology is contrary to traditional "subtractive manufacturing" technology whereby there is direct processing of materials according to the principle of "additive manufacturing" and layer-by-layer superposition [6]. This manufacturing process allows the precise control of the porous geometry and internal architecture of the 3D printed object. Importantly, 3DP techniques can incorporate imaging techniques, such as computed tomography (CT) and magnetic resonance imaging (MRI), to generate patient-specific 3D tissue models [7]. Such approaches can be used to provide a blueprint for fabricating customized bone scaffolds with accurate anatomical shapes used in oral and maxillofacial bone defects.

Most clinically used patient-specific implants for oral and maxillofacial reconstruction are composed of titanium, poly-ether-ether-ketone (PEEK), and other non-absorbable materials [6,8,9]. However, to achieve optimal scaffolding to facilitate regeneration of hard tissues, various scaffold properties, such as controlled biodegradability, architecture, mechanical property, biocompatibility, and osteoconductivity, should be considered. One type of commonly used polymer in oral and maxillofacial surgeries is poly lactic-co-glycolic acid (PLGA), which has been influential in tissue engineering and has been FDA-approved since 1986 [10]. PLGA-based applications include drug delivery systems, biodegradable sutures, and scaffolds for bone tissue regeneration [11]. However, the mechanical properties of PLGA lack the desired and required stability for optimal bone tissue engineering. Nevertheless, because of the dual organic and inorganic nature of bone, and thanks to its versatility, PLGA can be mixed with other materials to create a compound with increased stability and additional reinforcement, such as when combined with tricalcium phosphate (TCP) [12,13]. TCP is composed of calcium-phosphate, its chemical formula is $Ca_3(PO_4)_2$, and TCP naturally occurs inside the human body during the mineral phase for bone tissue [14]. Chen et al. [15] found that rhBMP-2 loaded 3D poly (lactic-co-glycolic acid)/β-tricalcium phosphate (3D-PLGA/TCP) scaffolds fabricated by low-temperature rapid prototyping technology repaired ulnar defects in rabbits. Abarrategi et al. [16] reported that the 3D β-tricalcium phosphate (3D-TCP) scaffold produced by 3DP performed a fully controllable and customizable structure and had good biocompatibility. It is evident that the existence of a balance between scaffold degradation and new bone formation is vital for better performance of scaffolds used in bone tissue engineering [17]. These are the main reasons why controlled degradation and better mechanical properties are needed to facilitate the development of usable advanced bone scaffolds, in parallel with innovations in bioresorbable materials.

Another essential aspect of a 3D printed scaffold is the seeding and co-culturing of the scaffolds with stem cells before implantation. To date, many studies have demonstrated that bone marrow mesenchymal stem cells (BMSCs) possess multilineage differentiation potential and can be widely used as seed cells for bone tissue engineering [18,19]. However, BMSCs are difficult to harvest, and its phenotypic behaviors are disabled during the culturing and expanding phases [20]. To counter these issues, in recent years, researchers have turned their attention to the use of human dental pulp stem cells (hDPSCs) instead. hDPSCs can be obtained from extracted wisdom teeth or teeth extracted due to orthodontic reasons, without additional injury. Some researchers have already isolated hDPSCs from adult human dental pulp and found that, like osteoblasts, hDPSCs expressed bone biomarkers such as type I collagen, alkaline phosphatase, and osteocalcin [18,21]. Furthermore, findings indicated that hDPSCs efficiently induced improvement in periodontal bone regeneration when implanted with conventionally made β-tricalcium phosphate (β-TCP) into swine [22]. Thus far, a lack of reporting of mechanical and biological comparison, especially with hDPSCs on different manufactured 3D-PLGA/TCP, 3D-TCP scaffolds, remains to be expanded.

In our current study, we utilized a preliminary approach to explore the feasibility of different 3D printed bioresorbable scaffolds to facilitate the reconstruction of patient-specific defects in oral and maxillofacial surgery. Thus, we sought to fabricate PLGA/TCP and β-TCP samples with the same morphologies, structures, and pore sizes (Figure 1). Besides, we also examined and compared the mechanical properties and biological behaviors of hDPSCs in these scaffolds in comparison to conventionally manufactured β-TCP scaffolds. We expect that our study could increase the understanding of the specific dental applications of 3D printed polymer composite and β-tricalcium phosphate scaffold in the field of oral and maxillofacial bone regeneration.

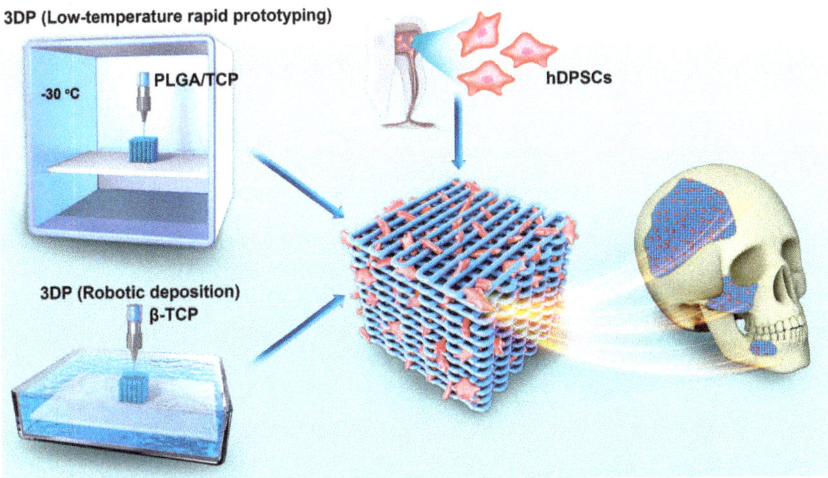

Figure 1. Overview of the application of two types of 3DP technologies used to fabricate scaffold incorporated with hDPSCs for oral and maxillofacial bone reconstruction.

2. Materials and Methods

2.1. Scaffold Preparation

3D-PLGA/TCP cube ($8 \times 8 \times 8$ mm^3) and cubic disk samples ($8 \times 8 \times 2$ mm^3) were fabricated with a low-temperature rapid prototyping 3D printer (Tissue Form II, Tsinghua University, Beijing, China) controlled by the printer's proprietary software program (Cark, Tsinghua University, Beijing, China). PLGA/TCP ink was prepared as described in a previous study [15]. Briefly, PLGA and β-TCP powder with a weight-based ratio of 75:25 was dissolved in 1,4-dioxane with magnetic stirring at 37 °C for 12 h. Then, the homogenized paste was added to the print head for subsequent printing. Table 1 lists the printing parameters we used for PLGA/TCP. Post-printing, the samples were dried in a vacuum freeze-dryer (LyoAlfa, Telstar, Terrassa, Spain) for solvent volatilization.

Table 1. The 3DP parameters for 3D-PLGA/TCP.

Description	Value
Layer height	375 μm
Pore diameter	300 μm
Nozzle diameter	400 μm
Printing speed	20 mm/s
Printing temperature	−30 °C

3D-TCP cube (8 × 8 × 8 mm^3) and cubic disk samples (8 × 8 × 2 mm^3) were fabricated with a robotic deposition 3D printer (3D Inks, Stillwater, MN, USA) controlled by Robocad 3.0 (3D Inks, Stillwater, MN, USA). β-TCP ink was prepared as described in a previous study [16]. Briefly, the β-TCP powder was mixed with deionized water, Darvan® C dispersant (Vanderbilt Minerals, Darvan C-N, CT, USA), hydroxypropyl methylcellulose, and flocculant in a concentrator overnight. After that, the β-TCP ink was added to a metal print head for printing. Table 2 lists the printing parameters we used for β-TCP. Finally, the samples were dried at room temperature for 24 h and were then sintered at 400 °C and 1200 °C respectively for 1 h to evaporate organic constituents.

Table 2. The 3DP parameters for 3D-TCP.

Description	Value
Layer height	375 μm
Pore diameter	300 μm
Nozzle diameter	400 μm
Printing speed	5 mm/s
Printing temperature	15 °C

A commercialized porous β-TCP (Bio-lu Biomaterials, Shanghai, China) was purchased and then cut into a cube (8 × 8 × 8 mm^3) and a cubic disk (8 × 8 × 2 mm^3) to serve as samples for the control group. These were conventionally fabricated by forming technology with a fully interoperable globular pore structure, an open porosity of 70 (±10)%, and a sphericity aperture of 400 (±50) μm. 3D β-TCP (3D-TCP) and commercialized β-TCP (C-TCP) were sterilized via autoclaving at 134 °C for 5 min, whereas 3D-PLGA/TCP samples were sterilized by gamma radiation of cobalt 60 under 30 kGy, after which samples were stored at room temperature.

2.2. *Characterization of Scaffolds*

The surface morphology and energy dispersive spectra (EDS) of the materials were examined with a scanning electron microscope (SEM; S-4800, Hitachi High-Technologies Co., Tokyo, Japan). A 20 nm thick Au-Pd film layer was uniformly sprayed on scaffolds surface prior to SEM analyses. Micro-CT (SkyScan 1172, Bruker, Belgium) was employed to qualitatively evaluate pore size and porosity with a scanning resolution of 15 μm (80 kV and 100 μA radiation source with a 0.5 mm aluminum filter). Volumetric reconstruction and porosity analyses were conducted separately with CTan 1.13 (NRecon 1.1, Bruker, Belgium).

The compressive mechanical properties of each sample were measured by a uniaxial compressive testing system (Electromechanical 3382, Instron, Norwood, MA, USA). C-TCP, 3D-PLGA/TCP, and 3D-TCP (N = 8) cubic samples (8 mm × 8 mm × 8 mm^3) were prepared on the holder and crosshead speed was set at 1 mm/min. The maximum applied load was recorded and compressive strength (MPa) was subsequently calculated by dividing the maximum applied load by the initial cross-sectional area of the samples.

2.3. *Biological Responses of hDPSCs*

2.3.1. Cell Culture and Seeding

The hDPSCs (Lonza, Walkersville, MD, USA) were cultured and expanded with Alpha-minimum eagle's medium (α-MEM) supplemented with 10% fetal bovine serum (FBS; Gibco, Thermo Fisher Scientific, Waltham, MA, USA) and were supplemented with 1% v/v penicillin-streptomycin (P/S) in physiological conditions held constant (37 °C air temperature, 5% CO_2 atmosphere). The mediums were exchanged every 3 days. Subculturing was conducted when samples reached 70%–80% confluency through dissociation induced with TrypLE™ Select (1×) (Gibco, Thermo Fisher Scientific, Waltham, MA, USA). Adherent cells on flask-bottoms were separated by 1.5 mL trypsin-EDTA

(0.05% trypsin/0.02% EDTA, Life Technologies Co., Waltham, MA, USA) for 5 min at 37 °C in an incubator.

hDPSCs were prepared into cell suspensions and we adjusted cell concentrations to 1×10^6 cells /mL. C-TCP, 3D-PLGA/TCP, and 3D-TCP (N = 8) samples were placed in a 24-well plate, and 15 μL of hDPSCs suspension was seeded onto each cubic disk for pre-culturing for 2 h. After cells were dropped to the scaffold, culture mediums were refilled.

2.3.2. Live/Dead Staining

After culturing for three days, live/dead staining (L3224, Thermo Fisher Scientific, Waltham, MA, USA) was performed to facilitate measurements of cell viability for each group (C-TCP, 3D-PLGA/TCP and 3D-TCP, N = 4). Scaffolds were stained with assay solution (0.2% v/v calcein AM, and 0.05% v/v ethidium homodimer-1 in phosphate-buffered saline (PBS) at room temperature for 45 min and were then imaged using fluorescence microscopy (Leica DM2500, Leica Microsystems AG, Wetzlar, Germany). The live and dead cells were manually counted in live and dead staining images with Leica software (LAS X, Leica Microsystems AG, Wetzlar, Germany), and the cell viability was reported as a percentage by dividing the number of live cells by the total cell count.

2.3.3. Cell Metabolic Activity

Cell viability reagent (AlamarBlue™, Thermo Fisher Scientific, Waltham, MA, USA) was employed to facilitate cell metabolic activity. After culturing for 1, 3, 5, and 7 days, three groups of scaffolds (N = 8 each group) were incubated in 10% v/v Alamar Blue dye diluted by culture medium at a constant temperature of 37 °C and with a constant 5% CO_2 atmosphere for 3 h following all manufacturer protocols. After sampling assay solutions in 100-μL sized aliquots, their fluorescence intensities (excitation: 544 nm/emission: 599 nm) were measured spectrophotometrically with a microplate reader (Synergy NEO2 Hybrid Multi-Mode Reader, Bio-Tek, Winooski, VT, USA). Then, the measured data were normalized relative to data collected on day 1. Finally, the culture mediums were renewed at the end of each measurement.

2.3.4. Osteogenic Differentiation

Alkaline phosphatase (ALP) activity was used to evaluate effects in different groups (C-TCP, 3D-PLGA/TCP and 3D-TCP, N = 8) on the differentiation of hDPSCs. After seeding and culturing for 24 h, culture mediums were replaced by osteogenic mediums (alpha-minimum eagle's medium supplemented with 10%, fetal bovine serum, 10 mM b-glyceraldehyde-3-phosphate, 50 mg/mL L-ascorbic acid, and 10 nM dexamethasone) as previously described [22]. The mediums were changed every 3 days, and ALP activity was calculated both on day 3, 7 and 14 with an ALP assay kit (BioVision, Milpitas, CA, USA). For quantitative analysis, scaffolds were washed using PBS and then lysed in 0.1% Triton X-100 for 40 min. Lysates were then centrifuged at 2500 rpm for 10 min at 4 °C. Supernatant was collected in a 96-well plate, and an equal volume of p-nitrophenylphosphate (pNPP) substrate was added, the samples incubated at 37 °C for 1 h to allow cleavage of the chromogenic substrate following manufacturer's protocol. The protein concentration of each sample was determined by the bicinchonic acid (BCA) protein assay kit (Best Bio, Shanghai, China) at optical density (OD) 540 nm and recorded according to the standard curve in order to normalize ALP activity. OD values of ALP activity were recorded at a wavelength of 405 nm. Finally, ALP activity was reported as ALP (Units/mg) = $(\frac{\text{measure OD}-\text{blank OD}}{\text{standard OD}-\text{blank OD}} \times \text{standard concentration } (0.1\ \text{mg/mL}))/P$, P (protein concentration).

2.4. Statistical Analysis

All data were presented as mean ± standard deviation (mean ± SD). Statistical analyses were performed using GraphPad Prism 7 (GraphPad Software, La Jolla, CA, USA). Statistical differences between two groups were assessed by using paired two-sided t tests. Statistical differences among multiple groups were evaluated by one-way analysis of variance (ANOVA) followed by Tukey's post-hoc tests. The statistical significance level was defined at $p < 0.05$.

3. Results

3.1. Characterization of Scaffolds

3.1.1. Structure and Surface

The structure and surface of C-TCP, 3D-PLGA/TCP, and 3D-TCP scaffolds were evaluated using SEM (Figure 2). Results indicated that all three groups of scaffolds possessed highly interconnected porous macro-structure and microporous structures on the surface. Compared with the C-TCP group, increasingly interconnected and homogeneous 3D pore structures were observed in the 3D-PLGA/TCP and 3D-TCP groups. Moreover, the 3D printed organic/inorganic PLGA/TCP compounds exhibited larger opening levels of connected micro-porosity on surfaces, compared with respective observations of rough surfaces for C-TCP and 3D-TCP groups. EDS-based results indicated that C-TCP and 3D-TCP scaffolds had similarly scaled presences of calcium (Ca) and phosphorus (P) peaks, whereas Ca and P peaks were decreased with corresponding decreased β-TCP proportions in the 3D-PLGA/TCP group.

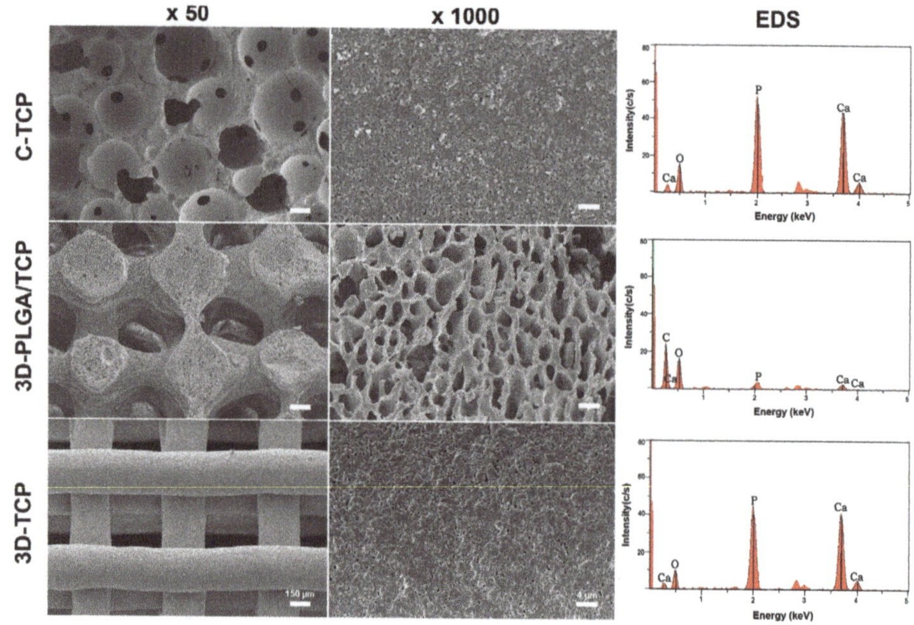

Figure 2. Characterizations of C-TCP, 3D-PLGA/TCP, and 3D-TCP scaffolds. SEM images showed the 3D interconnected structure and scaffold surface, and EDS-based assessments indicated the presence of β-TCP in these three scaffolds.

Table 3 shows pore sizes and porosities of different groups measured by micro-CT. The pore size of conventionally manufactured β-TCP scaffold was measured as 375 (±30.3) μm, which was larger than the pore size of 3D printed PLGA/TCP and β-TCP scaffolds each respectively measured as 362 (±16.5) and 345 (±9.1) μm. These three different scaffolds exhibited similarly to more than 60% porosity. The 3D-PLGA/TCP scaffolds possessed lower porosity = 65.6 (±5.0)%, whereas the porosity of the C-TCP and 3D-TCP scaffolds were 67.4 (±2.7)% and for 3D-TCP were 72.5 (±2.5)%.

These observations demonstrated that despite their differences in material composition, these three different scaffolds presented very similar pore sizes and porosities.

Table 3. Pore size and porosity.

Materials	Pore Size (μm)	Porosity (%)
C-TCP	375 ± 30.3	67.4 ± 2.7
3D-PLGA/TCP	362 ± 16.5	65.6 ± 5.0
3D-TCP	345 ± 9.1	72.5 ± 2.5

3.1.2. Mechanical Properties

Representative compressive strain–stress curves and modulus value for different groups of scaffolds are shown in Figure 3. Results indicated that the C-TCP and 3D-TCP scaffolds exhibited higher compressive strength than the 3D-PLGA/TCP scaffold, whereas the 3D-TCP scaffold presented the best compressive modulus among the tested groups. Moreover, the compressive modulus of the 3D-TCP scaffold increased significantly compared to the C-TCP scaffold, likely because of the 3D layer-by-layer structure and even being composed of the same materials. Primary consideration should be given to the occurrences of fractures, which were not observed in the 3D-PLGA/TCP group when they had experienced up to 80% levels of strain. These findings demonstrated that 3D-PLGA/TCP composite scaffold possessed excellent flexibility. The compressive modulus of the 3D-PLGA/TCP scaffold was calculated at a 20% strain, which was a significant decrease compared to the measures respective to the 3D-TCP scaffold.

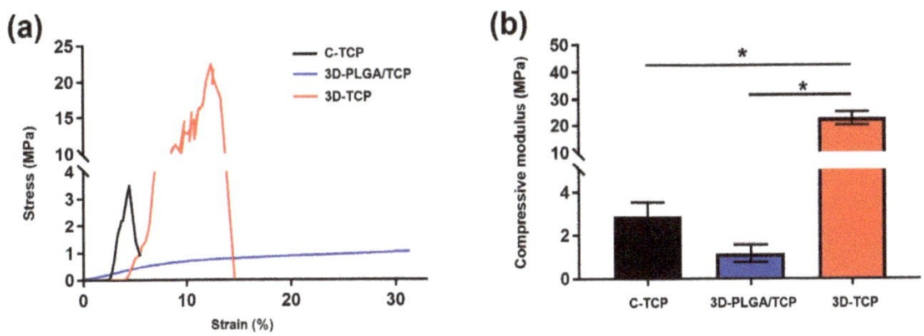

Figure 3. Mechanical properties of C-TCP, 3D-PLGA/TCP, and 3D-TCP scaffolds. (**a**) Compressive strain–stress curves indicated that 3D-PLGA/TCP possessed flexible mechanical properties. (**b**) Effects of 3DP and β-TCP amounts on the compressive modulus (* $p < 0.050$).

3.2. Biological Responses of hDPSCs

3.2.1. Live/Dead Staining

The adhesion morphology and viability of hDPSCs on different scaffolds were evaluated using fluorescent live/dead assays (Figure 4). Live hDPSCs (green-stained) attached on the surfaces of scaffolds, while only a few dead cells (red-stained) were observed on day 1 and 3. This suggested that the materials and designed structures possessed excellent cytocompatibility. At day 3, we can see that the hDPSCs adhered and proliferated deeper in 3D-PLGA/TCP and 3D-TCP scaffold, but the C-TCP material did not. This indicated that the well-connected and internal structure of the 3D printed material enhanced hDPSCs migration inside.

The viability of hDPSCs is shown in Figure 5. In our result, C-TCP and 3D-TCP group showed a consistent trend of excellent cell viability over time, reaching more than 90% after 3 days in culture.

Although hDPSCs viability of 3D-PLGA/TCP was significantly lower compared with 3D-TCP group, it is still higher than 80%.

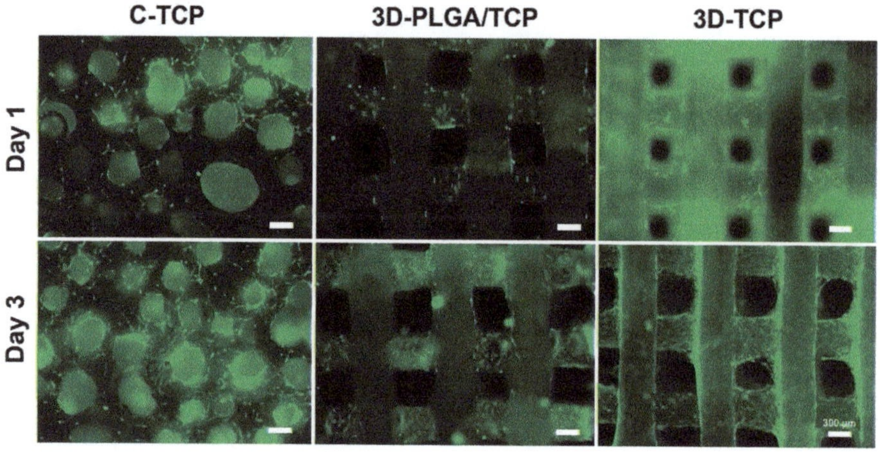

Figure 4. The effect of C-TCP, 3D-PLGA/TCP, and 3D-TCP scaffolds on hDPSCs viability. The live/dead assay results indicated that hDPSCs possessed excellent cell viability on the surfaces of all tested scaffolds (green: live cells; red: dead cells).

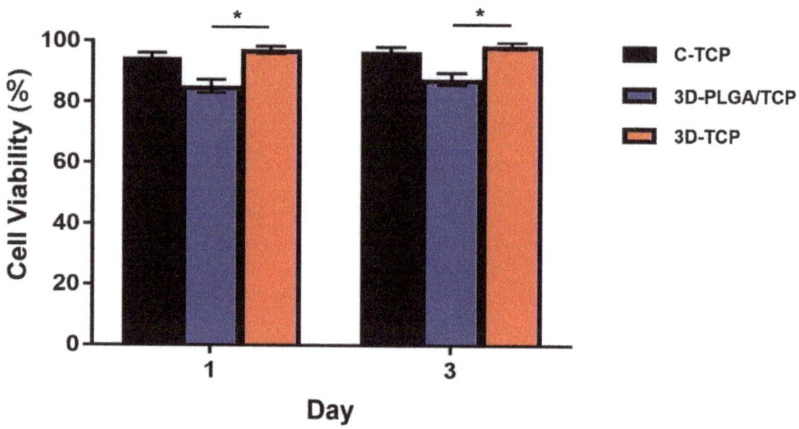

Figure 5. hDPSCs viability of C-TCP, 3D-PLGA/TCP, and 3D-TCP scaffolds. C-TCP and 3D-TCP scaffolds showed good cell viability over time, whereas 3D-PLGA/TCP scaffold had significantly lower cell viability than the other two groups (* $p < 0.050$).

3.2.2. Cell Metabolic Activity

The proliferation of hDPSCs on each group of scaffolds after 1, 3, 5, and 7 days of co-culturing are reported in Figure 6. In general, proliferation rates of hDPSCs in all groups increased over time. This result confirmed that C-TCP, 3D-PLGA/TCP, and 3D-TCP are quite feasible for use as carriers of hDPSCs. On day 1, there were no significant differences in these three groups. However, on day 3, the proliferation of 3D-PLGA/TCP and 3D-TCP groups were higher than of the C-TCP group. However, results also indicated that cell metabolic activity in the 3D-PLGA/TCP group was significantly lower than in the 3D-TCPgroup on days 3, 5, and 7. Additionally, a similar phenomenon was observed that the hDPSCs proliferation in the 3D-TCP group was higher after 3 days of co-culturing compared to C-TCP group.

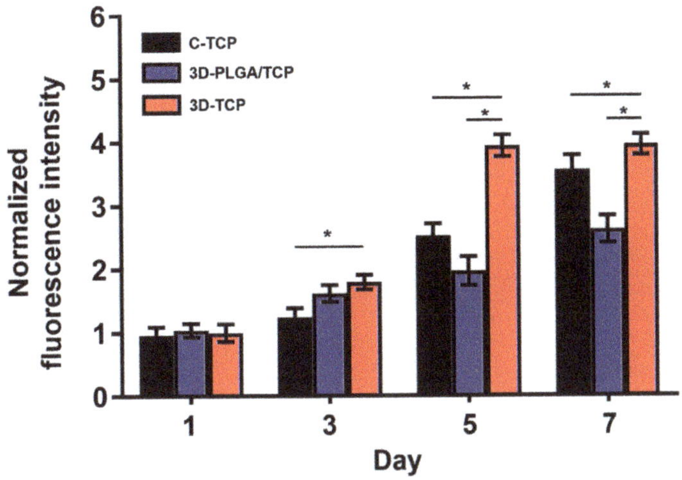

Figure 6. hDPSCs proliferation on C-TCP, 3D-PLGA/TCP, and 3D-TCP scaffolds. AlamarBlue assays indicated that all scaffolds significantly promoted the proliferation of hDPSCs (* $p < 0.050$).

3.2.3. Osteogenic Differentiation

BCA protein concentration (Figure S1) of each samples and quantitative ALP activity (Figure 7) indicated that there were no significant differences among all three groups and respective scaffolds on day 3. Furthermore, higher ALP activity values were revealed on the 3D-TCP scaffold compared to the 3D-PLGA/TCP and C-TCP scaffolds. However, the ALP activity of the 3D-PLGA/TCP group was significantly lower than in 3D-TCP group on day 7, and 14. Additionally, compared to the C-TCP scaffold, the 3D-TCP scaffold enhanced the expression of ALP activity. These results indicated that the osteogenic differentiation of hDPSCs favored β-TCP and 3D porous structure content.

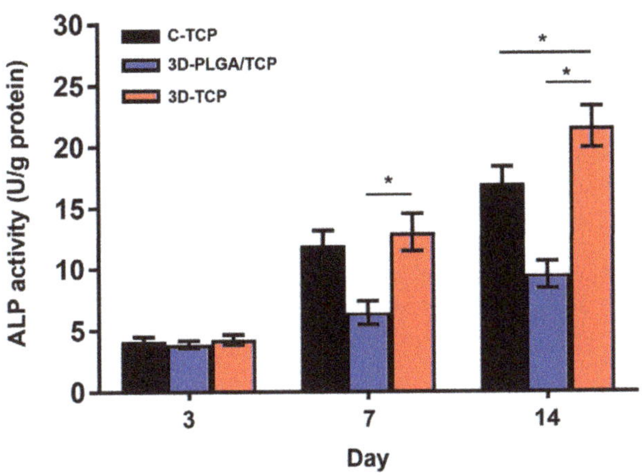

Figure 7. The effect of C-TCP, 3D-PLGA/TCP, and 3D-TCP scaffolds on ALP activity. The 3D interconnected structure and β-TCP amount enhanced the ALP activity on day 3, 7, and 14 (* $p < 0.050$).

4. Discussion

As a crucial issue in bone defect reconstruction, the mechanical and biological properties of PLGA/TCP and TCP scaffolds fabricated with two different printing technologies were assessed and compared in terms of specific oral and maxillofacial application. Once the chemical, physical, mechanical, and biological properties of the 3D printed biomaterials are well understood, then these biomaterials can be tailored to provide specific clinical applications. Comparison of differentially composed 3DP biomaterials with conventionally made biomaterials to facilitate examinations of mechanical property and biological responses on hDPSCs remains poorly investigated. In this study, we compared the mechanical properties of two 3D printed materials with a conventionally formed scaffold and assessed their biocompatibility and osteogenic differentiation on hDPSCs. The fact that rapid low-temperature prototyping and robocasting are extrusion-based and the widespread use of the layer-by-layer manufacturing process in 3DP helped to meet the needs of clinical applications [15,16]. Notably, in this regard, it can be seen in Figure 2 and Table 3 that the SEM and Micro-CT results indicated that two kinds of scaffolds with the same structures could be fabricated by each of the two 3DP technologies employed in this study. Besides, thanks to the advancement of 3DP technology, not only can the desired appearance be achieved, but also the internally controlled pore size and porosity can be achieved [3]. Our scaffold presented a macropore size of 300–400 μm, indicating that they were suitable for capillary formation, mineral deposition, and extracellular matrix secretion [13,15,16,23]. The in vitro results implied that 3D uniform architectures were an important contributing factor in achieving the desired levels of cell colonization, proliferation, and osteoconductivity. The highly porous and consistent structure also allowed for the 3D scaffold to be an appropriate carrier to facilitate the slow-release of drugs. This is an important consideration for future related research endeavors pursuant to our efforts.

Regarding targeting-based approaches for dental hard tissue regeneration, the mechanical behavior of the materials after 3DP has not been paid much attention. Weak mechanical properties of the scaffold are generally not desirable with respect to addressing bone defects in relatively large sections and in force bearing sites [16]. In this study, we found that the stiffness of 3D-TCP scaffold was highly improved in comparison with conventionally made C-TCP scaffold, even though they are the same material with a similar pore size and porosity. It is reported that the mechanical properties of the commercial heterogeneous bone "Bio-Oss®" used in oral and maxillofacial clinic are 17.93 ± 0.292 Mpa, which are lower than our 3D-TCP scaffold [24]. The mechanical results in our study suggested that 3D regular interconnected porous structures facilitated the desirable mechanical properties. The PLGA component, which consists of polymer materials, is known to degrade faster than the β-TCP component [11]. Previous research has also reported that the stiffness of PLGA is too weak to be applied alone in hard tissue engineering, but it would be improved as the incorporated β-TCP content is increased concomitantly [15]. In order to enhance the mechanical property of PLGA and accelerate the degradation of β-TCP, we 3D printed a polymer composite of PLGA/TCP for use to repair minor bone defects in dental application [11,23]. From the viewpoint of attempting to increase the effective reinforcement, polymer organic fillers were also applied with β-TCP to assess improvements in relation to flexibility [25,26]. Interestingly, we found that 3D-PLGA/TCP composite scaffold was not broken during the compression tests (Figure 3a). We also found that the compressive modulus was significantly decreased compared to C-TCP and 3D-TCP groups (Figure 3b). This implied that the 3D printed PLGA/TCP was not able to withstand the likely pressure to be experienced at loading sites or in critical areas of bone defects. Nevertheless, 3DP flexible reinforcement could be applied for personalized small bone defect reconstruction in periodontology and implantology [27,28].

The biological response of stem cells on materials is affected by many factors, such as material composition, macropore size, micro surface morphology, and so on [29,30]. For dentists, hDPSCs is present as mesenchymal stem cells in dental pulp tissue, which are easier to obtain than other cells, and have excellent osteogenic differentiation properties [21]. When materials were applied directly, hDPSCs cells were embedded into the materials, which provides advantageous biomimetic microenvironments for cell adhesion, proliferation, and migration [22]. However, the adhesion and proliferation of cells normally occur only on the surface of conventional materials and cells cannot migrate deeply into materials due to the lack of well-interconnected pores [19,31]. Approaches facilitated by the use of live/dead staining have results indicating that C-TCP, 3D-PLGA/TCP, and 3D-TCP are biocompatible materials and could be used to provide stable environment for hDPSCs. hDPSCs viability at early time-points provides limited information related to cellular metabolic activity and should be used in conjunction with AlamarBlue. Thus, these developed 3D structures and materials could be used to strengthen cell migration and to facilitate their osteointegration, which has been identified as a critical factor involved in bone regeneration in vivo and, therefore, should be investigated in further research efforts.

The evaluation of the microenvironmental response from different scaffolds has significance with hDPSCs behavior in hard tissue regeneration. Microenvironments that are important in the dynamics underlying cell proliferation and osteogenic differentiation are affected by elemental ions released from the scaffolds [32,33]. Thus, in this study, we used AlamarBlue analysis to evaluate the effects of C-TCP, 3D-PLGA/TCP, and 3D-TCP scaffolds on cell proliferation. In vitro results indicated that hDPSCs in the 3D-TCP group proliferated markedly faster than cells in the C-TCP group after three days of co-culturing. Studies that examined the mechanisms of interaction between materials and organisms demonstrated that the behavior of cells in tissues and organs was not only regulated by gene sequences and proteins, but was also affected by external environmental factors [34–36]. Thus, the reasons that may help to explain the increase in cell metabolic activity may be related to fact that 3D printed β-TCP has a larger surface area than otherwise conventionally formed β-TCP. 3D printed β-TCP increases contact area with the culture medium, and makes the pores more suitable for cell metabolism and circulation. Moreover, we noted that the proliferation of hDPSCs in 3D-PLGA/TCP scaffold was significantly lower than in the other two groups on day 5 and 7. PLGA is a hydrophobic material and its degradation could create acidic microenvironments, resulting in reduced adhesion of hDPSC on 3D-PLGA/TCP scaffold [37]. Thus, its incorporation with β-TCP would be an approach that improves this performance [13,17]. However, cell metabolic activity and differentiation were affected to a certain extent from the application of β-TCP [15,17]. Therefore, this adverse observation can be hypothesized to have affected our research so that the PLGA element caused the lower cell proliferation in the 3D-PLGA/TCP group. A notable observation in Figure 5 was that the 3D-TCP group presented a higher ALP activity compared to the other two groups. In support of our findings in hDPSCs proliferation and ALP activity, studies have reported that the mechanism by which Ca^{2+} ions impact cell behavior is promoting cell proliferation and differentiation by activating chimeric Ag receptor T cells [32,38]. Calcium and phosphorous concentrations can also significantly affect the proliferation, differentiation, and mineralization of hDPSCs [39]. Researchers exploring extracellular Ca^{2+} ions, which occurred through the activation of Ca^{2+} influx, found that there was a promotion of osteogenic differentiation of hDPSCs [37,38]. As previously mentioned, the 3D printed scaffold had a larger surface area and stronger levels of permeation into the medium than conventionally manufactured scaffold. Therefore, we speculate that this may be the reason for the stronger osteogenic capacity of the C-TCP and 3D-TCP scaffolds. However, calcium and phosphate ions from β-tricalcium phosphate of the C-TCP, 3D-TCP, and 3D-PLGA/TCP scaffolds were not investigated and compared in this study. To fully elucidate and to prove that these 3D printed scaffolds could have enhanced hDPSCs proliferation and osteoinduction, further calcium and phosphate ions release from scaffold and RNA quantification of osteogenic markers should be investigated.

5. Conclusions

PLGA/TCP and β-TCP scaffold manufactured by 3DP have a potentially broad dental application for personalized levels of treatments. In our preliminary study and efforts herein, we found that both 3D-PLGA/TCP and 3D-TCP scaffolds demonstrated a regular and widely interconnected porous structure that facilitated the increased in cell proliferation, migration, and osteogenic differentiation.

Thus, the introduction of 3D structure and β-TCP components not only contributed to better hDPSCs adhesion and proliferation, but also promoted osteogenic differentiation. Besides, compared to the C-TCP scaffold, we found that 3D-TCP scaffolds had higher mechanical properties which implied that the 3D network reinforces the compressive modulus. This is a crucial finding that can be used for customized reconstruction in critical bone defects. Moreover, this flexible feature of 3D-PLGA/TCP reinforcement could be applied for personalized bone augmentation in periodontology and implantology. Therefore, 3D-PLGA/TCP and 3D-TCP scaffolds incorporated with hDPSCs have a prospective potential in different clinical applications that can improve oral and maxillofacial bone regeneration.

Supplementary Materials: The following are available online at http://www.mdpi.com/1996-1944/13/14/3057/s1, Figure S1: Protein concentration of C-TCP, 3D-PLGA/TCP, and 3D-TCP scaffolds. (a) Standard curve of bovine serum albumin (BSA) protein. (b) BSA protein staining for calculating standard curve. (c) Quantified protein concentration of C-TCP, 3D-PLGA/TCP, and 3D-TCP scaffolds on day 3, 7, and 14.

Author Contributions: Conceptualization, F.M.T., H.-W.K. and S.C.; methodology, S.C., J.H. and N.S.; software, B.M. and W.J.; validation, S.C., J.H. and N.S.; formal analysis, J.S., S.C. and W.J.; investigation, S.C., J.H. and W.J.; data curation, S.C., J.H. and B.M.; writing—original draft preparation, S.C.; writing—review and editing, F.M.T., H.-W.K., J.H., N.S. and S.C.; supervision, C.K., F.M.T. and H.-W.K.; project administration, C.K., F.M.T. and H.-W.K. All authors have read and agreed to the published version of the manuscript.

Funding: This research was funded by Osteology Foundation, grant number 19-031, Bilateral Science and Technology cooperation programme with Asia, grant number IPG 01-112019, Leading Foreign Research Institute Recruitment Program through the National Research Foundation of Korea (NRF) funded by the Ministry of Education, Science and Technology (MEST) (NRF- 2018K1A4A3A01063890), the China Scholarship Council (CSC) for the financial support of Shuaishuai Cao (Grant 201708440260).

Conflicts of Interest: The authors declare no conflict of interest. The funders had no role in the design of the study; in the collection, analyses, or interpretation of data; in the writing of the manuscript, or in the decision to publish the results.

References

1. Warnke, P.H.; Springer, I.N.G.; Wiltfang, J.; Acil, Y.; Eufinger, H.; Wehmöller, M.; Russo, P.A.J.; Bolte, H.; Sherry, E.; Behrens, E.; et al. Growth and transplantation of a custom vascularised bone graft in a man. *Lancet* **2004**, *364*, 766–770. [CrossRef]
2. Ciocca, L.; Lesci, I.G.; Mezini, O.; Parrilli, A.; Ragazzini, S.; Rinnovati, R.; Romagnoli, N.; Roveri, N.; Scotti, R. Customized hybrid biomimetic hydroxyapatite scaffold for bone tissue regeneration. *J. Biomed. Mater. Res. B Appl. Biomater.* **2017**, *105*, 723–734. [CrossRef] [PubMed]
3. Cao, S.; Zhang, L.; Chen, Z.; Li, S.; Jiang, H.; Tian, Y.; Gu, W.; Zhou, M.; Chen, X. The Effect and Biocompatibility of Nanofibrous Nano-Hydroxyapatite/Polycaprolactone/Gelatin Scaffolds Multipurpose Membrane in Guiding Bone Regeneration. *J. Biomater. Tissue Eng.* **2017**, *7*, 721–729. [CrossRef]
4. Zhou, M.; Peng, X.; Mao, C.; Xu, F.; Hu, M.; Yu, G.Y. Primate mandibular reconstruction with prefabricated, vascularized tissue-engineered bone flaps and recombinant human bone morphogenetic protein-2 implanted in situ. *Biomaterials* **2010**, *31*, 4935–4943. [CrossRef]
5. Tang, D.; Tare, R.S.; Yang, L.Y.; Williams, D.F.; Ou, K.L.; Oreffo, R.O. Biofabrication of bone tissue: Approaches, challenges and translation for bone regeneration. *Biomaterials* **2016**, *83*, 363–382. [CrossRef]
6. Li, J.; Cui, X.; Hooper, G.J.; Lim, K.S.; Woodfield, T.B.F. Rational design, bio-functionalization and biological performance of hybrid additive manufactured titanium implants for orthopaedic applications: A review. *J. Mech. Behav. Biomed. Mater.* **2020**, *105*, 103671. [CrossRef]
7. Huotilainen, E.; Jaanimets, R.; Valasek, J.; Marcian, P.; Salmi, M.; Tuomi, J.; Makitie, A.; Wolff, J. Inaccuracies in additive manufactured medical skull models caused by the DICOM to STL conversion process. *J. Craniomaxillofac. Surg.* **2014**, *42*, e259–e265. [CrossRef]
8. Han, X.; Sharma, N.; Xu, Z.; Scheideler, L.; Geis-Gerstorfer, J.; Rupp, F.; Thieringer, F.M.; Spintzyk, S. An in vitro Study of Osteoblast Response on Fused-Filament Fabrication 3D Printed PEEK for Dental and Cranio-Maxillofacial Implants. *J. Clin. Med.* **2019**, *8*, 771. [CrossRef]
9. Ma, J.; Ma, L.; Wang, Z.; Zhu, X.; Wang, W. The use of 3D-printed titanium mesh tray in treating complex comminuted mandibular fractures: A case report. *Medicine* **2017**, *96*, e7250. [CrossRef]

10. Astete, C.E.; Sabliov, C.M. Synthesis and characterization of PLGA nanoparticles. *J. Biomater. Sci. Polym. Ed.* **2012**, *17*, 247–289. [CrossRef]
11. Gentile, P.; Chiono, V.; Carmagnola, I.; Hatton, P.V. An overview of poly(lactic-co-glycolic) acid (PLGA)-based biomaterials for bone tissue engineering. *Int. J. Mol. Sci.* **2014**, *15*, 3640–3659. [CrossRef] [PubMed]
12. Cvikl, B.; Hess, S.C.; Miron, R.J.; Agis, H.; Bosshardt, D.; Attin, T.; Schmidlin, P.R.; Lussi, A. Response of human dental pulp cells to a silver-containing PLGA/TCP-nanofabric as a potential antibacterial regenerative pulp-capping material. *BMC Oral Health* **2017**, *17*, 57. [CrossRef] [PubMed]
13. Yu, D.; Li, Q.; Mu, X.; Chang, T.; Xiong, Z. Bone regeneration of critical calvarial defect in goat model by PLGA/TCP/rhBMP-2 scaffolds prepared by low-temperature rapid-prototyping technology. *Int. J. Oral Maxillofac. Surg.* **2008**, *37*, 929–934. [CrossRef] [PubMed]
14. Bouler, J.M.; Pilet, P.; Gauthier, O.; Verron, E. Biphasic calcium phosphate ceramics for bone reconstruction: A review of biological response. *Acta Biomater.* **2017**, *53*, 1–12. [CrossRef]
15. Chen, S.H.; Lei, M.; Xie, X.H.; Zheng, L.Z.; Yao, D.; Wang, X.L.; Li, W.; Zhao, Z.; Kong, A.; Xiao, D.M.; et al. PLGA/TCP composite scaffold incorporating bioactive phytomolecule icaritin for enhancement of bone defect repair in rabbits. *Acta Biomater.* **2013**, *9*, 6711–6722. [CrossRef] [PubMed]
16. Abarrategi, A.; Moreno-Vicente, C.; Martinez-Vazquez, F.J.; Civantos, A.; Ramos, V.; Sanz-Casado, J.V.; Martinez-Corria, R.; Perera, F.H.; Mulero, F.; Miranda, P.; et al. Biological properties of solid free form designed ceramic scaffolds with BMP-2: In vitro and in vivo evaluation. *PLoS ONE* **2012**, *7*, e34117. [CrossRef]
17. Lai, Y.; Cao, H.; Wang, X.; Chen, S.; Zhang, M.; Wang, N.; Yao, Z.; Dai, Y.; Xie, X.; Zhang, P.; et al. Porous composite scaffold incorporating osteogenic phytomolecule icariin for promoting skeletal regeneration in challenging osteonecrotic bone in rabbits. *Biomaterials* **2018**, *153*, 1–13. [CrossRef]
18. Aguilar, I.N.; Olivos, D.J., 3rd; Brinker, A.; Alvarez, M.B.; Smith, L.J.; Chu, T.G.; Kacena, M.A.; Wagner, D.R. Scaffold-free bioprinting of mesenchymal stem cells using the Regenova printer: Spheroid characterization and osteogenic differentiation. *Bioprinting* **2019**, *15*. [CrossRef]
19. Jaquiery, C.; Schaeren, S.; Farhadi, J.; Mainil-Varlet, P.; Kunz, C.; Zeilhofer, H.F.; Heberer, M.; Martin, I. In vitro osteogenic differentiation and in vivo bone-forming capacity of human isogenic jaw periosteal cells and bone marrow stromal cells. *Ann. Surg.* **2005**, *242*, 859–867, discussion 867–858. [CrossRef] [PubMed]
20. Polymeri, A.; Giannobile, W.V.; Kaigler, D. Bone Marrow Stromal Stem Cells in Tissue Engineering and Regenerative Medicine. *Horm. Metab. Res.* **2016**, *48*, 700–713. [CrossRef]
21. Tatullo, M.; Marrelli, M.; Shakesheff, K.M.; White, L.J. Dental pulp stem cells: Function, isolation and applications in regenerative medicine. *J. Tissue Eng. Regen. Med.* **2015**, *9*, 1205–1216. [CrossRef] [PubMed]
22. Li, Y.; Nan, X.; Zhong, T.Y.; Li, T.; Li, A. Treatment of Periodontal Bone Defects with Stem Cells from Inflammatory Dental Pulp Tissues in Miniature Swine. *Tissue Eng. Regen. Med.* **2019**, *16*, 191–200. [CrossRef] [PubMed]
23. Kwon, D.Y.; Park, J.H.; Jang, S.H.; Park, J.Y.; Jang, J.W.; Min, B.H.; Kim, W.D.; Lee, H.B.; Lee, J.; Kim, M.S. Bone regeneration by means of a three-dimensional printed scaffold in a rat cranial defect. *J. Tissue Eng. Regen. Med.* **2018**, *12*, 516–528. [CrossRef]
24. Li, Q.; Wang, T.; Zhang, G.F.; Yu, X.; Zhang, J.; Zhou, G.; Tang, Z.H. A Comparative Evaluation of the Mechanical Properties of Two Calcium Phosphate/Collagen Composite Materials and Their Osteogenic Effects on Adipose-Derived Stem Cells. *Stem Cells Int.* **2016**, *2016*, 6409546. [CrossRef] [PubMed]
25. Nyberg, E.; Rindone, A.; Dorafshar, A.; Grayson, W.L. Comparison of 3D-Printed Poly-varepsilon-Caprolactone Scaffolds Functionalized with Tricalcium Phosphate, Hydroxyapatite, Bio-Oss, or Decellularized Bone Matrix. *Tissue Eng. Part A* **2017**, *23*, 503–514. [CrossRef] [PubMed]
26. Xie, X.H.; Wang, X.L.; Zhang, G.; He, Y.X.; Wang, X.H.; Liu, Z.; He, K.; Peng, J.; Leng, Y.; Qin, L. Structural and degradation characteristics of an innovative porous PLGA/TCP scaffold incorporated with bioactive molecular icaritin. *Biomed. Mater.* **2010**, *5*, 054109. [CrossRef]
27. Das, E.C.; Dhawan, S.; Babu, J.; Anil Kumar, P.R.; Kumary, T.V.; Haridas, V.; Komath, M. Self-assembling polymeric dendritic peptide as functional osteogenic matrix for periodontal regeneration scaffolds-an in vitro study. *J. Periodontal. Res.* **2019**, *54*, 468–480. [CrossRef]
28. Sunandhakumari, V.J.; Vidhyadharan, A.K.; Alim, A.; Kumar, D.; Ravindran, J.; Krishna, A.; Prasad, M. Fabrication and in vitro Characterization of Bioactive Glass/Nano Hydroxyapatite Reinforced Electrospun Poly(epsilon-Caprolactone) Composite Membranes for Guided Tissue Regeneration. *Bioengineering* **2018**, *5*, 54. [CrossRef]

29. Kowal, T.J.; Hahn, N.C.; Eider, S.; Marzillier, J.Y.; Fodera, D.M.; Thamma, U.; Jain, H.; Falk, M.M. New bioactive glass scaffolds with exceptional qualities for bone tissue regeneration: Response of osteoblasts and osteoclasts. *Biomed. Mater.* **2018**, *13*, 025005. [CrossRef]
30. Deliormanli, A.M.; Atmaca, H. Biological Response of Osteoblastic and Chondrogenic Cells to Graphene-Containing PCL/Bioactive Glass Bilayered Scaffolds for Osteochondral Tissue Engineering Applications. *Appl. Biochem. Biotechnol.* **2018**, *186*, 972–989. [CrossRef]
31. Zhang, Y.; Yu, W.; Ba, Z.; Cui, S.; Wei, J.; Li, H. 3D-printed scaffolds of mesoporous bioglass/gliadin/polycaprolactone ternary composite for enhancement of compressive strength, degradability, cell responses and new bone tissue ingrowth. *Int. J. Nanomed.* **2018**, *13*, 5433–5447. [CrossRef] [PubMed]
32. Sen, K.S.; Duarte Campos, D.F.; Kopf, M.; Blaeser, A.; Fischer, H. The Effect of Addition of Calcium Phosphate Particles to Hydrogel-Based Composite Materials on Stiffness and Differentiation of Mesenchymal Stromal Cells toward Osteogenesis. *Adv. Healthc. Mater.* **2018**, *7*, e1800343. [CrossRef] [PubMed]
33. Surmenev, R.A.; Surmeneva, M.A.; Ivanova, A.A. Significance of calcium phosphate coatings for the enhancement of new bone osteogenesis—A review. *Acta Biomater.* **2014**, *10*, 557–579. [CrossRef] [PubMed]
34. Zhang, X.; Ning, T.; Wang, H.; Xu, S.; Yu, H.; Luo, X.; Hao, C.; Wu, B.; Ma, D. Stathmin regulates the proliferation and odontoblastic/osteogenic differentiation of human dental pulp stem cells through Wnt/beta-catenin signaling pathway. *J. Proteom.* **2019**, *202*, 103364. [CrossRef] [PubMed]
35. Yang, W.; Xia, Y.; Qian, X.; Wang, M.; Zhang, X.; Li, Y.; Li, L. Co-expression network analysis identified key genes in association with mesenchymal stem cell osteogenic differentiation. *Cell Tissue Res.* **2019**, *378*, 513–529. [CrossRef] [PubMed]
36. Antebi, B.; Zhang, Z.; Wang, Y.; Lu, Z.; Chen, X.D.; Ling, J. Stromal-cell-derived extracellular matrix promotes the proliferation and retains the osteogenic differentiation capacity of mesenchymal stem cells on three-dimensional scaffolds. *Tissue Eng. Part C Methods* **2015**, *21*, 171–181. [CrossRef]
37. Xu, Y.; Kim, C.S.; Saylor, D.M.; Koo, D. Polymer degradation and drug delivery in PLGA-based drug-polymer applications: A review of experiments and theories. *J. Biomed. Mater. Res. B Appl. Biomater.* **2017**, *105*, 1692–1716. [CrossRef]
38. An, S.; Gao, Y.; Ling, J.; Wei, X.; Xiao, Y. Calcium ions promote osteogenic differentiation and mineralization of human dental pulp cells: Implications for pulp capping materials. *J. Mater. Sci. Mater. Med.* **2012**, *23*, 789–795. [CrossRef]
39. Alshemary, A.Z.; Pazarceviren, A.E.; Keskin, D.; Tezcaner, A.; Hussain, R.; Evis, Z. Porous clinoptilolite-nano biphasic calcium phosphate scaffolds loaded with human dental pulp stem cells for load bearing orthopedic applications. *Biomed. Mater.* **2019**, *14*, 055010. [CrossRef]

materials

MDPI

Article

Evaluation of Effective Condyle Positioning Assisted by 3D Surgical Guide in Mandibular Reconstruction Using Osteocutaneous Free Flap

Seong Ryoung Kim [1], Sam Jang [2], Kang-Min Ahn [1] and Jee-Ho Lee [1,*]

[1] Department of Oral and Maxillofacial Surgery, College of Medicine, University of Ulsan, ASAN MEDICAL CENTER, Seoul 05505, Korea; alwaysyouth37@gmail.com (S.R.K.); ahnkangmin@hanmail.net (K.-M.A.)

[2] Coreline Soft, Seoul 03991, Korea; semyeong.jang@corelinesoft.com

* Correspondence: jeehoman@amc.seoul.kr or jeehoman@gmail.com; Tel.: +82-2-3010-1757

Received: 21 April 2020; Accepted: 15 May 2020; Published: 19 May 2020

Abstract: In the present study, the reproducibility and postoperative stability of a 3D printed surgical guide were evaluated in mandibular reconstruction with an osteocutaneous free flap (OCFF), including a fibular free flap (FFF) and deep circumflex iliac artery free flap (DCIA). Fifteen patients were enrolled, and a 3D surgical guide was fabricated by simulation surgery using preoperative (T0) Computed tomography (CT) images. Mandibular reconstruction was performed with OCFF using the 3D surgical guide. Postoperative CTs were taken immediately, 1 week (T1), and 6 months (T2) after surgery, to evaluate the reproducibility of the 3D surgical guide and condyle stability. Error of the 3D surgical guide ranged from 0.85 to 2.56 mm. There were no differences in reproducibility according to flap type. Condylar error and error at mandible midpoint were significantly different in FFF. However, there was no difference in DCIA error between the condyle and mandible midpoint. Regarding condyle stability 6 months after surgery, condyles moved more than 2 mm (up to 2.85 mm) in FFF, whereas there were no significant movement in DCIA. Careful intraoperative flap fixation and closed postoperative observation should be considered for stable clinical outcome, especially in the case of FFF.

Keywords: three dimensional printing; microvascular flap; mandible reconstruction

1. Introduction

The mandible is an important structure in the maxillofacial area that functions in mastication, pronunciation, and organization of the lower facial contour [1,2]. Mandible resection is usually indicated in oral cancer, trauma, and severe osteomyelitis, which can eventually result in large composite tissue defect of tooth, oral mucosa, and mandibular bone [3,4]. Subsequent reconstruction of mandibular defects should consider the restoration of function and esthetics of maxillofacial structure, to improve patient quality of life [1]. Reconstruction of the mandible with vascularized osteocutaneous free flap (OCFF) has become the gold standard method for patients undergoing mandibular resection because it allows composite tissue reconstruction of wide mandibular defect. This technique maintains viability under postoperative radiation therapy and provides enough bone for future dental implant rehabilitation. There are several options for mandibular reconstruction with OCFF, including fibula free flap (FFF), deep circumflex iliac artery free flap (DCIA), and scapula free flap [5,6]. FFF and DCIA are popular options for mandible reconstruction [2,7]. FFF involves a long cortical bone shaft, which is suitable for wide resection of mandible. Moreover, it can be harvested with a wide skin paddle that can be used for oral mucosa or facial skin defect [8–10]. However, it has a smaller height than the mandibular body, and is relatively unfavorable for dental implant rehabilitation. DCIA has some advantages compared with FFF, which can have a similar height as the mandibular body, and provide sufficient bone for dental implant. In addition, its natural curve can reproduce the original contour of the mandible [2,7,11]. Lonie et al. recommended that DCIA is an option for mandible body or angle, whereas FFF should be considered for total or subtotal mandibulectomy [2].

With the advent of virtual surgery based on computer simulation software and 3D printing technology, 3D surgical guides for OCFF can be designed before performing surgery. Various surgical simulation processes and 3D printed surgical guides have been introduced for clinical applications in mandibular reconstruction [12–14]. Reconstructive surgery has been easily guided by the use of intraoperative 3D printed surgical guides [15–18]. De Maesschalck et al. reported that 3D print assisted reconstruction and conventional manual technique are comparable for mandibular reconstruction with FFF and provide satisfactory mandibular contour [17]. However, intraoperative condyle repositioning is a critical procedure for mandibular reconstruction with OCFF and repairing original mandible contour. Additionally, the mandibular condyle should maintain its own original position. Condyle displacement may induce temporomandibular joint problems, such as limited mouth opening, pain, clicking, malocclusion, or bone segment breakage, which threaten good clinical outcomes [19]. However, to our knowledge, there are few studies on microvascular reconstruction of the mandible using 3D surgical guides that focused on condylar stability after surgery. Therefore, the present study evaluated the reproducibility of original condyle position and postoperative stability in mandibular reconstruction with OCFF, using a 3D surgical guide.

2. Materials and Methods

2.1. Patients

Inclusion criteria in this retrospective study were mandibular reconstruction using vascularized OCFF 1) with 3D surgical guide, 2) defect within subcondyle and midline of mandible, and 3) without clinical complication for one year follow up. Two cases were excluded, as one was immediate failure of flap, due to venous thrombosis, and the other was early recurrence of malignancy. Fifteen patients met inclusion criteria among 27 patients who had mandibular reconstruction, due to head and neck cancer, osteomyelitis, or trauma from 2016 to 2018 in the department of oral and maxillofacial surgery of the Asan Medical Center (Table 1). The study protocol was reviewed and approved by the institutional review board of the Asan Medical Center, Seoul, Korea (IRB approval No. 2019-1448).

Table 1. Patient characteristics.

No.	Age	Gender	Diagnosis	Type of OCFF
1	26	F [1]	Ameloblastoma	DCIA
2	27	M [2]	Keratocystic odontogenic tumor	DCIA
3	40	M	Osteosarcoma	FFF
4	41	F	Ameloblastoma	DCIA
5	49	M	Osteomyelitis	DCIA
6	51	M	Ameloblastoma	DCIA
7	52	M	Ondontogenic myxoma	DCIA
8	57	M	Ameloblastoma	DCIA
9	59	M	Keratocystic odontogenic tumor	DCIA
10	65	M	MRONJ [3]	FFF
11	71	F	Squamous cell carcinoma	FFF
12	75	F	MRONJ	FFF
13	80	F	Osteomyelitis	DCIA
14	83	M	Squamous cell carcinoma	FFF
15	89	F	MRONJ	DCIA

[1] M: Male; [2] F: Female; [3] MRONJ: Medication related osteonecrosis of the jaw.

2.2. Fabrication of 3D Surgical Guide

Three dimensional Computed tomography (CT) images were taken before surgery. A 3D surgical guide composed of positioning guide, cutting guide, and anchoring unit was designed after original condyle position and occlusion were confirmed on the 3D modeling software platform using preoperative CT images (T0) (Aview(R) Modeler; Coreline Soft, Seoul, Korea or OnDemand3D®; Cybermed, Seoul, Korea). The 3D surgical guide was fabricated using 3D printing technology, Polyjet 3D printer (Stratasys Ltd., Eden Prairie, MN, USA). The material used for printing was MED610 (Stratasys Ltd., Eden Prairie, MN, USA), designed for surgical guides and approved for permanent skin and limited mucosal contact (Figure 1 and Supplementary Materials).

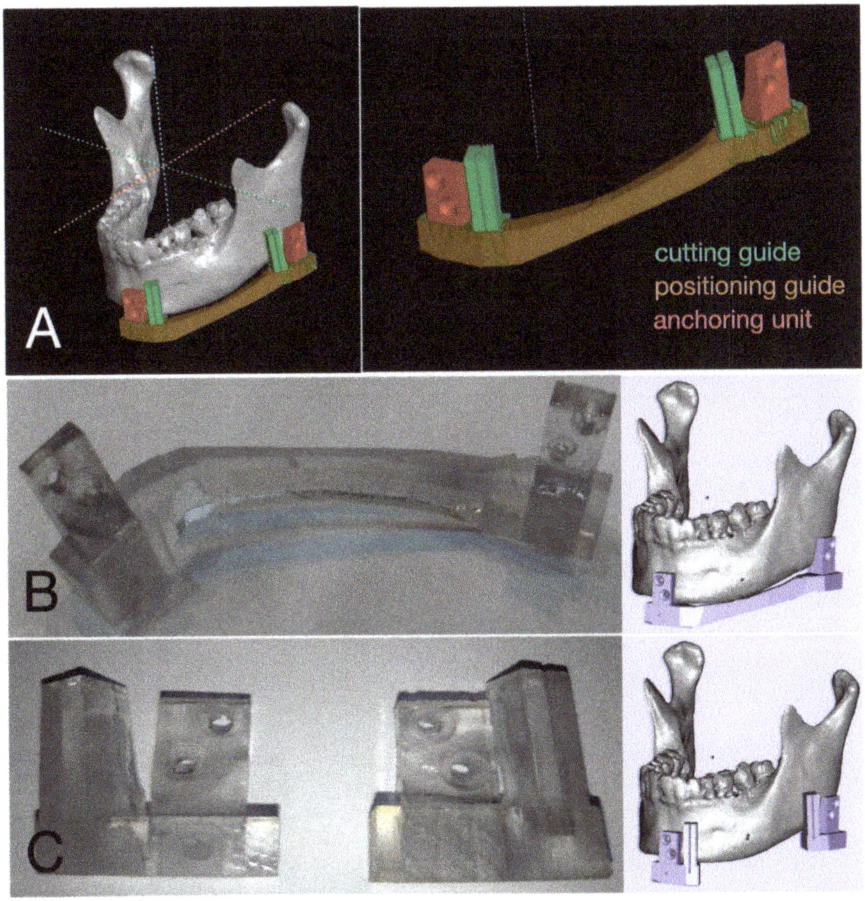

Figure 1. Virtual surgical planning and fabrication of 3D surgical guide. (**A**) Positioning and cutting guide were designed on virtual 3D model. (**B**) Positioning guide combined with anchoring units. (**C**) Cutting guide combined with anchoring units.

2.3. Surgical Technique

All cases of reconstruction included in this study were performed by single surgeon (J.-H.L.). The anchoring unit was intraoperatively fixed with temporary combination of the positioning guide on the mandible, to reproduce the original occlusion and condylar position at flap positioning. As the cutting guide was secured in the anchoring unit after removing the positioning guide, osteotomies were performed according to the cutting guide slot to reproduce the virtually planned mandibular resection line. An OCFF (FFF or DCIA) was carefully harvested and tailored, as planned, on a 3D virtual simulation. The flap was positioned into the mandible defect while being repositioned according to the positioning guide, to regain original occlusion and condylar positions. Microvascular anastomoses performed and semi rigid fixation of OCFF were completed using a mini plate system (Figure 2). One week after surgery, light guiding elastic was applied for 6 weeks to maintain original occlusion.

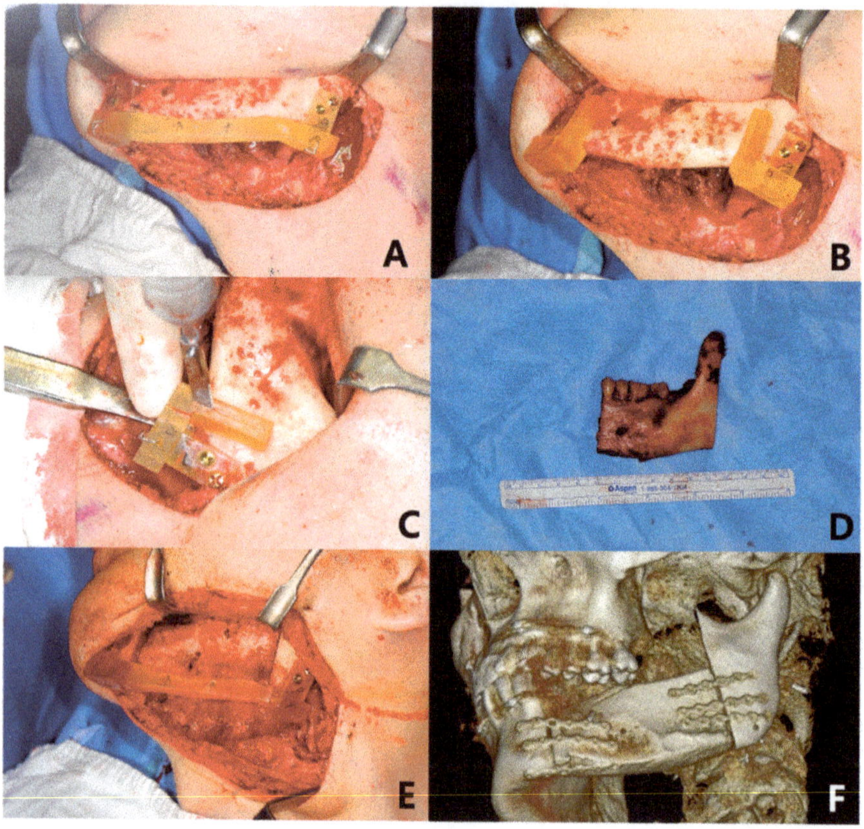

Figure 2. Mandibular reconstruction assisted by 3D surgical guide for case of deep circumflex iliac artery free flap (DCIA). (**A**) Mandibular positioning guide was temporarily fixed before mandibulectomy. (**B**) Cutting guide was engaged to cut mandible as planned on 3D virtual surgery after removal of positioning guide. (**C**) Sawing was performed according to cutting guide. (**D**) Body of mandible with tumor was removed. (**E**) Positioning guide was repositioned, and DCIA was set and fixed while original occlusion and condyle position were maintained. (**F**) Flap position was assessed by postoperative CT.

2.4. 3D Analysis for Reproducibility of 3D Surgical Guide and Stability of Condylar Position

Postoperative CTs were taken at 1 week (T1) and 6 months (T2) after surgery, respectively. The positions of each mandible landmark from CT images were recorded digitally as 3D coordinates (x, y, z) using simulation software (OnDemand3D®; Cybermed, Seoul, Korea). Positional changes according to time are presented as changes (mm) in coordinates (x: mediolateral direction, y: anteroposterior direction, z: superoinferior direction) and distance (mm, $D = \sqrt{x^2 + y^2 + z^2}$) (Figure 3A). Anatomic landmarks were selected and defined to estimate the stability of flaps as follows. CL (lateral pole of condylar head) was the most prominent point of the lateral surface of the mandibular condyle.

CM (medial pole of condylar head) was the most prominent point of the medial aspect of the mandibular condyle. CC (center of mandibular condyle) was the midpoint between CL and CM. ME (lowermost midpoint on lateral jaw projection) was the lowest point of the chin (Figure 3B).

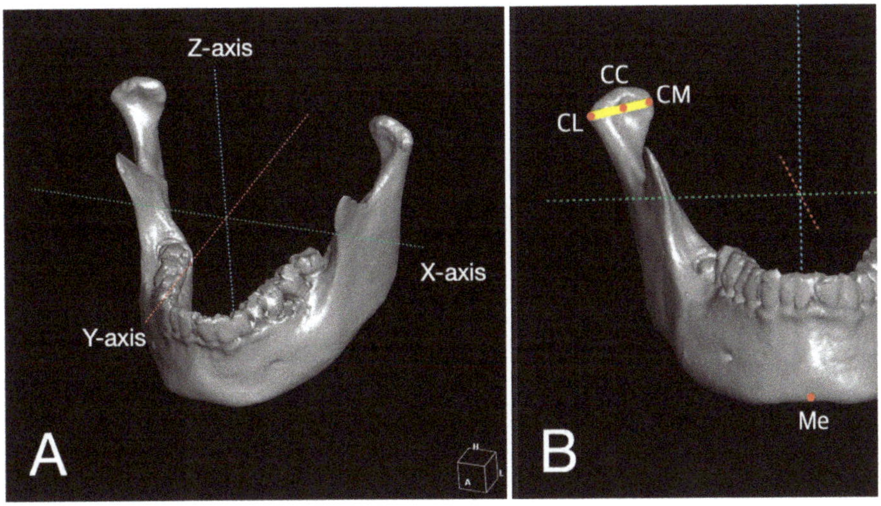

Figure 3. Schematic models of three-dimensional (3D) coordinated systems. (**A**) Positional changes of landmarks were presented as changes (mm) in coordinates (x: mediolateral direction, y: anteroposterior direction, z: superoinferior direction) and distance (mm) ($D = \sqrt{x^2 + y^2 + z^2}$). (**B**) Anatomic landmarks were defined on 3D model reconstructed using CT images in 3D coordinate system (CL = lateral pole of condylar head, CM = medial pole of condylar head, CC = center of mandibular condyle, Me = lowermost point on lateral jaw projection).

Spatial changes between immediate postoperative and preoperative (T1-T0) scans were calculated to assess the reproducibility of the surgical guide. The difference between T2-T0 (change 6 months after surgery) and T1-T0 (change immediately after surgery) was calculated to assess the stability of condylar position.

2.5. Statistical Analysis

All statistical analyses were performed using SPSS statistical software (Version 21, IBM Corp, Armonk, NY, USA). Results were presented as mean (standard deviation) in millimeters. The positional changes in landmarks between preoperative, immediate postoperative, and 6-month follow-up stages were assessed using the Wilcoxon signed rank test for continuous variables. A p-value < 0.05 was considered significant.

3. Results

The mean patient age was 50.1 ± 19.9 years in the DCIA group and 69.0 ± 15.6 years in the FFF group (Table 1). Male patients were more likely to undergo surgery than female patients in both groups (six vs. four in the DCIA group and three vs. two in the FFF group). However, there were no significant differences in gender and mean age between DCIA or FFF groups (p = 0.71 and 0.25, respectively). Designating landmarks was performed by one researcher (S.R.K.). Patients' information was not presented and time of CT taken (T0, T1, T2) was not informed either. Intra-rater and inter-rater reliability for designating landmarks were measured using the intraclass correlation coefficient, which showed that all values were over 0.979 (Table S1), indicating a high reliability of designating anatomic landmarks.

3.1. Reproducibility of 3D Surgical Guide

The amount of changes (*D*) between preoperative position (T0) and position immediately after surgery (T1) in the operated side of the mandible ranged from 0.85 mm for the menton with DCIA to 2.56 mm in the lateral pole of the condyle with FFF (Table 2). Although mean changes in FFF were more than those of OCFF and DCIA, there were no significant differences in directions (x, y, z) and the distances (*D*) between T1 and T0, according to the type of flaps in all landmarks ($p > 0.05$). However, condyle landmarks of CL and CM had significant differences with the menton (Me) in the mediolateral direction (x) for OCFF and condyle landmarks of CL, CM, and CC, with Me in distance (*D*) for FFF (Figure 4). In the intact side of the mandible, changes between preoperative (T0) and immediate position after surgery (T1) ranged from 0.79 mm in condyle center with DCIA, to 1.12 mm in lateral pole of condyle with FFF (Table S2), and there were no significant differences in landmarks and flap type ($p > 0.05$).

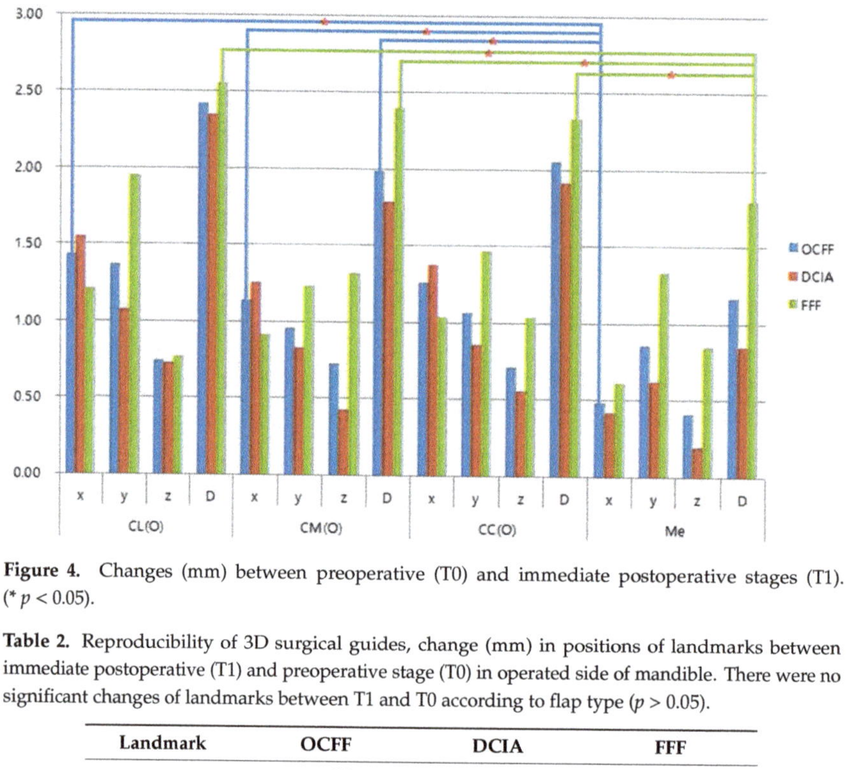

Figure 4. Changes (mm) between preoperative (T0) and immediate postoperative stages (T1). (* $p < 0.05$).

Table 2. Reproducibility of 3D surgical guides, change (mm) in positions of landmarks between immediate postoperative (T1) and preoperative stage (T0) in operated side of mandible. There were no significant changes of landmarks between T1 and T0 according to flap type ($p > 0.05$).

Landmark	OCFF	DCIA	FFF
	n = 15 Mean (SD)	n = 10 Mean (SD)	n = 5 Mean (SD)
CL			
x	1.44 (0.98)	1.55 (1.09)	1.21 (0.76)
y	1.37 (1.54)	1.08 (1.45)	1.95 (1.72)
z	0.74 (0.71)	0.73 (0.73)	0.77 (0.76)
D	2.42 (1.55)	2.35 (1.50)	2.56 (1.81)
CM			
x	1.14 (0.95)	1.25 (0.93)	0.92 (1.07)
y	0.96 (0.77)	0.83 (0.59)	1.23 (1.07)
z	0.73 (1.32)	0.43 (0.54)	1.32 (2.20)
D	1.99 (1.40)	1.79 (0.82)	2.40 (2.25)

Table 2. *Cont.*

Landmark	OCFF	DCIA	FFF
CC			
x	1.26 (0.89)	1.38 (0.90)	1.04 (0.93)
y	1.06 (1.02)	0.86 (0.75)	1.47 (1.44)
z	0.71 (0.84)	0.55 (0.43)	1.04 (1.36)
D	2.05 (1.22)	1.91 (0.86)	2.33 (1.83)
Me			
x	0.48 (0.47)	0.42 (0.41)	0.61 (0.60)
y	0.86 (1.20)	0.62 (0.98)	1.33 (1.58)
z	0.41 (0.58)	0.19 (0.22)	0.85 (0.83)
D	1.17 (1.32)	0.85 (1.02)	1.80 (1.74)

3.2. Stability of Condylar Position

With OCFF, the lateral pole of the condyle showed significant movement (1.44 mm) in the mediolateral direction, and the center of the condyle showed significant movement (1.82 mm) in distance (*D*) 6 months after surgery. There was no significant movement in all landmarks of DCIA. FFF has significant movement in all landmarks except the lateral pole of the condyle. This included the mediolateral direction (2.2 mm) in condylar medial pole, mediolateral direction (2.18 mm) and distance (2.85 mm) in center of condyle, and superoinferior direction (1.56 mm) in the menton (Table 3).

Table 3. Stability of condylar position, changes between immediate postoperative stage and six months after surgery in operated side of mandible. Positional changes of landmarks between T2-T0 [a] and T1-T0 [b] to assess condylar stability.

Landmark	OCFF	DCIA	FFF
	n = 15 Mean (SD)	n = 10 Mean (SD)	n = 5 Mean (SD)
CL			
x	1.44 (1.87) *	1.07 (1.43)	2.18 (2.57)
y	0.98 (1.25)	0.52 (0.74)	1.90 (1.63)
z	0.27 (0.33)	0.24 (0.33)	0.35 (0.34)
D	2.03 (2.02)	1.33 (1.54)	3.42 (2.31)
CM			
x	1.56 (1.70)	1.25 (1.31)	2.20 (2.35) *
y	0.60 (0.62)	0.56 (0.44)	0.69 (0.94)
z	0.38 (0.48)	0.35 (0.52)	0.42 (0.42)
D	1.95 (1.61)	1.56 (1.29)	2.71 (2.06)
CC			
x	1.45 (1.8)	1.08 (1.39)	2.18 (2.44) *
y	0.68 (0.91)	0.48 (0.56)	1.08 (1.39)
z	0.3 (0.28)	0.27 (0.28)	0.36 (0.31)
D	1.82 (1.85) *	1.31 (1.43)	2.85 (2.32) *
Me			
x	0.36 (0.45)	0.23 (0.19)	0.61 (0.70)
y	0.99 (1.77)	0.47 (0.39)	2.02 (2.95)
z	1.12 (1.53)	0.91 (1.07)	1.56 (2.30) *
D	1.74 (2.23)	1.13 (1.07)	2.97 (3.47)

[a] Between 6-month follow-up and preoperative stages; [b] Between immediate postoperative and preoperative stages; * $p < 0.05$

4. Discussion

Osteocutaneous free flaps have been widely used for mandible reconstruction, and FFF and DCIA are usually chosen as appropriate options [2,12,13]. Elaborate surgical planning for accurate flap positioning should be considered to ensure a successful clinical outcome. However, it is difficult to accurately reproduce the contour and position of the original mandible, because of its three-dimensional structure, movable temporomandibular joint, and complicated occlusion [20,21]. With the recent development of 3D simulation and printing technology, virtual surgical planning for mandibular reconstruction using OCFF has become a safe and reliable technique to increase the accuracy of mandible positioning [20,22–24]. A previous systematic review by Rodby et al. reported that the accuracy of reconstruction improved in 93% of cases when comparing virtual and actual osteotomy positions and contours [4]. A virtual surgical plan can optimize surgical results and minimize surgical time. Avraham et al. reported improved surgical outcomes and increased dental rehabilitation rates in cases using a virtual surgical plan for mandibular reconstruction [21]. Prefabricated cutting and positioning guides allow creation of a more accurate OCFF contour to reproduce the original mandible. However, repositioning of the mandibular condyle after mandible resection or splitting is also an important factor for a successful clinical outcome. This factor depends on appropriate removal of the bone interference and reproducing the original position of the mandible [11,16,25,26]. In the present study, mandible reconstructions were performed using 3D printed surgical guides composed of cutting, positioning guides, and anchoring units based on virtual surgical simulation. The accuracy of 3D surgical guides was assessed based on stability of the mandibular condyle. Changes in the positions of anatomic landmarks between the planning stage (T0), and immediately after surgery (T1), were defined as reproducibility of the surgical guide for mandibular reconstruction. There were no significant differences between T0 and T1, according to flap type, in reproducing the original position of the mandibular condyle and midline. However, two points (CL and CM) on the condyle showed significantly more change, compared to the midpoint of the mandible (Me), especially in the mediolateral direction for OCFF and in distance (*D*) for FFF. In FFF, Me showed less than 2 mm of error, compared with the planned position, whereas the condyle showed more than 2 mm of error (Table 2 and Figure 4). For intraoperative positioning of the OCFF in mandibular defect, the flap was fixed at a maximum intercuspation of occlusion that could be easily assessed. Conversely, the condylar position could not be thoroughly confirmed, due to limited visual accessibility. Therefore, in our cases, there might be enlarged error on the condyle compared with the midline of the mandible caused by intraoperative intermaxillary fixation for flap positioning. In addition, the slender dimension of FFF might result in more prominent error than the DCIA group.

Overall, OCFF was displaced in the mediolateral direction of the condyle lateral pole for 6 months after surgery, but significant movement of the entire condyle center was within 2 mm. DCIA maintained landmark positions for six months. However, significant movements were observed in most landmarks with FFF. This was especially true in the center of the condyle, up to 2.85 mm, and midpoint of the mandible, 1.56 mm in superoinferior direction (Table 3). In the present study, condyles of the FFF group had moved in the mediolateral direction 6 months after surgery. Several factors explain this finding. Displacement can be affected by both the position and placement of the segment [16]. Masticatory muscles that are resected or peeled off during surgery can interfere with balance of the muscular system. Excessive fibula shaping can lead to bone deficiency, and the condyle may be pulled forward to fill the gap. The remaining condyle is small and deep, which poses a great challenge to fixation [11]. In addition, excessive manipulation can cause edema in the temporomandibular joint [25]. Bone interference between osteotomy gaps may be another factor contributing to condyle displacement in a relaxed state under general anesthesia [3,27].

Displacement of the mandibular condyle may occur as healing progresses between bone segments. Moreover, the force generated by mandibular function induces bone movement that bends and breaks the metal plate. Condylar position can also be severely displaced during healing after reconstruction with FFF [11,28,29]. In contrast, DCIA has an advantage in contours similar to the natural shape of the hemimandible, and is suitable for use in the ipsilateral reconstruction of the mandibular angle or body defects [7,10]. Chen et al. reported that DCIA provides a larger amount of bone that could match with the original mandible dimensions to allow for faster bony union and later osteointegration compared to FFF [3]. Kang et al. suggested that thickness should be considered when using OCFF for mandible reconstruction. DCIA is an alternative option to FFF when there is instability from severe discordance in dimensions between FFF and the original mandible [11]. In our results, DCIA is superior in reproducibility of 3D surgical guide and postoperative stability compared to FFF. The advantageous dimension of DCIA will be helpful to reproduce the original mandible position using a 3D surgical guide, and the condylar position can be stably maintained due its larger dimensions than FFF.

Han et al. reported condyles were laterally displaced about 1.3 mm after sagittal split ramus osteotomy of mandibles, but they effectively regained their original position with semi rigid fixation [26]. They concluded that semi rigid fixation provides micromovement between bone segments to allow functional adjustment of the condylar position. Although SSRO and mandible reconstruction with OCFF differ in the extent of intraoperative condyle manipulation, the result of Han et al.'s study indicates that condylar displacement in DCIA ranged from 1.31 to 1.56 mm, which might be physiologically adjusted during the functional period. However, in FFF with more than 2 mm of condylar displacement, careful intraoperative flap fixation should be taken in addition to closed observation for complications that may occur during mastication, such as plate fatigue fracture, segment breakage, and condyle sagging [11,29].

There are some limitations in this study. The sample size was relatively small and assignment of patients to each group was haphazard under retrospective study design. Therefore, in the present study, it cannot be easily concluded which type of flap would be advantageous in mandible reconstruction using 3D surgical guide, and whether the use of 3D surgical guide would be more accurate compared with cases without 3D guide. Further prospective study is required with a greater sample size and a comparison of other cases without a 3D guide for widespread clinical application of the 3D surgical guide.

5. Conclusions

In the present study, total condyle errors were significantly larger than those of the midpoint of the mandible with OCFF. DCIA was superior to FFF in condyle position and midpoint after 6 months of healing, and had advantageous dimensions for the reproducibility of the 3D surgical guides for mandible reconstruction. However, further study should be considered for the clinical application of the 3D surgical guide. Additionally, special consideration should be given in all stages of intraoperative fixation and functional loading when reconstructing mandibles with FFF.

Supplementary Materials: The following are available online at http://www.mdpi.com/1996-1944/13/10/2333/s1, Table S1: Intra-rater and inter-rater reliability, Table S2: Changes (mm) in positions of landmarks between immediate postoperative (T1) and preoperative stage (T0) in intact side of mandible.

Author Contributions: Conceptualization, J.-H.L.; Formal analysis, S.R.K.; Investigation, K.-M.A.; Methodology, S.J. and J.-H.L.; Resources, K.-M.A. and J.-H.L.; Software, S.J.; Supervision, J.-H.L.; Writing—original draft, S.R.K.; Writing—review & editing, J.-H.L. All authors have read and agreed to the published version of the manuscript.

Funding: This research received no external funding.

Acknowledgments: All statistical analyses were consulted to an independent statistician, Jimi Choi affiliated to Department of Biostatistics, College of Medicine, Korea University, Korea.

Conflicts of Interest: The authors declare no conflict of interest.

References

1. Urken, M.L.; Buchbinder, D.; Weinberg, H.; Vickery, C.; Sheiner, A.; Parker, R.; Schaefer, J.; Som, P.; Shapiro, A.; Lawson, W.; et al. Functional evaluation following microvascular oromandibular reconstruction of the oral cancer patient: A comparative study of reconstructed and nonreconstructed patients. *Laryngoscope* **1991**, *101*, 935–950. [CrossRef]
2. Lonie, S.; Herle, P.; Paddle, A.; Pradhan, N.; Birch, T.; Shayan, R. Mandibular reconstruction: Meta-analysis of iliac-versus fibula-free flaps. *ANZ J. Surg.* **2016**, *86*, 337–342. [CrossRef]

3. Chen, S.H.; Chen, H.C.; Horng, S.Y.; Tai, H.C.; Hsieh, J.H.; Yeong, E.K.; Cheng, N.C.; Hsieh, T.M.; Chien, H.F.; Tang, Y.B. Reconstruction for osteoradionecrosis of the mandible: Superiority of free iliac bone flap to fibula flap in postoperative infection and healing. *Ann. Plast. Surg.* **2014**, *73*, S18–S26. [CrossRef]
4. Powcharoen, W.; Yang, W.F.; Yan Li, K.; Zhu, W.; Su, Y.X. Computer-Assisted versus Conventional Freehand Mandibular Reconstruction with Fibula Free Flap: A Systematic Review and Meta-Analysis. *Plast. Reconstr. Surg.* **2019**, *144*, 1417–1428. [CrossRef]
5. Goh, B.T.; Lee, S.; Tideman, H.; Stoelinga, P.J. Mandibular reconstruction in adults: A review. *Int. J. Oral Maxillofac. Surg.* **2008**, *37*, 597–605. [CrossRef]
6. van Gemert, J.T.; van Es, R.J.; Rosenberg, A.J.; van der Bilt, A.; Koole, R.; Van Cann, E.M. Free vascularized flaps for reconstruction of the mandible: Complications, success, and dental rehabilitation. *J. Oral Maxillofac. Surg.* **2012**, *70*, 1692–1698. [CrossRef]
7. Bisase, B.; Sloane, J.; Coombes, D.M.; Norris, P.M. The deep circumflex iliac artery perforator flap (DCIAP)–a reconstructive option for the large composite oro-mandibular cutaneous defect. *Br. J. Oral Maxillofac. Surg.* **2013**, *51*, 962–964. [CrossRef]
8. Cordeiro, P.G.; Disa, J.J.; Hidalgo, D.A.; Hu, Q.Y. Reconstruction of the mandible with osseous free flaps: A 10-year experience with 150 consecutive patients. *Plast. Reconstr. Surg.* **1999**, *104*, 1314–1320. [CrossRef]
9. Strackee, S.D.; Kroon, F.H.; Jaspers, J.E.; Bos, K.E. Modeling a fibula transplant in mandibular reconstructions: Evaluation of the effects of a minimal number of osteotomies on the contour of the jaw. *Plast. Reconstr. Surg.* **2001**, *108*, 1915–1921; discussion 1922-3. [CrossRef]
10. Takushima, A.; Harii, K.; Asato, H.; Nakatsuka, T.; Kimata, Y. Mandibular reconstruction using microvascular free flaps: A statistical analysis of 178 cases. *Plast. Reconstr. Surg.* **2001**, *108*, 1555–1563. [CrossRef]
11. Kang, S.H.; Lee, S.; Nam, W. Condyle dislocation following mandibular reconstruction using a fibula free flap: Complication cases. *Maxillofac. Plast. Reconstr. Surg.* **2019**, *41*, 14. [CrossRef] [PubMed]
12. Chao, A.H.; Weimer, K.; Raczkowsky, J.; Zhang, Y.; Kunze, M.; Cody, D.; Selber, J.C.; Hanasono, M.M.; Skoracki, R.J. Pre-programmed robotic osteotomies for fibula free flap mandible reconstruction: A preclinical investigation. *Microsurgery* **2016**, *36*, 246–249. [CrossRef] [PubMed]
13. Hidalgo, D.A. Reply: Long-Term Operative Outcomes of Preoperative Computed Tomography-Guided Virtual Surgical Planning for Osteocutaneous Free Flap Mandible Reconstruction. *Plast. Reconstr. Surg.* **2016**, *138*, 560e. [CrossRef]
14. Ritschl, L.M.; Mucke, T.; Fichter, A.; Gull, F.D.; Schmid, C.; Duc, J.M.P.; Kesting, M.R.; Wolff, K.D.; Loeffelbein, D.J. Functional Outcome of CAD/CAM-Assisted versus Conventional Microvascular, Fibular Free Flap Reconstruction of the Mandible: A Retrospective Study of 30 Cases. *J. Reconstr. Microsurg.* **2017**, *33*, 281–291. [PubMed]
15. Pauchet, D.; Pigot, J.L.; Chabolle, F.; Bach, C.A. Prefabricated fibula free flap with dental implants for mandibular reconstruction. *Eur. Ann. Otorhinolaryngol. Head Neck Dis.* **2018**, *135*, 279–282. [CrossRef] [PubMed]
16. Sawh-Martinez, R.; Parsaei, Y.; Wu, R.; Lin, A.; Metzler, P.; DeSesa, C.; Steinbacher, D.M. Improved Temporomandibular Joint Position after 3-Dimensional Planned Mandibular Reconstruction. *J. Oral Maxillofac. Surg.* **2017**, *75*, 197–206. [CrossRef]
17. De Maesschalck, T.; Courvoisier, D.S.; Scolozzi, P. Computer-assisted versus traditional freehand technique in fibular free flap mandibular reconstruction: A morphological comparative study. *Eur. Arch. Otorhinolaryngol.* **2017**, *274*, 517–526. [CrossRef]
18. Yuan, X.; Xuan, M.; Tian, W.; Long, J. Application of digital surgical guides in mandibular resection and reconstruction with fibula flaps. *Int. J. Oral Maxillofac. Surg.* **2016**, *45*, 1406–1409. [CrossRef]
19. Nahabedian, M.Y.; Tufaro, A.; Manson, P.N. Improved mandible function after hemimandibulectomy, condylar head preservation, and vascularized fibular reconstruction. *Ann. Plast. Surg.* **2001**, *46*, 506–510. [CrossRef]
20. Antony, A.K.; Chen, W.F.; Kolokythas, A.; Weimer, K.A.; Cohen, M.N. Use of virtual surgery and stereolithography-guided osteotomy for mandibular reconstruction with the free fibula. *Plast. Reconstr. Surg.* **2011**, *128*, 1080–1084. [CrossRef]
21. Avraham, T.; Franco, P.; Brecht, L.E.; Ceradini, D.J.; Saadeh, P.B.; Hirsch, D.L.; Levine, J.P. Functional outcomes of virtually planned free fibula flap reconstruction of the mandible. *Plast. Reconstr. Surg.* **2014**, *134*, 628e–634e. [CrossRef] [PubMed]

22. Eckardt, A.; Swennen, G.R. Virtual planning of composite mandibular reconstruction with free fibula bone graft. *J. Craniofac. Surg.* **2005**, *16*, 1137–1140. [CrossRef] [PubMed]
23. Hirsch, D.L.; Garfein, E.S.; Christensen, A.M.; Weimer, K.A.; Saddeh, P.B.; Levine, J.P. Use of computer-aided design and computer-aided manufacturing to produce orthognathically ideal surgical outcomes: A paradigm shift in head and Neck. reconstruction. *J. Oral Maxillofac. Surg.* **2009**, *67*, 2115–2122. [CrossRef] [PubMed]
24. Toto, J.M.; Chang, E.I.; Agag, R.; Devarajan, K.; Patel, S.A.; Topham, N.S. Improved operative efficiency of free fibula flap mandible reconstruction with patient-specific, computer-guided preoperative planning. *Head Neck* **2015**, *37*, 1660–1664. [CrossRef] [PubMed]
25. Ueki, K.; Moroi, A.; Sotobori, M.; Ishihara, Y.; Marukawa, K.; Yoshizawa, K.; Kato, K.; Kawashiri, S. Changes in temporomandibular joint and ramus after sagittal split ramus osteotomy in mandibular prognathism patients with and without asymmetry. *J. CranioMaxillofac. Surg.* **2012**, *40*, 821–827. [CrossRef] [PubMed]
26. Han, J.J.; Hwang, S.J. Three-dimensional analysis of postoperative returning movement of perioperative condylar displacement after bilateral sagittal split ramus osteotomy for mandibular setback with different fixation methods. *J. CranioMaxillofac. Surg.* **2015**, *43*, 1918–1925. [CrossRef]
27. Mendez-Manjon, I.; Guijarro-Martinez, R.; Valls-Ontanon, A.; Hernandez-Alfaro, F. Early changes in condylar position after mandibular advancement: A three-dimensional analysis. *Int. J. Oral Maxillofac. Surg.* **2016**, *45*, 787–792. [CrossRef]
28. Geusens, J.; Sun, Y.; Luebbers, H.T.; Bila, M.; Darche, V.; Politis, C. Accuracy of Computer-Aided Design/Computer-Aided Manufacturing-Assisted Mandibular Reconstruction with a Fibula Free Flap. *J. Craniofac. Surg.* **2019**, *30*, 2319–2323. [CrossRef]
29. Goormans, F.; Sun, Y.; Bila, M.; Schoenaers, J.; Geusens, J.; Lubbers, H.T.; Coucke, W.; Politis, C. Accuracy of computer-assisted mandibular reconstructions with free fibula flap: Results of a single-center series. *Oral Oncol.* **2019**, *97*, 69–75. [CrossRef]

materials

MDPI

Review

Reliability of Metal 3D Printing with Respect to the Marginal Fit of Fixed Dental Prostheses: A Systematic Review and Meta-Analysis

Soohyun Bae [1], Min-Ho Hong [2], Hyunwoo Lee [3], Cheong-Hee Lee [1], Mihee Hong [4], Jaesik Lee [5] and Du-Hyeong Lee [1,6,*]

1 Department of Prosthodontics, School of Dentistry, Kyungpook National University, Daegu 41940, Korea; hyun5601@knu.ac.kr (S.B.); chlee@mail.knu.ac.kr (C.-H.L.)
2 Department of Dental Laboratory Science, College of Health Sciences, Catholic University of Pusan, Busan 46252, Korea; mhhong@cup.ac.kr
3 Department of Dental Clinic, National Medical Center, Seoul 04564, Korea; surgeonlee@nmc.or.kr
4 Department of Orthodontics, School of Dentistry, Kyungpook National University, Daegu 41940, Korea; mhhong1208@knu.ac.kr
5 Department of Pediatric Dentistry, School of Dentistry, Kyungpook National University, Daegu 41940, Korea; leejs@knu.ac.kr
6 Institute for Translational Research in Dentistry, Kyungpook National University, Daegu 41940, Korea
* Correspondence: deweylee@knu.ac.kr; Tel.: +82-53-600-7676

Received: 15 September 2020; Accepted: 19 October 2020; Published: 26 October 2020

Abstract: Three-dimensional (3D) printing technologies have been widely used to manufacture crowns and frameworks for fixed dental prostheses. This systematic review and meta-analysis aimed to assess the reliability of the marginal fit of 3D-printed cobalt-chromium-based fixed dental prostheses in comparison to conventional casting methods. Articles published until 25 June 2020, reporting the marginal fit of fixed prostheses fabricated with metal 3D printing, were searched using electronic literature databases. After the screening and quality assessment, 21 eligible peer-reviewed articles were selected. Meta-analysis revealed that the marginal gap of the prostheses manufactured using 3D printing was significantly smaller compared to that manufactured using casting methods (standard mean difference (95% CI): −0.92 (−1.45, −0.38); $Z = -3.37$; $p = 0.0008$). The estimated difference between the single and multi-unit types did not differ significantly ($p = 0.3573$). In the subgroup analysis for the measurement methods, the tendency of marginal discrepancy between the 3D printing and casting groups was significantly different between articles that used direct observation and those that used the silicone replica technique ($p < 0.001$). Metal 3D printing technologies appear reliable as an alternative to casting methods in terms of the fit of the fixed dental prostheses. In order to analyze the factors influencing manufacturing and confirm the results of this review, further controlled laboratory and clinical studies are required.

Keywords: metal; 3D printing; reliability; marginal fit; fixed dental prosthesis; systematic review; meta-analysis

1. Introduction

Three-dimensional (3D) printing is a process wherein a product is manufactured using layering materials from 3D digital data [1,2]. This process enables the fabrication of sophisticated customized products without complicated laboratory manual works, unlike conventional manufacturing methods [3]. Powder bed fusion is a form of a 3D printing technology commonly used for metal 3D printing [4,5]. This technology is also referred to as selective laser sintering (SLS), selective laser melting (SLM), direct metal laser sintering (DMLS), or electron beam melting (EBM) in the literature [6,7].

During the procedure of powder bed fusion, a high-powered laser beam is directed at the layer of metal powder following the design of an object and fuses the powder particles sequentially until the 3D object is completely formed [8]. The main differences between the metal 3D printing technologies are operational parameters and post-treatment processes [9,10].

Cobalt-chromium (Co-Cr) alloys are primarily viable for metal 3D printing in dental prostheses [4]. These alloys demonstrate good tensile strength, elasticity, fatigue resistance, or corrosion resistance [11]. The major constituents of the powder are cobalt and chromium; however, molybdenum, tungsten, silicon, manganese, niobium, cerium, iron, and carbon are also included to improve the properties of the material [9]. Chromium increases corrosion resistance by forming a passivation film; molybdenum influences the grain size and decreases the susceptibility to pitting corrosion; tungsten causes solid solution strengthening with molybdenum; silicon and manganese are inserted to enhance the alloy's fluidity; and niobium affects the intermetallic phase formation and solution strengthening. Generally, the particles used in the powder bed fusion must be approximately 3–14 μm in size [10], and the products are characterized by the anisotropic γ-phase and ε-phase [12]. Gold and titanium alloys can be processed with the powder bed fusion technology; however, this method is rarely used in dental prostheses owing to the higher cost and mechanical properties [8].

Metal 3D printing technologies have been increasingly used in the field of dentistry for the manufacturing of crowns and frameworks of fixed dental prostheses; however, the accuracy of 3D-printed dental prostheses has not been fully elucidated. Although previous experimental and review trials have compared the accuracy of 3D printing and conventional fabrication methods, the comparisons were limited to individual settings and descriptive analyses [6,7,13]. In the evaluation of the prognosis of fixed prostheses, an acceptable marginal fit is considered a key criterion that influences the clinical success of prostheses [14]. A large marginal discrepancy can influence the cement dissolution and plaque accumulation along the margins, potentially causing secondary caries, inflammatory marginal gingivitis, or prosthesis loosening [15]. The purpose of this systematic review and meta-analysis was to review the reliability of the marginal fit of the Co-Cr based fixed dental prostheses fabricated using metal 3D printing technologies in comparison with conventional casting methods.

2. Materials and Methods

2.1. Search Strategy

This systematic review was designed as per the "Preferred Reporting Items for Systematic Reviews and Meta-Analyses" (PRISMA) guidelines [16]. The review was processed to answer the primary population, intervention, comparison, and outcome question [17]: in the fabrication of fixed dental prostheses (P), are the 3D printing methods (I) as reliable as the conventional casting method (C) in terms of marginal fit (O)?

The electronic search was performed on 25 June 2020, using the following databases: PubMed, Scopus, Cochrane, and Science Direct, and were limited to articles published in English only. The formulated search strategy included the use of Medical Subject Heading terms and free-text words with Boolean operators (AND or OR): ("metal"[tiab] OR "alloy"[tiab]) AND ("3D printing"[tiab] OR "additive manufacturing"[tiab] OR "SLS"[tiab] OR "DMLS"[tiab] OR "SLM"[tiab]) AND ("accuracy"[tiab] OR "fit"[tiab] OR "adaptation"[tiab]). A direct online search was performed in order to identify additional articles on Google Scholar.

2.2. Inclusion and Exclusion Criteria

In the present review, we included original studies that evaluated the marginal fit of the Co-Cr-based complete-coverage prostheses, including single and multiple units. The eligible studies included in vitro, in vivo, and clinical studies, irrespective of the experimental design. The studies were required to have quantitative results of the marginal fit that were recorded as the marginal gap and the absolute marginal discrepancy. The studies that evaluated partial-coverage prostheses, different materials, and other 3D-printed objects, such as dental implants, removable dentures, and artificial bones, were excluded. Narrative reviews, case reports, and studies that did not include a control group with a casting method were excluded as well. The inclusion and exclusion criteria used in this meta-analysis are described in Table 1.

Table 1. Inclusion and exclusion criteria used in the meta-analysis.

Inclusion Criteria	Exclusion Criteria
Study Design	**Study Design**
In vitro study	Case report
In vivo study	Animal studies
Clinical trial	Narrative review
Comparative study	Only charts and questionnaires
Evaluation study	No control group
Contents	**Contents**
Assessing marginal fit	Assessing only the whole or internal fit
Complete-coverage prostheses	Direct restorations and partial-coverage prostheses
3D printing using cobalt-chromium alloy	3D printing of dental implants, removable dentures, and artificial bones 3D printing using titanium and gold alloys

2.3. *Study Selection and Data Extraction*

Two independent reviewers (S.B., and D.-H.L.) screened the studies as per the aforementioned inclusion and exclusion criteria. A calibration exercise with the two reviewers was conducted to increase the reliability of data collection. First, the searched articles were screened as per their titles and abstracts; thereafter, the full text was read after both the reviewers had agreed to the relevance of an article. Disagreements between the reviewers were resolved via discussion. The Cohen kappa coefficient was calculated to determine the final agreement between the reviewers. Subsequently, the characteristics of the eligible studies were extracted from the studies and tabulated in a spreadsheet (Excel; Microsoft, Redmond, WA, USA). The following details were recorded: name of the first author, year of publication, 3D printing device, material, abutment type, prosthesis type, cementation space between the prosthesis and abutment, measurement parameter, measurement method for the marginal gap, sample size, and the value for the marginal fit. While collecting the marginal fit data, the absolute marginal discrepancy (the distance between the most external point of the prosthesis margin and the finish line of the abutment) was first determined as the outcome parameter. When the value was not provided, the marginal gap (the perpendicular measurement from the internal surface of the crown to the margin of the abutment) was recorded.

2.4. *Quality Assessment*

The quality of the included studies was assessed using the Quality Assessment Tool for Diagnostic Accuracy Studies-2 (QUADAS-2) [18]. The four domains for risk of bias assessment were as follows: patient selection, index test, reference standard, and flow and timing. When at least one domain was rated as high risk, the study was considered to have a high risk of bias in its overall judgment. When more than two domains were scored as unclear, the study was regarded as having an unclear bias risk. The traffic-light plots of the specific domain judgments for each study were drawn within each bias domain using the ROBVIS package for R (R software v.3.6.0; R Foundation for Statistical Computing Platform, Vienna, Austria) [19].

2.5. Data Analyses

The standard mean difference (SMD) between the prostheses fabricated using 3D printing and those fabricated using casting methods in each study was calculated with the following equation:

$$\text{SMD} = \frac{\text{Difference in the mean values of the groups}}{\text{Standard deviation of the measurements}}$$

A value of 0 for the SMD indicated that the two fabrication methods produced the prostheses with the same marginal accuracy.

The heterogeneity among the studies was evaluated using the I^2 statistic, τ^2, and p value ($\alpha = 0.05$; $I^2 > 50\%$ was considered to indicate heterogeneity). Based on the resulting heterogeneity, a fixed or random effects model was selected for the meta-analyses of the SMD data. The overall estimate of the SMDs was computed with the inverse variance weighted method, and the effect size estimates were adjusted as per the Hedges method [20]. Subgroup analyses of the SMDs were performed for the different types of prostheses (single and multi-unit) and the measurement methods for the marginal fit (direct observation and silicone replica technique). Publication bias was first assessed by inspecting the asymmetry of the meta-analysis results in a funnel plot. Egger's linear regression test of the funnel plot was then contacted to calculate the statistical value of publication bias. All the meta-analyses were performed using the Meta package for R (R software v.3.6.0; R Foundation for Statistical Computing Platform, Vienna, Austria).

3. Results

3.1. Search Results

The database and manual search initially identified 142 articles. After excluding 12 duplicate articles, 130 articles were screened by reviewing their titles and abstracts. After the exclusion of 91 irrelevant articles, 38 studies were then evaluated for further eligibility. With full-text reading, 17 articles were further excluded as per the inclusion and exclusion criteria; thus, finally, 21 articles were included in the meta-analysis [21–41]. The strength of the inter-reviewer agreement for the whole screening process was moderate ($\kappa = 0.463$, $p = 0.010$). The search results are described in the PRISMA flow diagram (Figure 1).

3.2. Characteristics of the Included Studies

The characteristics of the 21 included studies are summarized in Table 2. In most of the articles, the fit accuracy was investigated on tooth-like abutments; however, there were three studies that used implant abutments. Sixteen studies investigated the fit of single crowns, and five evaluated the fit of a multi-unit fixed dental prosthesis. The mean cement space setting was 35.5 µm (range: 20–70 µm) in 16 studies, excluding the studies that did not provide the set value. In the measurement parameter, two studies showed both the absolute marginal discrepancy and marginal gap values; the other studies showed the marginal gap value alone. In terms of the measurement method for the marginal fit, 11 studies used the silicone replica technique, seven used direction observation, two used mechanical sectioning, and one used a computer-aided digital technique. The sample size in each group was about 10–20 in most studies, except one study that used 110 specimens.

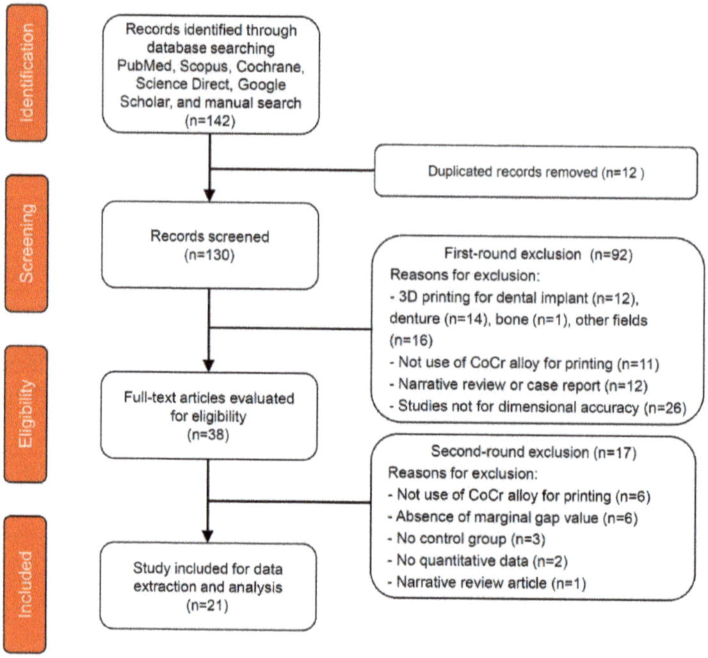

Figure 1. PRISMA flow diagram of the literature search.

Table 2. Characteristics of the included studies (n = 21).

	3D Printing			Prosthesis		Measurement		
Study	**Device**	**Material**	**Ab**	**Type**	**Space**	**Gap**	**Way**	**N**
Chang 2019 [24]	EOSINT M270, EOS	Wirobond C+, Bego	T	S	30	MG	CD	10
Yildirim 2019 [21]	EOSINT M270, EOS	EOS CoCr SP2, EOS	I	S	25	MG	SR	12
James 2018 [25]	EOSINT M270, EOS	EOS CoCr SP2, EOS	T	S	25	MG	SR	10
Ullattuthodi 2017 [27]	EOSINT M270, EOS	N/P	T	S	50	MG	DO	10
Kocaağaoğlu 2016 [30]	EOSINT M270, EOS	EOS CoCr SP2, EOS	T	S	30	MG	SR	10
Park 2015 [35]	EOSINT M270, EOS	EOS CoCr SP2, EOS	T	S	25	MG	SR	10
Tamac 2014 [37]	EOSINT M270, EOS	EOS CoCr SP2, EOS	T	S	30	MG	SR	20
Kim 2013 [39]	EOSINT M270, EOS	EOS CoCr SP2, EOS	T	S	30	MG	SR	10
Kaleli 2017 [29]	EOSINT M270, EOS	Keramit N/P-S, Nobil Metal	T	M	20	MG	DO	24
Kim 2013 [38]	EOSINT M270, EOS	EOS CoCr SP2, EOS	T	M	30	MG, AMD	SR	10
Hong 2019 [23]	M1, CL	Remanium Star CL, CL	I	S	N/P	MG, AMD	SR	20
Gunsoy 2016 [31]	M1, CL	N/P	T	S	50	MG	DO	16
Lövgren 2017 [28]	Mlab cusing, CL	N/P	T	S	50	MG	SR	12
Presotto 2019 [22]	Mlab cusing, CL	Remanium Star CL, CL	I	M	N/P	MG	DO	10
Ates 2016 [32]	N/P, CL	N/P, Dentaurum	T	S	30	MG	DO	10
Huang 2015 [36]	Medifacturing System, Bego	Wirobond C+, Bego	T	S	70	MG	SR	110
Zeng 2015 [33]	Medifacturing System, Bego	Wirobond C+, Bego	T	S	N/P	MG	SR	15
Arora 2018 [26]	Pro X, 100DP	N/P	T	S	N/P	MG	DO	10
Pompa 2015 [34]	N/P, DeguDent	Starloy LS, DeguDent	T	M	20	MG	MS	20
Castillo-de-Oyagüe 2012 [40]	PM100 Dental, Phenix System	ST2724G, Sint-Tech	T	S	N/P	MG	DO	10
Örtorp 2011 [41]	N/P, Biomain AB	N/P	T	M	50	MG	MS	8

Ab—abutment; CL—concept laser; I—implant; T—tooth; S—single; M—multi; MG—marginal gap; AMD—absolute marginal discrepancy; SR—silicone replica technique; DO—direct observation; MS—mechanical sectioning; CD—computer-aided digital technique; N/P—not provided; N— number of specimen.

3.3. Quality Assessment and Applicability Concerns

Figure 2 shows the results of the quality assessment using QUADAS-2. Of the 21 articles, 10 exhibited a low risk of bias [21,24,28–30,32,34,36–38], and 11 articles showed some level of unclear risk of bias [22,23,25–27,31,33,35,39–41]. All the included studies had a clearly stated purpose and included a control group for the evaluation of the marginal fit. There was major bias in patient selection due to the high number of studies that did not clearly justify the sample size calculation and random sampling. Randomization was not considered necessary because both 3D printing and casting methods were applied to identical specimens, preventing an increase in selection bias. With respect to the index and reference test domains, most studies provided adequate detailed information about the fabrication procedures, parameters, and devices. However, several studies did not explicitly provide the product name of the alloy [26,27,31,32,41] and the setting of cementation space [22,23,26,33,40]. With respect to the flow and timing domain, all the studies clearly reported the measurement methods, positions, and the number of measurement points per specimen. Strategies for achieving measurement reproducibility [24,26,29,30,32,38,40] and blinding tests [22,36,37,40] were provided in several studies to mitigate bias opportunities.

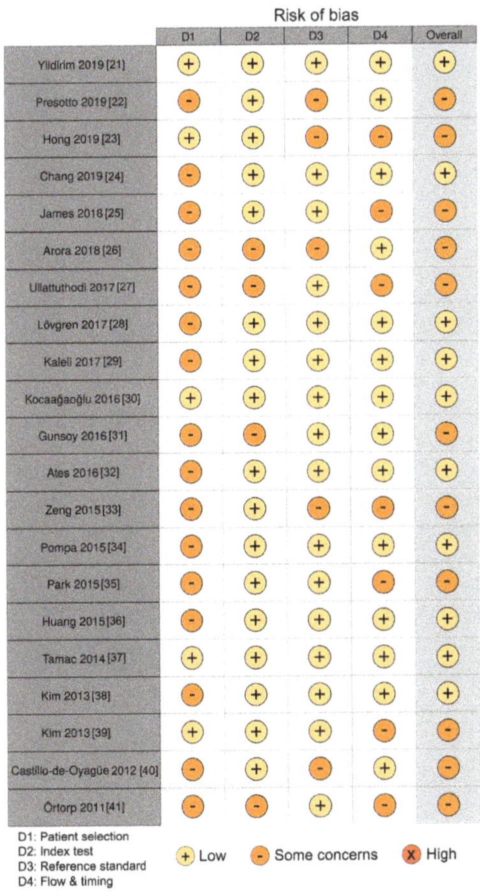

Figure 2. Quality assessment results according to the Quality Assessment Tool for Diagnostic Accuracy Studies-2 (QUADAS-2).

3.4. Meta-Analysis

In the global analysis, a random effects model was applied to analyze the outcomes of all the studies, considering the heterogeneity among them. The overall SMDs of the marginal gap for two fabrication methods are shown in Figure 3. Pooled analysis revealed that the value of the marginal gap was significantly smaller in the prostheses fabricated with 3D printing methods rather than those made using the casting methods [SMD (95% CI): −0.92 (−1.45, −0.38); Z = −3.37; $p = 0.0008$].

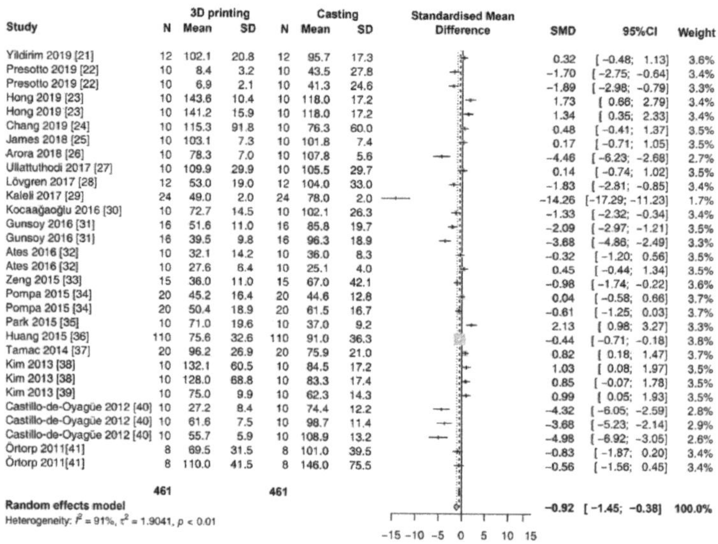

Figure 3. Global meta-analysis on the marginal gap of prostheses fabricated with 3D printing versus casting methods.

The first subgroup analysis was performed for different types of prosthesis. There was no significant difference noted in the estimated SMD between single and multi-unit types ($p = 0.3573$). Within the subgroups, the results in the random effects model are as follows (Figure 4): single type [SMD (95% CI): −0.7700 (−1.3871, −0.1529); Z = −2.45; $p = 0.0145$] and multi-unit type [SMD (95% CI): −1.3938 (−2.5697, −0.2178); Z = −2.32; $p = 0.0202$].

The second subgroup analysis was conducted for the different measurement methods of the marginal fit. There was a significant difference between the subgroups of the direct observation and the silicone replica technique ($p < 0.001$). Within the subgroups, results in the random effects model yielded the following data (Figure 5): direct observation [SMD (95% CI): −3.0735 (−4.3947, −1.7523); Z = −4.56; $p < 0.001$] and the silicone replica technique [SMD (95% CI): 0.3379 (−0.2331, −0.9088); Z = 1.16; $p = 0.2461$].

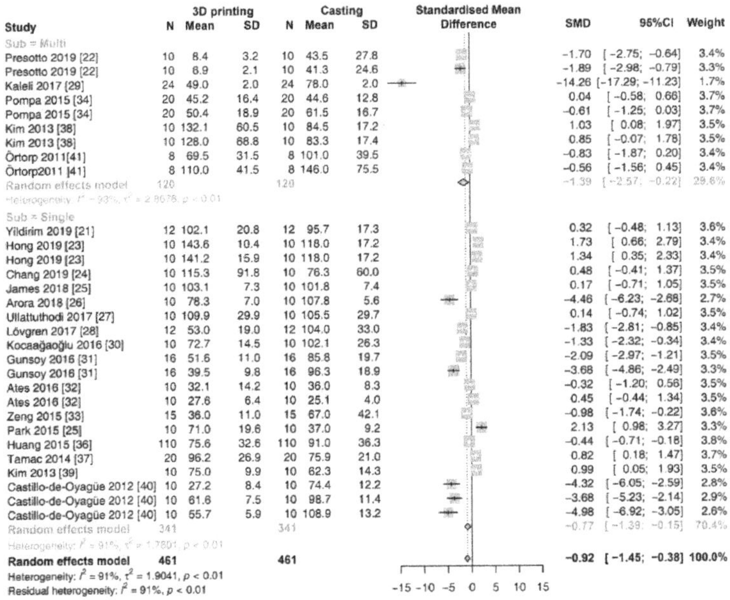

Figure 4. Subgroup meta-analysis for the different prosthesis types on the marginal gap between 3D printing and casting methods.

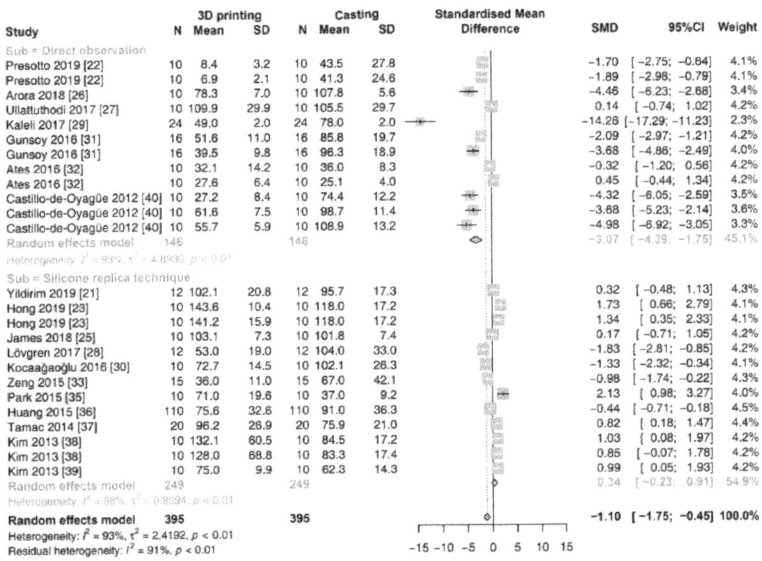

Figure 5. Subgroup meta-analysis for the different measurement methods on the marginal gap between 3D printing and casting methods.

Funnel plotting and Egger's regression test showed a moderate risk of publication bias for both global analyses (p = 0.0528) (Figure 6). Accordingly, a random effects model was used to evaluate the SMD results.

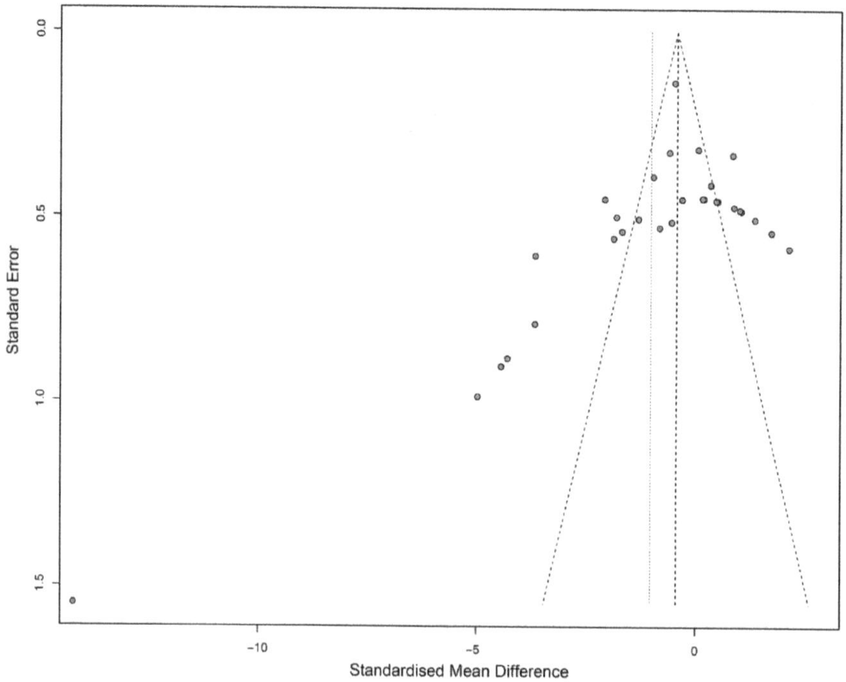

Figure 6. Funnel plot showing publication bias assessment.

4. Discussion

This review is aimed at assessing the marginal fit of 3D-printed Co-Cr fixed dental prostheses based on previous original articles. Studies that discussed both 3D printing and conventional casting were systematically selected for a comparative analysis, and statistical meta-analyses were then performed. The results from this review reveal that the marginal gap values of prostheses manufactured with 3D printing were significantly smaller than those of prostheses fabricated using casting methods. Thus, 3D printing technology appears to be capable of providing results comparable or even better than those achieved using prostheses utilizing established fabrication techniques in terms of the marginal accuracy; thus, 3D printing technology can be used as an alternative manufacturing modality. The present results correspond well with earlier narrative reviews wherein the marginal fit of metal frameworks fabricated using 3D printing was within the clinically accepted range [6,7]. To our knowledge, this is the first meta-analysis to compare the 3D printing methods with conventional methods for evaluating the fit of fixed dental prostheses.

The subgroup meta-analysis on the different types of prosthesis presented no significant difference in terms of the estimated SMD between single crowns and multi-unit prostheses. Thus, the 3D-printed prostheses had a better marginal fit than the prostheses fabricated using casting methods, irrespective of the size. Meanwhile, in the subgroup meta-analysis on the measurement methods, the tendency of marginal discrepancy between the 3D printing and casting groups was significantly different between articles that used the direct observation and the silicone replica technique. In the articles with the direct observation, large differences in the misfit were found between the 3D printing and casting groups (SMD = −3.0735, $p < 0.001$). However, within the comparison of the articles with the silicone replica technique, the difference in the misfit between the 3D printing and casting groups was non-significant (SMD = 0.3379, $p = 0.2461$). This finding might be related to the measurement procedure and reliability in the testing methods of the studies [42]. The silicone replica technique is the most commonly used nondestructive method that is applicable in the clinical setting; however, its major drawback is its susceptibility to error [43]. The thin silicone layer in the margin area can be torn or distorted during silicone replica formation. The sectioning of the silicone replica could also be problematic because of human error when the cutting position is inconsistent or the cutting is conducted in oblique planes. When the section is not standardized, the measurements are unreliable [44]. Specific sectioning strategies, such as the use of fiducial markers or cutting devices, have been suggested in several studies to help reduce the possibility of sectioning error [26,29,32,38,40]. Reading error is another issue among observers during the manual selection of measurement points to measure the marginal gap in the acquired images [45]. Thus, suitable standardized procedures are necessary to increase the reliability and reproducibility of the outcomes of individual experiment studies and minimize the bias risk in the meta-analysis performed on the studies.

The fabrication of prostheses via 3D printing begins with the process of digitizing the surface of the prepared abutments with laboratory-based or intraoral optical scanners [46,47]. The scanned image is transferred to a computer design software where the prosthesis is designed. Thereafter, the design is virtually sliced and placed with support structures within the build platform in the computer manufacturing software. In the printing phase, the final prosthesis is manufactured using a stepwise metal powder supply and a laser fusion process. Finally, heat treatment is performed to relieve the internal stress caused by thermal gradients during the whole 3D printing process [48]. The final misfit of 3D-printed prostheses represents the summation of the errors involved in all the steps from the image acquisition to the post-treatment process. Compared to conventional methods, although the digital workflow allows the elimination of inherent inaccuracies related to laboratory manual works, different devices and parameters can highly influence the dimensional accuracy of outcome products [9]. The quality of optical scanners and scan protocols also affect the accuracy of digitization. Technical parameters defined in printing, such as energy source, energy power, laser beam absorption/reflection coefficients, chamber condition, build orientation, layer thickness, and support generation, are all important [10]. The diversity in the manufacturing parameters makes it difficult to make assertive conclusions in the review. Thus, a detailed protocol that discloses all the manufacturing parameters of 3D printing process should be provided to analyze the reliability of a specific 3D printing method, because these factors are commonly interrelated and determine the product quality.

Powder bed fusion technologies use a high-power laser that selectively melts the pre-alloyed powders, following the design of the product, and then partially melts the previous powder layer [2]. The consecutive melting and solidifying of material powders enables interlayer fusion for the completion of the product [8]. Powders for the powder bed fusion are typically produced using gas atomization processes [49]. Spherical particles with a smooth surface and Gaussian size distribution are especially recommended because the spherical shape increases the powder flowability, resulting in higher uniformity and density of powder beds [50]. As the laser beam is shone over the powders, solidification structures such as cells or dendrites are formed in fine and anisotropic microstructures due to the high scanning speeds and small melt pools [51]. Altogether, the particle morphology, particle size distribution, and voids between the powders affect the absorption, reflection, and penetration of the laser radiation [52–54]. Consequently, the characteristics of the powder are related to the shape of melt pools and lattice structure. Because the surface roughness and subsequent surface treatment could influence the adaptation of the printed fixed dental prostheses [55,56], it may be necessary to appropriately select powders for the fabrication of dental prostheses.

Close adaptation between mechanical components of implant is essential to minimize biologic and prosthetic complications. The micro gap at the implant–abutment connection is also an important factor that could cause peri-implantitis, and the relationship between the implant–abutment connection and bacterial leakage has been reported in a review [57]. Further meta-analysis on the micro gap and resultant complications might be recommended. In the present review, a meta-analysis on the effects of scanning, printing, and post-treatment conditions could not be performed because the related information was not sufficiently described in the included studies. Most studies reporting on the accuracy of 3D-printed metal frameworks were in vitro studies that involved a bias risk in the justification of the sample size and the random allocation of specimens. We could identify few eligible clinical studies. Therefore, randomized controlled clinical trials will be needed to strengthen the power of review articles. Moreover, considering the rapid development in the fields of technology and material, further original studies with newly developed devices and materials need to be continuously pursued to establish knowledge as per the present times.

5. Conclusions

Within the limitations of this systematic review and meta-analysis, the following conclusions were drawn:

1. Metal 3D printing technologies are reliable for fabricating Co-Cr-based fixed dental prostheses with an accurate marginal fit, as compared to conventional casting methods.
2. The difference in methodology for evaluating the marginal fit could influence the results in comparative studies.
3. Further controlled laboratory and clinical studies with a detailed protocol that discloses all the manufacturing parameters are needed to statistically analyze the factors affecting the accuracy of 3D-printed prostheses.

Author Contributions: Conceptualization, S.B. and D.-H.L.; methodology, M.-H.H. and H.L.; data curation, S.B., J.L., C.-H.L. and M.H.; formal analysis, H.L. and J.L.; investigation, M.-H.H., C.-H.L., M.H. and D.-H.L.; writing—original draft preparation, S.B.; writing—review and editing, M.-H.H., H.L., C.-H.L., M.H., J.L. and D.-H.L.; supervision, D.-H.L. All authors have read and agreed to the published version of the manuscript.

Funding: This research received no external funding.

Conflicts of Interest: The authors declare no conflict of interest.

References

1. Korner, M.E.H.; Lambán, M.P.; Albajez, J.A.; Santolaria, J.; Ng Corrales, L.D.C.; Royo, J. Systematic Literature Review: Integration of Additive Manufacturing and Industry 4.0. *Metals* **2020**, *10*, 1061. [CrossRef]
2. Akhila, A.S.; Nandakishore, B.; Miriam, M.; Anil, S.K.; Abhinav, M.; Fares, A. Rapid prototyping: An innovative technique in prosthodontics. *Int. J. Prev. Clin. Dent. Res.* **2019**, *6*, 46. [CrossRef]
3. Fan, D.; Li, Y.; Wang, X.; Zhu, T.; Wang, Q.; Cai, H.; Li, W.; Tian, Y.; Liu, Z. Progressive 3D Printing Technology and Its Application in Medical Materials. *Front. Pharmacol.* **2020**, *11*, 122. [CrossRef] [PubMed]
4. Wang, H.; Lim, J.Y. Metal-ceramic bond strength of a cobalt chromium alloy for dental prosthetic restorations with a porous structure using metal 3D printing. *Comput. Biol. Med.* **2019**, *112*, 103364. [CrossRef] [PubMed]
5. Razavykia, A.; Brusa, E.; Delprete, C.; Yavari, R. An Overview of Additive Manufacturing Technologies—A Review to Technical Synthesis in Numerical Study of Selective Laser Melting. *Materials* **2020**, *13*, 3895. [CrossRef]
6. Revilla-León, M.; Meyer, M.J.; Özcan, M. Metal additive manufacturing technologies: Literature review of current status and prosthodontic applications. *Int. J. Comput. Dent.* **2019**, *22*, 55–67.
7. Alharbi, N.; Wismeijer, D.; Osman, R.B. Additive Manufacturing Techniques in Prosthodontics: Where Do We Currently Stand? A Critical Review. *Int. J. Prosthodont.* **2017**, *30*, 474–484. [CrossRef]
8. Revilla-León, M.; Sadeghpour, M.; Özcan, M. A Review of the Applications of Additive Manufacturing Technologies Used to Fabricate Metals in Implant Dentistry. *J. Prosthodont.* **2020**, *29*, 579–593. [CrossRef]
9. Konieczny, B.; Szczesio-Wlodarczyk, A.; Sokolowski, J.; Bociong, K. Challenges of Co–Cr Alloy Additive Manufacturing Methods in Dentistry—The Current State of Knowledge (Systematic Review). *Materials* **2020**, *13*, 3524. [CrossRef]
10. Koutsoukis, T.; Zinelis, S.; Eliades, G.; Al-Wazzan, K.; Al Rifaiy, M.; Al Jabbari, Y.S. Selective Laser Melting Technique of Co-Cr Dental Alloys: A Review of Structure and Properties and Comparative Analysis with Other Available Techniques. *J. Prosthodont.* **2015**, *24*, 303–312. [CrossRef]
11. Wang, J.-H.; Ren, J.; Liu, W.; Wu, X.-Y.; Gao, M.-X.; Bai, P. Effect of Selective Laser Melting Process Parameters on Microstructure and Properties of Co-Cr Alloy. *Materials* **2018**, *11*, 1546. [CrossRef]

12. Takaichi, A.; Suyalatu; Nakamoto, T.; Joko, N.; Nomura, N.; Tsutsumi, Y.; Migita, S.; Doi, H.; Kurosu, S.; Chiba, A.; et al. Microstructures and mechanical properties of Co–29Cr–6Mo alloy fabricated by selective laser melting process for dental applications. *J. Mech. Behav. Biomed. Mater.* **2013**, *21*, 67–76. [CrossRef]
13. Svanborg, P.; Hjalmarsson, L. A systematic review on the accuracy of manufacturing techniques for cobalt chromium fixed dental prostheses. *Biomater. Investig. Dent.* **2020**, *7*, 31–40. [CrossRef]
14. Nascimento, C.D.; Ikeda, L.N.; Pita, M.S.; E Silva, R.C.P.; Pedrazzi, V.; de Albuquerque Junior, R.F.; Ribeiro, R.F. Marginal fit and microbial leakage along the implant-abutment interface of fixed partial prostheses: An in vitro analysis using Checkerboard DNA-DNA hybridization. *J. Prosthet. Dent.* **2015**, *114*, 831–838. [CrossRef] [PubMed]
15. Rossetti, P.H.O.; Valle, A.L.D.; De Carvalho, R.M.; De Goes, M.F.; Pegoraro, L.F. Correlation between margin fit and microleakage in complete crowns cemented with three luting agents. *J. Appl. Oral Sci.* **2008**, *16*, 64–69. [CrossRef] [PubMed]
16. Moher, D.; Liberati, A.; Tetzlaff, J.; Altman, D.G.; The PRISMA Group. Preferred Reporting Items for Systematic Reviews and Meta-Analyses: The PRISMA Statement. *PLoS Med.* **2009**, *6*, e1000097. [CrossRef]
17. Phillips, B.; X, H.; J, L.; D, D.-F. Faculty Opinions recommendation of Evaluation of PICO as a knowledge representation for clinical questions. *Fac. Opin. Post-Publ. Peer Rev. Biomed. Lit.* **2007**, *2006*, 359–363. [CrossRef]
18. Whiting, P.F.; Rutjes, A.W.; Westwood, M.E.; Mallett, S.; Deeks, J.J.; Reitsma, J.B.; Leeflang, M.M.; Sterne, J.A.; Bossuyt, P.M.M. QUADAS-2: A Revised Tool for the Quality Assessment of Diagnostic Accuracy Studies. *Ann. Intern. Med.* **2011**, *155*, 529–536. [CrossRef]
19. McGuinness, L.A.; Higgins, J.P.T. Risk-of-bias VISualization (robvis): An R package and Shiny web app for visualizing risk-of-bias assessments. *Res. Synth. Methods* **2020**. [CrossRef] [PubMed]
20. Borenstein, M.; Hedges, L.V.; Higgins, J.P.T.; Rothstein, H.R. *Introduction to Meta-Analysis*; Wiley: Hoboken, NJ, USA, 2009; pp. 311–319.
21. Yildirim, B.; Paken, G. Evaluation of the Marginal and Internal Fit of Implant-Supported Metal Copings Fabricated with 3 Different Techniques: An In Vitro Study. *J. Prosthodont.* **2019**, *28*, 315–320. [CrossRef]
22. Presotto, A.G.C.; Barão, V.A.R.; Bhering, C.L.B.; Mesquita, M.F. Dimensional precision of implant-supported frameworks fabricated by 3D printing. *J. Prosthet. Dent.* **2019**, *122*, 38–45. [CrossRef] [PubMed]
23. Hong, M.-H.; Min, B.K.; Lee, D.-H.; Kwon, T.-Y. Marginal fit of metal-ceramic crowns fabricated by using a casting and two selective laser melting processes before and after ceramic firing. *J. Prosthet. Dent.* **2019**, *122*, 475–481. [CrossRef]
24. Chang, H.-S.; Peng, Y.-T.; Hung, W.-L.; Hsu, M.-L. Evaluation of marginal adaptation of Co-Cr-Mo metal crowns fabricated by traditional method and computer-aided technologies. *J. Dent. Sci.* **2019**, *14*, 288–294. [CrossRef] [PubMed]
25. James, A.E.; Umamaheswari, B.; Lakshmi, C.B.S. Comparative Evaluation of Marginal Accuracy of Metal Copings Fabricated using Direct Metal Laser Sintering, Computer-Aided Milling, Ringless Casting, and Traditional Casting Techniques: An In vitro Study. Contemp. *Clin. Dent.* **2018**, *9*, 421–426. [CrossRef]
26. Yadav, A.; Arora, A.; Upadhyaya, V.; Jain, P.; Verma, M. Comparison of marginal and internal adaptation of copings fabricated from three different fabrication techniques: An in vitro study. *J. Indian Prosthodont. Soc.* **2018**, *18*, 102. [CrossRef] [PubMed]
27. Ullattuthodi, S.; Cherian, K.P.; Anandkumar, R.; Nambiar, M.S. Marginal and internal fit of cobalt-chromium copings fabricated using the conventional and the direct metal laser sintering techniques: A comparative in vitro study. *J. Indian Prosthodont. Soc.* **2017**, *17*, 373–380. [CrossRef]
28. Lövgren, N.; Roxner, R.; Klemendz, S.; Larsson, C. Effect of production method on surface roughness, marginal and internal fit, and retention of cobalt-chromium single crowns. *J. Prosthet. Dent.* **2017**, *118*, 95–101. [CrossRef]
29. Kaleli, N.; Saraç, D. Influence of porcelain firing and cementation on the marginal adaptation of metal-ceramic restorations prepared by different methods. *J. Prosthet. Dent.* **2016**, *117*, 656–661. [CrossRef]
30. Kocaağaoğlu, H.; Kılınç, H.I.; Albayrak, H.; Kara, M. In vitro evaluation of marginal, axial, and occlusal discrepancies in metal ceramic restorations produced with new technologies. *J. Prosthet. Dent.* **2016**, *116*, 368–374. [CrossRef]

31. Gunsoy, S.; Ulusoy, M. Evaluation of marginal/internal fit of chrome-cobalt crowns: Direct laser metal sintering versus computer-aided design and computer-aided manufacturing. *Niger. J. Clin. Pr.* **2016**, *19*, 636–644. [CrossRef]
32. Ates, S.M.; Duymus, Z.Y. Influence of Tooth Preparation Design on Fitting Accuracy of CAD-CAM Based Restorations. *J. Esthet. Restor. Dent.* **2016**, *28*, 238–246. [CrossRef] [PubMed]
33. Zeng, L.; Zhang, Y.; Liu, Z.; Wei, B. Effects of repeated firing on the marginal accuracy of Co-Cr copings fabricated by selective laser melting. *J. Prosthet. Dent.* **2015**, *113*, 135–139. [CrossRef] [PubMed]
34. Pompa, G.; Di Carlo, S.; De Angelis, F.; Cristalli, M.P.; Annibali, S. Comparison of Conventional Methods and Laser-Assisted Rapid Prototyping for Manufacturing Fixed Dental Prostheses: An In Vitro Study. *BioMed Res. Int.* **2015**, *2015*, 1–7. [CrossRef]
35. Park, J.-K.; Lee, W.-S.; Kim, H.-Y.; Kim, W.-C.; Kim, J.-H. Accuracy evaluation of metal copings fabricated by computer-aided milling and direct metal laser sintering systems. *J. Adv. Prosthodont.* **2015**, *7*, 122–128. [CrossRef] [PubMed]
36. Huang, Z.; Zhang, L.; Zhu, J.; Zhao, Y.; Zhang, X. Clinical Marginal and Internal Fit of Crowns Fabricated Using Different CAD/CAM Technologies. *J. Prosthodont.* **2014**, *24*, 291–295. [CrossRef] [PubMed]
37. Tamac, E.; Toksavul, S.; Toman, M. Clinical marginal and internal adaptation of CAD/CAM milling, laser sintering, and cast metal ceramic crowns. *J. Prosthet. Dent.* **2014**, *112*, 909–913. [CrossRef]
38. Kim, K.-B.; Kim, W.-C.; Kim, H.-Y.; Kim, J.-H. An evaluation of marginal fit of three-unit fixed dental prostheses fabricated by direct metal laser sintering system. *Dent. Mater.* **2013**, *29*, e91–e96. [CrossRef]
39. Kim, K.-B.; Kim, J.-H.; Kim, W.-C.; Kim, H.-Y.; Kim, J.-H. Evaluation of the marginal and internal gap of metal-ceramic crown fabricated with a selective laser sintering technology: Two- and three-dimensional replica techniques. *J. Adv. Prosthodont.* **2013**, *5*, 179–186. [CrossRef]
40. Castillo-Oyagüe, R.; Turrión, A.S.; Lozano, J.F.L.; Albaladejo, A.; Torres-Lagares, D.; Montero, J.; Suárez-García, M.-J. Vertical misfit of laser-sintered and vacuum-cast implant-supported crown copings luted with definitive and temporary luting agents. *Med. Oral Patol. Oral Cir. Bucal* **2012**, *17*, e610–e617. [CrossRef]
41. Örtorp, A.; Jönsson, D.; Mouhsen, A.; Von Steyern, P.V. The fit of cobalt–chromium three-unit fixed dental prostheses fabricated with four different techniques: A comparative in vitro study. *Dent. Mater.* **2011**, *27*, 356–363. [CrossRef]
42. Nawafleh, N.A.; Mack, F.; Evans, J.; Mackay, J.; Hatamleh, M.M. Accuracy and Reliability of Methods to Measure Marginal Adaptation of Crowns and FDPs: A Literature Review. *J. Prosthodont.* **2013**, *22*, 419–428. [CrossRef]
43. Lee, D.-H. Digital approach to assessing the 3-dimensional misfit of fixed dental prostheses. *J. Prosthet. Dent.* **2016**, *116*, 836–839. [CrossRef] [PubMed]
44. Schlenz, M.A.; Vogler, J.A.H.; Schmidt, A.; Rehmann, P.; Wöstmann, B. Chairside measurement of the marginal and internal fit of crowns: A new intraoral scan–based approach. *Clin. Oral Investig.* **2019**, *24*, 2459–2468. [CrossRef] [PubMed]
45. Mai, H.-N.; Lee, K.E.; Ha, J.-H.; Lee, D.-H. Effects of image and education on the precision of the measurement method for evaluating prosthesis misfit. *J. Prosthet. Dent.* **2018**, *119*, 600–605. [CrossRef]
46. Barrios-Muriel, J.; Romero-Sánchez, F.; Alonso, F.J.; Salgado, D.R. Advances in Orthotic and Prosthetic Manufacturing: A Technology Review. *Materials* **2020**, *13*, 295. [CrossRef]
47. Oropallo, W.; Piegl, L.A. Ten challenges in 3D printing. *Eng. Comput.* **2015**, *32*, 135–148. [CrossRef]
48. Huang, Z.; Zhang, X.; Zhu, J.; Zhang, X. Clinical marginal and internal fit of metal ceramic crowns fabricated with a selective laser melting technology. *J. Prosthet. Dent.* **2015**, *113*, 623–627. [CrossRef]
49. Franz, H.; Plöchl, L.; Schimansky, F.-P. Recent advances of titanium alloy powder production by ceramic-free inert gas atomization. In Proceedings of the 24th Annual International Titanium Associaction Conference Titatnium 2008, Las Vesgas, NV, USA, 21–24 September 2008.
50. Gu, D.; Meiners, W.; Wissenbach, K.; Poprawe, R. Laser additive manufacturing of metallic components: Materials, processes and mechanisms. *Int. Mater. Rev.* **2012**, *57*, 133–164. [CrossRef]
51. Murr, L.E.; Gaytan, S.M.; Ramirez, D.A.; Martinez, E.; Hernandez, J.; Amato, K.N.; Shindo, P.W.; Medina, F.R.; Wicker, R.B. Metal Fabrication by Additive Manufacturing Using Laser and Electron Beam Melting Technologies. *J. Mater. Sci. Technol.* **2012**, *28*, 1–14. [CrossRef]

52. Gusarov, A.V.; Yadroitsev, I.; Bertrand, P.; Smurov, I. Model of Radiation and Heat Transfer in Laser-Powder Interaction Zone at Selective Laser Melting. *J. Heat Transf.* **2009**, *131*, 072101. [CrossRef]
53. Heeling, T.; Cloots, M.; Wegener, K. Melt pool simulation for the evaluation of process parameters in selective laser melting. *Addit. Manuf.* **2017**, *14*, 116–125. [CrossRef]
54. Meier, C.; Penny, R.W.; Zou, Y.; Gibbs, J.S.; Hart, A.J. Thermophysical Phenomena in Metal Additive Manufacturing by Selective Laser Melting: Fundamentals, Modeling, Simulation, and Experimentation. *Annu. Rev. Heat Transf.* **2017**, *20*, 241–316. [CrossRef]
55. Mitteramskogler, G.; Gmeiner, R.; Felzmann, R.; Gruber, S.; Hofstetter, C.; Stampfl, J.; Ebert, J.; Wachter, W.; Laubersheimer, J. Light curing strategies for lithography-based additive manufacturing of customized ceramics. *Addit. Manuf.* **2014**, 110–118. [CrossRef]
56. Wilkes, J.; Hagedorn, Y.; Meiners, W.; Wissenbach, K. Additive manufacturing of ZrO2-Al2O3ceramic components by selective laser melting. *Rapid Prototyp. J.* **2013**, *19*, 51–57. [CrossRef]
57. Candotto, V.; Gabrione, F.; Oberti, L.; Lento, D.; Severino, M. The role of implant-abutment connection in preventing bacterial leakage: A review. *J. Biol. Regul Homeost. Agents.* **2019**, *33*, 129–134. [PubMed]

materials

MDPI

Review

Challenges of Co–Cr Alloy Additive Manufacturing Methods in Dentistry—The Current State of Knowledge (Systematic Review)

Bartłomiej Konieczny [1,*], Agata Szczesio-Wlodarczyk [1], Jerzy Sokolowski [2] and Kinga Bociong [1]

[1] University Laboratory of Materials Research, Medical University of Lodz, ul. Pomorska 251, 92-213 Lodz, Poland; agata.szczesio@umed.lodz.pl (A.S.-W.); kinga.bociong@umed.lodz.pl (K.B.)

[2] Department of General Dentistry, Medical University of Lodz, ul. Pomorska 251, 92-213 Lodz, Poland; jerzy.sokolowski@umed.lodz.pl

* Correspondence: bartlomiej.konieczny@umed.lodz.pl; Tel.: +48-42-272-57-66

Received: 18 June 2020; Accepted: 4 August 2020; Published: 10 August 2020

Abstract: Complex dental components which are individually tailored to the patient can be obtained due to new additive manufacturing technology. This paper reviews the metallic powders used in dental applications, the fabrication process (build orientation, process parameters) and post-processing processes (stress relieving, surface finishing). A review of the literature was performed using PubMed, ScienceDirect, Mendeley and Google Scholar. Over eighty articles were selected based on relevance to this review. This paper attempts to include the latest research from 2010 until 2020, however, older manuscripts (10 articles) were also selected. Over 1200 records were identified through the search; these were screened for title and/or summary. Over eighty articles were selected based on relevance to this review. In order to obtain a product which can be used in clinical applications, the appropriate manufacturing parameters should be selected. A discussion was made on optimal selective laser melting (SLM) parameters in dentistry. In addition, this paper includes a critical review of applied thermal treatment methods for Co–Cr alloys used in dentistry.

Keywords: powder bed fusion; selective laser sintering; selective laser melting; electron beam melting; process parameters; stress relieving; heat treatment; cobalt–chromium; dentistry

1. Introduction

CoCr-based alloys are commonly used in dentistry because of their excellent corrosion resistance and outstanding mechanical properties, such as high stiffness. Since its development in 1907, lost wax casting is still the dominant method of dental metal processing [1]. Unfortunately, this technique has some limitations, one of which is the fact that metal shrinks during its transition from the liquid to the solid phase, and this shrinkage should be taken into account when preparing the part for casting. Additionally, pores and other defects are usually present in the structure of the cast element [2,3], the process is time-consuming and requires certain skills for the operators [4], and CoCr alloys are difficult to treat and process because of their high hardness [5].

Nowadays, metallic materials are processed by computer-aided design and computer-aided manufacturing (CAD–CAM) (Table 1) that allows 3D structures to be produced based on data (appropriate conversed–segmented) regarding individual organs, bones or blood vessels obtained from medical imaging devices such as magnetic resonance imaging (MRI), computed tomography (CT), cone beam tomography (CBCT) or ultrasound (USG). Segmentation and analysis software is available as open source versions (e.g., InVesalius or 3D Slicer) and as a paid version with extended functionality (Materialize Mimics, Amira or Dolphin 3d). Three-dimensional models can also be obtained using

3D scanning; this is the most common type of solution used in Dentistry (i.e., in prosthetics and orthodontics), using optical scanners employing photogrammetry or scanning with structured light. The 3D data obtained in this way are used for the design of prosthetic restorations, orthodontic appliances, surgical templates or individualized implants using dedicated CAD software [6–9].

CAD–CAM technology encompasses two main categories: subtractive manufacturing processes like milling, and additive manufacturing (AM) processes like powder bed fusion [10,11]. Milling uses tools (saws, lathes, grinders, drill presses) to mechanically cut a block to a desired geometry and this process is controlled by software. Compared to the casting method, this technique can reduce flaws and pores because the blanks are made under high industrial standards [12,13]. However, the process is associated with a greater waste of materials and some limitations in complex projects compared to casting and AM [10]. AM technologies, more popularly known as 'three-dimensional (3D) printing', build physical objects in a single stage directly from their computer-aided design. With this technology, the products are formed through the addition of the materials layer by layer, based on sliced data from the 3D design [14,15]. Therefore, this method is used for producing complex products and has opened new possibilities in dentistry [16]. AM can use polymers, ceramics, metal alloys and composites. New approaches are focused on the development of biological ink [15,17]. Some common uses of AM techniques in dentistry are stereolithography (SLA), fused deposition modeling (FDM), powder bed fusion (PBF) and ink-jet printing (IJP) [18]. Of these, powder bed fusion (PBF) is commonly employed for metal processing in dentistry [19,20]. Powder bed fusion uses a heat source to consolidate metallic powder to form a 3D object (layer by layer), according to CAD. This techniques offer cost-effective customization and reduced assembly [21].

Table 1. Computer-aided design/computer-aided manufacturing (CAD/CAM) processes currently upgraded into dentistry.

Process	Technology	Ref.
Digital impression	It is a non-invasive method to obtain a virtual model of the hard and soft tissue of the patient's oral cavity. This involves the use of an intraoral scanner which records a series of snapshots of the oral cavity of the patient.	[22]
Prosthetic designing	Scanner data are evaluated and processed by the dental laboratory using special software. The digital prosthetic model is individually tailored to the patient.	[22]
Manufacturing process	Milling (subtractive manufacturing): a prepared prosthetic design is mechanically cut from a metal block. This process is controlled by software. Milling units in the last decade were optimized—large angulations of the fourth and fifth axes (>30 degrees), dry or wet grinding.	[5]
	Sintering (subtractive manufacturing): technology developed by Amann Girrbach. The prepared prosthetic is mechanically cut from metal blanks with a wax-like texture. The process is controlled by software. The blocks are made from unsintered metal powder held together by a binder. After the milling process, the structure is subjected to sintering in a special furnace.	
	Powder bed fusion (PBF, additive manufacturing): the prepared prosthetic is formed by the thermal consolidation of a metal powder (layer by layer). The process is controlled by software. Selective laser sintering (SLS), selective laser melting (SLM) and electron beam melting (EBM) are three methods classified as PBF.	

2. Materials and Methods

An electronic search was performed in the databases PubMed, ScienceDirect, Mendeley and Google Scholar. A manual search of citations from relevant articles was also conducted. The following keywords were used: powder bed fusion (or PBF), selective laser sintering (or SLS), selective laser melting (or SLM), electron beam melting (or EBM), inclination angle, stress relieving, heat treatment, cobalt–chromium (or Co–Cr), dental. This paper attempts to include the latest research from the last 10 years (2010–2020), however, older manuscripts were also selected. Over 1200 records were identified through the search; these were screened for title and/or summary. Over eighty articles were selected based on their relevance to this review. The exclusion criteria included non-dental (or non-medical) applications and the articles on 3D printing of metal alloys other than Co–Cr. The results were based on a descriptive analysis of the techniques and materials of additive manufacturing, fabrication process and post-processing strategies.

3. Powder Bed Fusion (PBF)

Powder bed fusion can be subdivided into three methods: selective laser sintering (SLS), selective laser melting (SLM) and electron beam melting (EBM). In SLS, metal powder compacts are transformed into coherent solids at temperatures below their melting point. In SLM and EBM, the metal powder is fully melted, however, the two methods use different ways to achieve their melting point [23].

3.1. Selective Laser Sintering (SLS)

Carl Deckard and Joe Beaman developed and patented in 1989 selective laser sintering (SLS) technology [24]. In this method, a high-power laser is focused onto a thin layer of metal powder. The layer is heated, and next bonding processes between metal particles is started. This step requires the transport of material from inside the powder to points and areas where particles are in contact with each other. There are five different transport mechanisms possible: volume diffusion, grain-boundary diffusion, surface diffusion, viscous or plastic flow. Elements made by SLS technique are characterized by high porosity. It is crucial to correctly select the parameters of the SLS process (temperature, time, geometrical structure of the powder particles, composition of the powder mix, density of the powder compact, composition of the protective atmosphere in the sintering furnace) [25]. Unfortunately, the complete elimination of porosities is not possible due to the partial melting and sintering caused by the melting point not being reached [26].

3.2. Selective Laser Melting (SLM)

It is possible to melt metal powder using powerful, high-quality lasers. In 1995, commercial machines using SLM technology were launched on the market. Selective laser melting printers use CO_2 lasers or fiber lasers (Nd:YAG or Yb:YAG) [27]. The laser beam is focused onto the powder, and the energy supplied by the laser is able to melt it. The melting process can be adjusted by varying the wavelength, laser source and power. The resulting products are characterized by a lower occurrence of blisters and a better superficial finish than those made by SLS. Unfortunately, high internal stresses are found in materials, caused by the thermal gradients induced during manufacturing. To reduce these stresses, additional heat treatment is required [19,28,29]. Selective laser melting technology is the most popular approach to metal processing in Dentistry (Table 1).

3.3. Electron Beam Melting (EBM)

This technology is very similar to SLM. However, EBM technology uses a focused electron beam in a vacuum environment to melt the layers of powder. During EBM processing, a tungsten filament is heated, and this gives off electrons which are accelerated into a beam by two magnetic coils. The beam strikes the metal powder, which is melted by the transmission of kinetic energy [30,31].

4. Metallurgy

The most commonly used alloys for PBF in dental applications are cobalt–chromium (Co–Cr) and Titanium (Ti). Other metals are also added to improve the strength properties of the material. Co–Cr-based alloys are the hardest known biocompatible materials that are commonly used in medicine and dentistry. They demonstrate good fatigue resistance, tensile strength, elasticity or corrosion resistance, and are suitable for use in medical implants, partial skeletal denture frameworks and for crown and bridge substructure restorations in dentistry [31,32]. Chromium forms a solid solution with cobalt and increases corrosion resistance by surface passivation; however, a chromium content greater than 30% results in difficulty in casting and the formation of a brittle σ phase. Molybdenum (Mo) and wolfram (W) cause solid solution strengthening, and the formation of M6C, MC type carbides and Co3M intermetallic phase (M represents a metal element). Molybdenum affects the grain size and reduces the susceptibility to pitting corrosion. Silicon (Si) and manganese (Mn) are added to improve the alloy's fluidity, while niobium (Nb) affects the solution strengthening, intermetallic phase formation and MC type carbides. The cobalt-based alloys used in dentistry have a low carbon (C) content. The addition of carbon has a very significant impact on mechanical properties, and especially on plasticity, even in small quantities. High strength and creep resistance (resistance to plastic flow) are obtained at a carbon content of 0.3–1.0%. Due to the presence of carbide-forming additives (with a significant carbon content), carbides with a complex structure e.g., M23C6 type, are formed in interdendritic spaces during the heat treatment [33,34].

Powder compositions and mechanical properties are summarized in Tables 2 and 3. Differences can be seen between Co–Cr alloys. Only SLM technology is used to manufacture Co–Cr dental prosthetics [19].

Table 2. Brands and chemical composition of CoCr alloys for dental (DA) and medical (MA) applications. Data from reference [19].

Brand	PBF System	Chemical Composition (wt.%)
EOS CoCr SP2 (DA)	DMLS (direct metal laser solidification) = SLM	Co: 63.8; Cr: 24.7; Mo: 5.1; W: 5.4; Si: 1.0; Fe: ≤0.50; Mn: ≤0.10 Free of Ni, Be, Cd and Pb
EOS CoCr MP1(MA)	DMLS (direct metal laser solidification) = SLM	Co: 60–65; Cr: 26–30; Mo: 5–7; Si: ≤1.0; Mn: ≤1.0; Fe: ≤0.75; C: ≤0.16; Ni: ≤0.10
Renishaw CoCr DG1(DA)	SLM	Co: 63.9; Cr: 24.7; Mo: 5.0; W: 5.4; Si: 1.0 Free of Ni, Be, Cd and Pb
SLM Solutions MediDent (DA)	SLM	Co: Balance; Cr: 22.7–26.7; Mo: 4–6; W: 4.4–6.4; Si: 2; Fe: 0.5; Mn: 0.10; C: 0.02; Ni: 0.10; B, S: 0.10
SLM Solutions CoCr28Mo6 (MA)	SLM	Co: Balance; Cr: 27–30; Mo: 5–7; W: 0.20; Si: 1; Al: 0.10; Fe: 0.75; Mn: 1; C: 0.35; N: 0.25; Ni: 0.5 Ti: 0.1; B, S: 0.01
3D systems LaserForm CoCr(A,B,C) ASTM F75(DA and MA)	SLM	Co Bal., Cr 28.00–30.00, Mo 5.00–6.00, Ni 0.00–0.10, Fe 0.00–0.50, C 0.00–0.02, Si 0.00–1.00, Mn 0.00–1.00, Cd 0.00–0.02, Be 0.00–0.02, Pb 0.00–0.02
Concept Laser Remanium star CL	DMLM (direct metal laser melting)	Co: 60.5; Cr: 28; W: 9; Si: 1.5; Other elements <1: Mn, N, Nb, Fe. free from nickel, beryllium and gallium
BEGO Wirobond C+	SLM	Co: 63.9; Cr: 24.7; W: 5.4; Mo: 5.0; Si: <1
Scheftner Starbond COS	SLM	Co: 59; Cr: 25; W: 9.5; Mo: 3.5; Si: 1; C,Fe,Mn,N: <1%
Scheftner Starbond Easy 30	SLM	Co: 61; Cr: 27.5; W: 8.5; Si: 1,6; C,Fe,Mn: <1

Table 3. Physical and mechanical properties of 3D printed CoCr (after stress relief) provided by their manufacturers after heat treatment. NA: Not available. Data from Reference [19].

Property	OS SP2	EOS MP1	Renisaw DG1	SLM MediDent	SLM CoCr28Mo6	LaserForm CoCr (B)	Concept Laser Remanium Star CL	BEGO Wirobond C+	Scheftner Starbond COS	Scheftner Starbond Easy 30
Density (g/cm^3)	8.5	8.3	8.3	NA	NA	8.3	8.6	8.6	8.8	8.5
Tensile strength (MPa)	1350	1100	1076	1415	1215	1445 +/− 50	1030	1315	990–1250	1090
Elongation at break (%)	3	Min. 20	2.7	4	21	34 +/− 6	10		2–10	15
Young's Modulus (GPa)	approx. 200	200	224	245	205	230 +/− 40	230	215	195–200	225
Hardness	420 HV	approx. 35–45 HRC	430 HV	NA/375 HV as built	385 HV	26 +/− 5 Rockwell C	NA	NA	345–490 HV 10	425 HV 10
Coefficient of thermal expansion	14.3 × 10^{-6} m/m °C	13.6 × 10^{-6} m/m °C– 15.1 × 10^{-6} m/m °C	14.1	NA	NA	14	14.1 (500 °C)	14.3 (RT-500 °C) 14.5 (RT-600 °C)	14.4 (600 °C)	14.5 (500 °C) 14.7(600 °C)
Melting interval (°C)	1410–1450	1350–1430	1375–1405	NA	NA	1350–1430	1320–1420	1380–1420	1305–1400	1310–1410

5. Fabrication Process

The properties of the final product depend on a number of factors. The key element is the choice of powder; however, the optimization of the process parameters is equally important. The most important factors include the development of a model in a computer program, the determination of its build orientation and the selection of machine parameters [18,29,35–37].

5.1. Build Orientation

The building orientation is generally defined as the acute angle between the longitudinal axis of a given sample and the vertical axis of the building platform. Microstructure, texture and residual stress concentration are dependent on the building orientation [38]. The thermal fluctuations occurring during the manufacturing process have the greatest effect on the orientations of the formed grains: in general, the grain grows from a cooler (building platform) to a warmer region (top surface) [39,40].

Selective laser melting manufactured parts are characterized by anisotropic γ-phase, i.e., face-centered cubic (fcc) and ε-phase, i.e., hexagonal close-packed (hcp). The Fcc phase is dominant [41]. Additionally, precipitates were observed to align along the build direction [42]. The anisotropic structure influences the mechanical properties of SLM products. Figure 1 presents a scheme of fabricated layers in SLM samples according to different building orientations. At 45° and 0°, there are more layers, which result in more molten pool boundaries. Fractures in SLM parts can be initiated at the molten pool boundaries and cracks may be observed along the boundaries of tensile fracture extensions. For samples built at 0° orientations, the fracture surface is almost parallel to the molten pool boundaries and cracks may easily propagate along them. Hence, molten pool boundaries appear to have some impact on the anisotropy behavior of SLM builds [43].

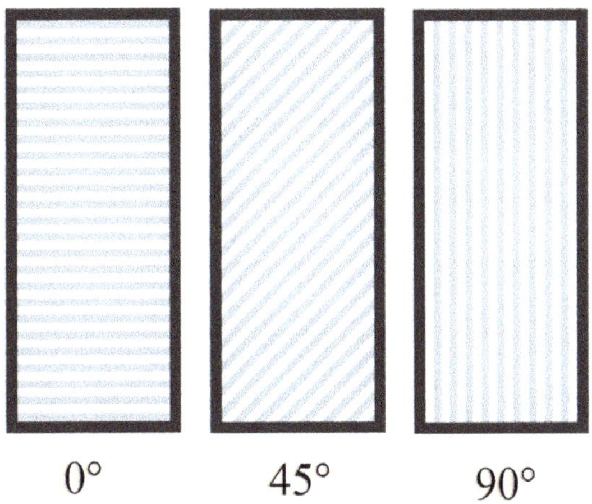

Figure 1. Scheme of the fabricated layers in the SLM samples according to the different building orientations—0°, 45° or 90°.

Materials prepared by PBF exhibited comparable (or even higher) mechanical properties (yield strength, tensile strength) as those prepared by casting. Higher yield strength and lower elongation were observed at 45° or 90° building orientations [41,44]. Samples built at 0° and 45° had lower fatigue strength than the cast samples, but the samples manufactured at 90° have the highest fatigue strength. These properties can be affected by anisotropic microstructure, crystal orientation, surface roughness and residual stress [43,45]. The fatigue strength of metal AM parts can be improved through post-heat treatment [5]. The anisotropy in PBF parts may affect clinical performance. It is essential to apply a proper post-processing treatment to ensure the reliable usage of manufactured products.

5.2. Process Parameters

A layer-by-layer manufacturing process results in complex, time-dependent temperature profiles. Each metallic layer may repeatedly transform between phases (e.g., $\alpha \rightarrow \beta$) and states (from solid to liquid). Such frequent thermal cycling effects the microstructure of the material [46]. Temperature profiles are dependent upon a number of variables, including the AM equipment, the time between passes, and the size of the part being fabricated.

The quality and effects of the metal SLM process is influenced by laser power, scanning speed, laser beam size and layer thickness; these are responsible for the melting energy and penetration depth of alloy powder, which translates into the density of the melted material [47]. As the laser power increases, the amount of powder melted increases per unit of time. Although the width and depth of the molten pool increase, they decrease when we increase the speed of the laser beam feed, while maintaining the same power. Scan line spacing (scanning pitch) i.e., the distance between two adjacent laser scanning trajectories, also influences the characteristics of the molten pool [32,48]. A large scanning pitch may result in a large number of voids, and lowered density, while a small pitch may cause the formation of a coarse grain structure, which affects the performance of the product [32]. Energy input, calculated as P/V, where P is laser power and V scanning speed, is also a determining factor. When the energy input is below 0.36 J/s, the density of the products increases with an increase in energy input. With an increase in energy input, metal powders tend to be completely melted and a full metallurgical bond is achieved between particles. Above 0.36 J/s, the density begins to reduce due to a vaporization of melt pools [49].

These process parameters have a significant impact on product performance [50]. The tensile strength and yield strength of the sample increase as the laser power increases and the scanning pitch decreases. However, increasing the scanning speed deceases the tensile strength and yield strength. To achieve the best properties of cobalt–chromium alloys in the SLM process, the optimal parameters seem to be a laser power of 160 W, a scanning speed of 1100 mm/s, and a scan line spacing of 0.05 mm [32].

Laser energy density (LED) or volume energy is an established characteristic, which combines four major process parameters, namely laser power P (W), scanning velocity v (mm s^{-1}), distance between two consequent laser scans h (mm) and layer thickness d (mm) (Equation (1)):

$$LED = \frac{P}{v \cdot h \cdot d} \left[\frac{J}{mm^3} \right] \tag{1}$$

This metric correlates well with the hardness, microstructure and surface morphology. LED values of 150–200 J mm^{-3} are optimal for obtaining high quality $Co_{28}Cr_6Mo$ SLM parts [51].

6. Post-Processing Strategies

After the fabrication process, there are a few steps required to obtain the final product. Unprocessed loose powder particles and needless support structures are removed. Following this, the object is prepared for heat treatment. Final processes like surface finishing and sterilization are often used [27].

6.1. Stress Relieving

In SLM, a high gradient of temperature and build orientation have a profound influence on microstructures, textures, roughness and residual stress occurrence. As a result, the fabricated object has anisotropic properties dependent on build-up orientation [52,53]. Due to the complex structure of dental prosthesis and various stress directions during mastication, anisotropy and residual stress should be eliminated. Post-processing heat treatment is considered necessary to ensure the reliable use of PFB-built parts in practical applications. The main phases of Co–Cr–Mo alloys are the γ-phase, i.e., the face-centered cubic (fcc) and ε-phase, i.e., hexagonal close-packed (hcp). The γ-phase is stable at a high temperature and the ε-phase at low temperature. The hcp structure is formed while the alloy is cooled from high temperatures. The phase diagram for the Co–Cr alloys shows that $\gamma \rightarrow \varepsilon$ transformation takes place around 900 °C. The differences in temperature may be due to a different elemental composition [54,55].

Table 4 presents the main conditions of heat treatment for PFB-built parts.

Table 4. Heat treatment procedures of 3D printed CoCr.

Procedure	Note	References
Under an argon atmosphere. 1. Heat furnace from room temperature to 450 °C in 60 min and hold at this temperature for 45 min. 3. Heat furnace to 750 °C in 45 min and hold at this temperature for 60 min (holding temperature and time tolerance inside the box: 740 °C +/− 10 °C, 60 min +/− 20 min). 5. Switch off the heating. 6. When temperature has dropped down to approx. 600 °C, open the furnace door. 7. When furnace has cooled down to approx. 300 °C, remove the protective gas box from furnace and shut down the argon flow.	Instructions for use material: EOS CobaltChrome SP2. Longer holding time, utilization of higher stress-relieving temperature or forced cooling may lead to increased brittleness of restorations.	[56]
Post-process stress relieving at 1150 °C for six hours.	Instructions for use material: EOS CoCr MP1 for medical applications.	[57]
Under an argon atmosphere. Hold at 750 °C temperature for 60 min and allowed to cool naturally.	Instructions for use Renishaw CoCr DG1.	[58]
I. First heating process 1. Heat furnace from room temperature to 500 °C (a ramp rate of 8 °C/min) and hold at this temperature for 45 min. 2. Heat furnace to 880 °C in 60 min, and hold at this temperature for 60 min. 3. Switch off the heating. 4. When temperature has dropped down to approx. 600 °C, open the furnace door. 5. Remove specimens from the furnace when the temperature has dropped to 300 °C. II. Second heating process 1. Heat furnace from room temperature to 1100 °C (a ramp rate of 8 °C/min) and hold at this temperature for 30 min. 2. Switch off the heating. 3. When temperature has dropped down to approx. 600 °C, open the furnace door. 4. Remove specimens from the furnace when the temperature has dropped to 300 °C.	Heat treated SLM-fabricated samples (at 880 °C and 1100 °C) exhibited mechanical properties that exceeded the minimum requirements according to ISO standard (ISO 22674:2016.8). The heat treatment at 1100 °C was more efficient for relieving residual stress.	[55]
1. Heat furnace from room temperature to 1150 °C and hold at this temperature for 60 min. 2. Cool samples in water (water quenching) 3. Half of the samples were additionally subjected to isothermal heat treatment at 800 °C for four hours 4. Cool samples in water (water quenching)	The elimination of dendritic microstructure and micro-segregation was achieved after heat treatment at 1150 °C. Increased tensile strength and yield stress were achieved by isothermal heat treatment at 800 °C and water quenching due to a diffusely formed hcp ε phase, finely distributed in the fcc γ matrix. Crack initiation and propagation occur preferentially at the ε martensite.	[59]
Under an argon atmosphere. 1. Heat furnace from room temperature to 750, 900, 1050, or 1150 °C (a ramp rate of 60 °C/min) and hold at the specified temperature for six hours. 2. Switch off the heating. 3. When temperature has dropped down to approx. 300 °C, open the furnace door.	Heat treatment at temperatures below 1050 °C was insufficient to eliminate the anisotropic columnar grains, fiber texture and residual stress. Recrystallization via heat treatment at 1150 °C homogenizes the microstructure, eliminate residual stress and enables reduction of the anisotropic mechanical properties. Increasing the heat-treatment temperature from 750 °C to 1150 °C increased the ductility of the alloy and decreased its 0.2% offset yield strength and Vickers hardness.	[60,61]
The three heat treatment cycles were used: I. One hour at 1220 °C; II. Four hours preheating at 815 °C and then two hours at 1220 °C; III. Four hours at 1220 °C. Rapid quenching in water at room temperature was done at the end of preheating and solution treatment.	After heat treatment, both the ultimate tensile strength and yield strength of SLM CoCrMo decreased due to the homogenization of microstructure and texture. The microstructure analysis concluded carbides formation.	[62]
Under an argon atmosphere. 1. Heat furnace from room temperature to 600 °C (a ramp rate of 10 °C/min) and hold at this temperature for 30 min. 2. Heat furnace to 1150 °C and hold at this temperature for one or six hours. 3. After one or six hours switch off the heating. 4. Cool samples slowly to room temperature in a furnace.	Heat treatment at 1150 °C for one and six hours allowed the homogenization of microstructure and texture. Higher fatigue strength was observed after 1 h treatment compared with control groups (as built 0° and 45° building angulations). Six hours heat treatment created large precipitates and a thick oxide layer associated with a decrease in fatigue strength.	[45,63]

It was shown that the heat treatment up to 1050 °C for six hours was insufficient to eliminate anisotropy and residual stress. However, the dendritic structures and number of sub-grains decreased while increasing the heat-treatment temperature (from 750 °C to 1050 °C) compared with the as-built samples [60]. During the recovery process, the deformed grains reduced their stored energy through the removal or rearrangement of defects in their crystal structure [64]. In PFB samples, some defects occurred during manufacturing which may initiate a recovery process. Dislocations were rearranged during recovery and subsequently transformed into LABs (low-angle boundaries), leading to the formation of sub-grains [61]. Heating samples at 1150 °C even for one hour causes the microstructure to undergo homogenization. Anisotropic columnar grains, dendritic structures, and sub-grains for samples with all build angles were transformed into uniform equiaxed grains with no apparent internal disorientation. The residual strain inside the grains was relieved [63] as a result of thermally induced recrystallization, which is likely driven by the strain energy stored in the microstructure by differential thermal contractions during the PBF process [65,66]. High dislocation densities are present at the boundaries of the cellular dendritic structures, observed in the finished PBF products, which result in stored energy in these regions. The structure of the recrystallized grains depend on the level of accumulated (residual) stress in the region [65]. Due to recrystallization, the heat-treated (1150 °C) samples display new equiaxed grains containing a number of $\Sigma3$ annealing twin boundaries with new crystal orientations and the residual plastic strain inside the grains was drastically relieved. This process results in grains with uniformly-distributed crystal orientations and a homogenous isotropic microstructure [61].

It should be emphasized that the products manufactured by casting also have some defects which significantly affect alloy ductility. Thermal processing has been commonly used in casted Co–Cr alloys to improve their final properties. In addition to structure homogenization, the formation of metal carbides is known to influence Co-based alloy (comparable to standard specification ASTM F75) performance [67,68]. Carbides inside the grains strengthen the alloy matrix, acting as obstacles in dislocations while they prevent grain boundary sliding and migration at the grain boundaries [62,69]. The main factors which influence the size and amount of carbides are the heat-treatment temperature and the cooling rates. The dissolution of carbides into matrix occurs above 1200 °C [70]. After this heat treatment, slow cooling rates promote the development of a lamellar eutectic structure with carbides at the grain boundaries [71]. The use of strong cooling (e.g., water quenching from heat treatment temperature) causes the formation of fine primary carbide which are more homogenously distributed in the matrix [72]. By increasing the cooling rate, the size of the carbides formed decreases [73]. Moreover, in PBF materials subjected to heat treatment, there are precipitations that occur both in the grains and on their boundaries. The amount, size and distribution of the precipitations will depend mainly on the temperature, heating time and cooling method. Furnace cooling contributes to the formation of larger precipitates at the grain boundary regions. Water quenching promotes the formation of smaller precipitates and carbide dissolution into the matrix [74,75].

Increasing the heat-treatment temperature decreased by 0.2% the yield strength, ultimate tensile strength and Vickers hardness of the CoCr alloy specimens but enhanced the ductility. Recovery processes, which occurred in the heat treatment under 1050 °C, resulted in a reduced dislocation density and the volume fraction of the ε phase. This explains the reduction in material strength and an increase in the ductility. Elongation is an important factor, especially in the removal partial dentures. Denture parts characterized by low elongation can fracture more easily than those with high elongation. The reduction of the ε phase in alloys results in sample elongation. Considering the characteristics of loads that occur in the oral environment, one of the key properties of prosthetic components is fatigue resistance. The fatigue strength of SLM samples was improved after heat treatment at 1150 °C [63]. However, in one study, controls with 90° building angulations exhibited longer fatigue life than the heat-treated groups [45]. It was explained due to fine cellular or columnar dendritic structures which have a function as obstacles for the dislocation motion. Samples with 0° and 45° building angulations showed a lower fatigue life than the heat-treated groups due to the occurrence of molten pool boundaries and Schmid factor [45]. Extended heat treatment (six hours) resulted in large precipitates (large blocky carbides formed at the grain boundaries) and a thick oxide layer which decreased fatigue strength [45]. The optimization of the heat-treatment conditions for improving the mechanical properties remains a major challenge in SLM.

6.2. Surface Finishing

One significant challenge to the commercialization of 3D printed dental products is the variable surface finish, which can compromise the aesthetic, technical function and the achievable tolerances. The surface roughness of PBF products is dependent on the process parameters, the position and orientation to the building direction and the choice of the supports [18,28]. Traditional polishing methods (mechanical, ultrasonic, ion-beam, and chemical) have some limitations in processing PBF parts. Recent studies have focused on surface modification using lasers to satisfy strict surface requirements in medical applications. The surface quality of additive manufactured parts can be significantly improve by laser polishing [76,77]. Additionally, some studies show that the surface microstructure and corrosion resistance was improved by controlling the hexagonal close packed structures and the formed oxides [78].

The sterilization of medical products is a vital step before their clinical use. It can be managed by using irradiation (Gamma and E-beam), plasma and chemicals (peracetic acid). These methods are efficient but expensive. Dry heat and steam (autoclave) sterilization both proved to be efficient in the case of dental implants produced by SLM (even with a porous structure) [79].

7. Summary

Additive manufacturing processes have opened new possibilities, allowing the production of complex components, individually tailored to the patient. In dentistry, SLM is the most popular of all powder bed fusion technologies. Seemingly, this method seems to be less complicated than casting. However, the CAD–CAM specialist should have the knowledge to choose the right process parameters as well as post-processing methods. Without this ability, the resulting product may not be suitable for reliable use in practical applications.

The following conclusions can be drawn from the literature review:

1. PBF-manufactured parts are characterized by an anisotropic γ-phase (face-centered cubic (fcc)) and ε-phase (hexagonal close-packed (hcp)). The microstructure, roughness and properties of the samples depend on build orientation. Parts built at 0° were characterized by the worst mechanical properties.
2. Basic parameters, such as the laser power, scanning speed, laser beam size and layer thickness, are connected and they influence the density of the melted material. These parameters determine the material properties. In the SLM processes, energy input values above 0.36 J/s result in reduced sample density. The optimized range of laser energy density (LED) for $Co_{28}Cr_6Mo$ SLM parts is 150–200 J mm^{-3}.
3. Post-processing heat treatment is considered necessary to ensure the reliable use of PFB-built parts in practical applications. Heat-treatment up to 1050 °C (even for six hours) is insufficient to eliminate anisotropy and residual stress. As heat-treatment temperatures increase from 750 °C to 1050 °C, homogenization also increases, compared with the as-built samples. Heating samples at 1150 °C for one hour causes the total homogenization of the sample's microstructure.
4. Optimization of the heat-treatment conditions for improving the mechanical properties (especially fatigue properties) remains a major challenge in SLM.
5. Surface finishing of PFB-built parts is necessary.

Author Contributions: B.K.—investigation, conceptualization, writing—original draft, writing—review and editing, A.S.-W.—investigation, writing—review and editing, J.S.—conceptualization, resources, supervision, K.B.—writing—review and editing, project administration, supervision. All authors have read and agreed to the published version of the manuscript.

Funding: This research received no external funding.

Conflicts of Interest: The authors declare no conflict of interest.

References

1. Myszka, D.; Skrodzki, M. Comparison of Dental Prostheses Cast and Sintered by SLM from Co-Cr-Mo-W Alloy. *Arch. Foundry Eng.* **2016**, *16*, 201–207. [CrossRef]
2. Craig, R.G. *Materiały Stomatologiczne*, 12th ed.; Powers, J.M., Sakaguchi, R.L., Shaw, H., Shaw, J.G., Eds.; Edra Urban and Partner: Wrocław, Poland, 2008; ISBN 9780323081085.
3. Anusavice, K.; Shen, C.; Rawls, H.R. *Phillips' Science of Dental Materials*, 12th ed.; Saunders: St. Louis, MO, USA, 2012.
4. Antanasova, M.; Kocjan, A.; Kovač, J.; Žužek, B.; Jevnikar, P. Influence of thermo-mechanical cycling on porcelain bonding to cobalt–chromium and titanium dental alloys fabricated by casting, milling, and selective laser melting. *J. Prosthodont. Res.* **2018**, *62*, 184–194. [CrossRef]
5. Reclaru, L.; Ardelean, L.C. *Current Alternatives for Processing CoCr Dental Alloys Lucien*; Elsevier Inc.: Cambridge, MA, USA, 2018; Volume 1–3, ISBN 9780128051443.
6. Ferraiuoli, P.; Taylor, J.C.; Martin, E.; Fenner, J.W.; Narracott, A.J. The accuracy of 3D optical reconstruction and additive manufacturing processes in reproducing detailed subject-specific anatomy. *J. Imaging* **2017**, *3*, 45. [CrossRef]
7. Hasan, H.A.; Alam, M.K.; Yusof, A.; Matsuda, S.; Shoumura, M.; Osuga, N. Accuracy of three dimensional CT craniofacial measurements using mimics and InVesalius software programs. *J. Hard Tissue Biol.* **2016**, *25*, 219–224. [CrossRef]
8. Haleem, A.; Javaid, M. 3D scanning applications in medical field: A literature-based review. *Clin. Epidemiol. Glob. Health* **2019**, *7*, 199–210. [CrossRef]
9. Javaid, M.; Haleem, A.; Kumar, L. Current status and applications of 3D scanning in dentistry. *Clin. Epidemiol. Glob. Health* **2019**, *7*, 228–233. [CrossRef]
10. Strub, J.R.; Rekow, E.D.; Witkowski, S. Computer-aided design and fabrication of dental restorations: Current systems and future possibilities. *J. Am. Dent. Assoc.* **2006**, *137*, 1289–1296. [CrossRef]
11. Sahasrabudhe, H.; Bose, S.; Bandyopadhyay, A. Laser-Based Additive Manufacturing Processes. In *Advances in Laser Materials Processing*; Lawrence, J., Ed.; Woodhead Publishing: Coventry, UK, 2018; pp. 507–539. ISBN 9780081012529.
12. Han, X.; Sawada, T.; Schille, C.; Schweizer, E.; Scheideler, L.; Geis-Gerstorfer, J.; Rupp, F.; Spintzyk, S. Comparative analysis of mechanical properties and metal-ceramic bond strength of Co-Cr dental alloy fabricated by different manufacturing processes. *Materials (Basel)* **2018**, *11*, 1801. [CrossRef]
13. Egea, A.J.S.; Martynenko, V.; Krahmer, D.M.; de Lacalle, L.N.L.; Benítez, A.; Genovese, G. On the cutting performance of segmented diamond blades when dry-cutting concrete. *Materials (Basel)* **2018**, *11*, 264. [CrossRef]
14. Chhaya, M.P.; Poh, P.S.P.; Balmayor, E.R.; Van Griensven, M.; Schantz, J.T.; Hutmacher, D.W. Additive manufacturing in biomedical sciences and the need for definitions and norms. *Expert Rev. Med. Devices* **2015**, *12*, 537–543. [CrossRef]
15. Singh, A.V.; Dad Ansari, M.H.; Wang, S.; Laux, P.; Luch, A.; Kumar, A.; Patil, R.; Nussberger, S. The adoption of three-dimensional additive manufacturing from biomedical material design to 3D organ printing. *Appl. Sci.* **2019**, *9*, 811. [CrossRef]
16. Dobrzański, L.A.; Dobrzański, L.B. Dentistry 4.0 concept in the design and manufacturing of prosthetic dental restorations. *Processes* **2020**, *8*, 525. [CrossRef]
17. Ngo, T.D.; Kashani, A.; Imbalzano, G.; Nguyen, K.T.Q.; Hui, D. Additive manufacturing (3D printing): A review of materials, methods, applications and challenges. *Compos. Part B Eng.* **2018**, *143*, 172–196. [CrossRef]

18. Dikova, T. Properties of Co-Cr Dental Alloys Fabricated Using Additive Technologies. In *Biomaterials in Regenerative Medicine*; Dobrzański, L.A., Ed.; IntechOpen: London, UK, 2018; pp. 141–159.
19. Revilla-León, M.; Özcan, M. Additive Manufacturing Technologies Used for 3D Metal Printing in Dentistry. *Curr. Oral Health Rep.* **2017**, *4*, 201–208. [CrossRef]
20. Oliveira, T.T.; Reis, A.C. Fabrication of dental implants by the additive manufacturing method: A systematic review. *J. Prosthet. Dent.* **2019**, *122*, 270–274. [CrossRef]
21. Okazaki, Y.; Ishino, A.; Higuchi, S. Chemical, physical, and mechanical properties and microstructures of laser-sintered Co-25Cr-5Mo-5W (SP2) and W-Free Co-28Cr-6Mo alloys for dental applications. *Materials (Basel)* **2019**, *12*, 4039. [CrossRef]
22. Gabor, A.-G.; Zaharia, C.; Stan, A.T.; Gavrilovici, A.M.; Negruțiu, M.-L.; Sinescu, C. Digital Dentistry—Digital Impression and CAD/CAM System Applications. *J. Interdiscip. Med.* **2017**, *2*, 54–57. [CrossRef]
23. Revilla-León, M.; Klemm, I.M.; García-Arranz, J.; Özcan, M. 3D Metal Printing–Additive Manufacturing Technologies for Frameworks of Implant- Borne Fixed Dental Prosthesis. *Eur. J. Prosthodont. Restor. Dent.* **2017**, *25*, 143–147. [CrossRef]
24. Beaman, J.J.; Deckard, C.R. Selective Laser Sinterng with Assisted Powder Handlng. U.S. Patent 4,938,816, 3 July 1990.
25. Höganäs, A.B. Höganäs Handbook for Sintered Components. Available online: https://www.hoganas.com/globalassets/download-media/sharepoint/handbooks---all-documents/handbook-2_production_of_sintered_components_december_2013_0675hog_interactive.pdf. (accessed on 20 June 2020).
26. Anestiev, L.A.; Froyen, L. Model of the primary rearrangement processes at liquid phase sintering and selective laser sintering due to biparticle interactions. *J. Appl. Phys.* **1999**, *86*, 4008–4017. [CrossRef]
27. Alageel, O.; Wazirian, B.; Almufleh, B.; Tamimi, F. Fabrication of Dental Restorations Using Digital Technologies: Techniques and Materials. In *Digital Restorative Dentistry: A Guide to Materials, Equipment, and Clinical Procedures*; Tamimi, F., Hirayama, H., Eds.; Springer: Cham, Switzerland, 2019; pp. 55–91.
28. Vandenbroucke, B.; Kruth, J.P. Selective laser melting of biocompatible metals for rapid manufacturing of medical parts. *Rapid Prototyp. J.* **2007**, *13*, 196–203. [CrossRef]
29. Yap, C.Y.; Chua, C.K.; Dong, Z.L.; Liu, Z.H.; Zhang, D.Q.; Loh, L.E.; Sing, S.L. Review of selective laser melting: Materials and applications. *Appl. Phys. Rev.* **2015**, *2*, 1–21. [CrossRef]
30. Murr, L.E.; Gaytan, S.M.; Ramirez, D.A.; Martinez, E.; Hernandez, J.; Amato, K.N.; Shindo, P.W.; Medina, F.R.; Wicker, R.B. Metal Fabrication by Additive Manufacturing Using Laser and Electron Beam Melting Technologies. *J. Mater. Sci. Technol.* **2012**, *28*, 1–14. [CrossRef]
31. Singh, R.; Singh, S.; Hashmi, M.S.J. *Implant Materials and Their Processing Technologies*; Elsevier Ltd.: Amsterdam, The Netherlands, 2016; ISBN 9780128035818.
32. Wang, J.; Ren, J.; Liu, W.; Wu, X.; Gao, M.; Bai, P. Effect of Selective Laser Melting Process Parameters on Microstructure and Properties of Co-Cr Alloy. *Materials (Basel)* **2018**, *11*, 1546. [CrossRef] [PubMed]
33. Szczurek, A. Struktura i własności stopów dentystycznych na bazie kobaltu stosowanych do wykonywania protez szkieletowych. *Inżynieria Mater.* **2013**, *XXXIV*, 116–120.
34. Mróz, A.; Jakubowicz, J.; Gierzyńska-dolna, M.; Wiśniewski, T.; Wendland, J. Wpływ technologii wytwarzania wyrobów ze stopu Co28Cr6Mo na ich właściwości fizyczne, mechaniczne i odporność korozyjną. *Inżynieria Mater.* **2015**, *1*, 2–8. [CrossRef]
35. Fatemi, A.; Molaei, R.; Fatemi, A. Fatigue Design with Additive Manufactured Metals: Issues to Consider and Perspective for Future Research. *Procedia Eng.* **2018**, *213*, 5–16. [CrossRef]
36. Kok, Y.; Tan, X.P.; Wang, P.; Nai, M.L.S.; Loh, N.H.; Liu, E.; Tor, S.B. Anisotropy and heterogeneity of microstructure and mechanical properties in metal additive manufacturing: A critical review. *Mater. Des.* **2017**, *139*, 565–586. [CrossRef]
37. Kajima, Y.; Takaichi, A.; Nakamoto, T.; Kimura, T.; Kittikundecha, N.; Tsutsumi, Y.; Nomura, N.; Kawasaki, A.; Takahashi, H.; Hanawa, T.; et al. Effect of adding support structures for overhanging part on fatigue strength in selective laser melting. *J. Mech. Behav. Biomed. Mater.* **2018**, *78*, 1–9. [CrossRef]
38. Harun, W.; Sharuzi, W.; Kadirgama, K.; Samykano, M.; Ramasamy, D.; Ahmad, I.; Moradi, M. Mechanical behavior of selective laser melting-produced metallic biomaterials. In *Mechanical Behavior of Biomaterials*; Davim, J.P., Ed.; Woodhead Publishing: Cambridge, UK, 2019; pp. 101–116. ISBN 9780081021743.

39. Shifeng, W.; Shuai, L.; Qingsong, W.; Yan, C.; Sheng, Z.; Yusheng, S. Effect of molten pool boundaries on the mechanical properties of selective laser melting parts. *J. Mater. Process. Technol.* **2014**, *214*, 2660–2667. [CrossRef]
40. Hanzl, P.; Zetek, M.; Bakša, T.; Kroupa, T. The influence of processing parameters on the mechanical properties of SLM parts. *Procedia Eng.* **2015**, *100*, 1405–1413. [CrossRef]
41. Takaichi, A.; Suyalatu; Nakamoto, T.; Joko, N.; Nomura, N.; Tsutsumi, Y.; Migita, S.; Doi, H.; Kurosu, S.; Chiba, A.; et al. Microstructures and mechanical properties of Co-29Cr-6Mo alloy fabricated by selective laser melting process for dental applications. *J. Mech. Behav. Biomed. Mater.* **2013**, *21*, 67–76. [CrossRef] [PubMed]
42. Sun, S.H.; Koizumi, Y.; Kurosu, S.; Li, Y.P.; Matsumoto, H.; Chiba, A. Build direction dependence of microstructure and high-temperature tensile property of Co-Cr-Mo alloy fabricated by electron beam melting. *Acta Mater.* **2014**, *64*, 154–168. [CrossRef]
43. Kajima, Y.; Takaichi, A.; Nakamoto, T.; Kimura, T.; Yogo, Y.; Ashida, M.; Doi, H.; Nomura, N.; Takahashi, H.; Hanawa, T.; et al. Fatigue strength of Co-Cr-Mo alloy clasps prepared by selective laser melting. *J. Mech. Behav. Biomed. Mater.* **2016**, *59*, 446–458. [CrossRef] [PubMed]
44. Øilo, M.; Nesse, H.; Lundberg, O.J.; Gjerdet, N.R. Mechanical properties of cobalt-chromium 3-unit fi xed dental prostheses fabricated by casting, milling, and additive manufacturing. *J. Prosthet. Dent.* **2015**, *120*, 1–7. [CrossRef]
45. Kittikundecha, N.; Kajima, Y.; Takaichi, A.; Htoot, H.; Cho, W. Fatigue properties of removable partial denture clasps fabricated by selective laser melting followed by heat treatment. *J. Mech. Behav. Biomed. Mater.* **2019**, *98*, 79–89. [CrossRef] [PubMed]
46. Frazier, W.E. Metal Additive Manufacturing: A Review. *J. Mater. Eng. Perform.* **2014**, *23*, 1917–1928. [CrossRef]
47. Averyanova, M.; Bertrand, P.; Verquin, B. Manufacture of Co-Cr dental crowns and bridges by selective laser Melting technology: This paper presents the successful application of the selective laser melting technology in dental frameworks manufacturing from Co-Cr alloy using Phenix PM 100T dental. *Virtual Phys. Prototyp.* **2011**, *6*, 179–185. [CrossRef]
48. Gu, D.; Shi, Q.; Lin, K.; Xi, L. Microstructure and performance evolution and underlying thermal mechanisms of Ni-based parts fabricated by selective laser melting. *Addit. Manuf.* **2018**, *22*, 265–278. [CrossRef]
49. Song, C.; Yang, Y.; Wang, Y.; Wang, D.; Yu, J. Research on rapid manufacturing of Co-Cr-Mo alloy femoral component based on selective laser melting. *Int. J. Adv. Manuf. Technol.* **2014**, *75*, 445–453. [CrossRef]
50. Lu, Y.; Wu, S.; Gan, Y.; Li, J.; Zhao, C.; Zhuo, D.; Lin, J. Investigation on the microstructure, mechanical property and corrosion behavior of the selective laser melted Co-Cr-W alloy for dental application. *Mater. Sci. Eng. C* **2015**, *49*, 517–525. [CrossRef]
51. Tonelli, L.; Fortunato, A.; Ceschini, L. Co-Cr alloy processed by Selective Laser Melting (SLM): Effect of Laser Energy Density on microstructure, surface morphology, and hardness. *J. Manuf. Process.* **2020**, *52*, 106–119. [CrossRef]
52. Popovich, V.A.; Borisov, E.V.; Popovich, A.A.; Su, V.S.; Masaylo, D.V.; Alzina, L. Functionally graded Inconel 718 processed by additive manufacturing: Crystallographic texture, anisotropy of microstructure and mechanical properties. *Mater. Des.* **2016**, *114*, 441–449. [CrossRef]
53. Xie, W.; Zheng, M.; Wang, J.; Li, X. The effect of build orientation on the microstructure and properties of selective laser melting Ti-6Al-4V for removable partial denture clasps. *J. Prosthet. Dent.* **2020**, *123*, 163–172. [CrossRef] [PubMed]
54. Ishida, B.K.; NIshizawa, T. The Co-Cr (Cobalt-Chromium) System. *Bull. Alloy Phase Diagrams* **1990**, *11*, 357–370. [CrossRef]
55. Yan, X.; Lin, H.; Wu, Y.; Bai, W. Effect of two heat treatments on mechanical properties of selective-laser-melted Co-Cr metal-ceramic alloys for application in thin removable partial dentures. *J. Prosthet. Dent.* **2018**, *119*, 1028.e1–1028.e6. [CrossRef] [PubMed]
56. Instructions for Use EOS CobaltChrome SP2. Available online: http://webcache.googleusercontent.com/search?q=cache:ltA3cJm7RRAJ:ip-saas-eos-cms.s3.amazonaws.com/public/32ff6c9b7964c1c9/7c73a9305d8007c47dec2e65196f09e5/EOS_CobaltChrome_SP2_en.pdf+&cd=1&hl=pl&ct=clnk&gl=pl&lr=lang_en%7Clang_pl&client=firefox-b-d (accessed on 6 May 2020).

57. Material Data Sheet EOS CobaltChrome MP1. Available online: https://webcache.googleusercontent.com/search?q=cache:FU463ZFb7_cJ:https://ip-saas-eos-cms.s3.amazonaws.com/public/4b839242298b3d77/721463526ca053889c9784ec989f3c88/EOS_CobaltChrome_MP1_en.pdf+&cd=1&hl=pl&ct=clnk&gl=pl&lr=lang_en%7Clang_pl&client=firefox- (accessed on 6 May 2020).
58. Instructions for Use Renishaw Co-Cr DG1. Available online: http://webcache.googleusercontent.com/search?q=cache:_eQiV5qm-rMJ:resources.renishaw.com/en/download/instructions-for-use-cocr-dg1--96951+&cd=1&hl=pl&ct=clnk&gl=pl&lr=lang_en%7Clang_pl&client=firefox-b-d (accessed on 6 May 2020).
59. Béreš, M.; Silva, C.C.; Sarvezuk, P.W.C.; Wu, L.; Antunes, L.H.M.; Jardini, A.L.; Feitosa, A.L.M.; Žilková, J.; de Abreu, H.F.G.; Filho, R.M. Mechanical and phase transformation behaviour of biomedical Co-Cr-Mo alloy fabricated by direct metal laser sintering. *Mater. Sci. Eng. A* **2018**, *714*, 36–42. [CrossRef]
60. Takaichi, A.; Kajima, Y.; Kittikundecha, N.; Linn, H.; Htoot, H.; Cho, W.; Hanawa, T.; Yoneyama, T.; Wakabayashi, N. Effect of heat treatment on the anisotropic microstructural and mechanical properties of Co-Cr-Mo alloys produced by selective laser melting. *J. Mech. Behav. Biomed. Mater.* **2020**, *102*, 103496. [CrossRef]
61. Kajima, Y.; Takaichi, A.; Kittikundecha, N.; Nakamoto, T.; Kimura, T.; Nomura, N.; Kawasaki, A.; Hanawa, T.; Takahash, H.; Wakabayashi, N. Effect of heat-treatment temperature on microstructures and mechanical properties of Co-Cr-Mo alloys fabricated by selective laser melting. *Mater. Sci. Eng. A* **2018**, *726*, 21–31. [CrossRef]
62. Sing, S.L.; Huang, S.; Yeong, W.Y. Effect of solution heat treatment on microstructure and mechanical properties of laser powder bed fusion produced cobalt-28chromium-6molybdenum. *Mater. Sci. Eng. A* **2020**, *769*, 138511. [CrossRef]
63. Seki, E.; Kajima, Y.; Takaichi, A.; Kittikundecha, N.; Htoot, H.; Cho, W.; Linn, H.; Doi, H.; Hanawa, T.; Wakabayashi, N. Effect of heat treatment on the microstructure and fatigue strength of Co-Cr-Mo alloys fabricated by selective laser melting. *Mater. Lett.* **2019**, *245*, 53–56. [CrossRef]
64. Doherty, R.D.; Hughes, D.A.; Humphreys, F.J.; Jonas, J.J.; Juul Jensen, D.; Kassner, M.E.; King, W.E.; McNelley, T.R.; McQueen, H.J.; Rollett, A.D. Current issues in recrystallization: A review. *Mater. Sci. Eng. A* **1997**, *238*, 219–274. [CrossRef]
65. Liu, F.; Lin, X.; Yang, G.; Song, M.; Chen, J.; Huang, W. Microstructure and residual stress of laser rapid formed Inconel 718 nickel-base superalloy. *Opt. Laser Technol.* **2011**, *43*, 208–213. [CrossRef]
66. Song, B.; Dong, S.; Liu, Q.; Liao, H.; Coddet, C. Vacuum heat treatment of iron parts produced by selective laser melting: Microstructure, residual stress and tensile behavior. *Mater. Des.* **2014**, *54*, 727–733. [CrossRef]
67. Bedolla-Gil, Y.; Hernandez-Rodriguez, M.A.L. Tribological Behavior of a Heat-Treated Cobalt-Based Alloy. *J. Mater. Eng. Perform.* **2013**, *22*, 541–547. [CrossRef]
68. Montero-Ocampo, C.; Talavera, M.; Lopez, H. Effect of Alloy Preheating on the Mechanical Properties of As-Cast Co-Cr-Mo-C Alloys. *Metall. Mater. Trans. A* **1999**, *30*, 611–620. [CrossRef]
69. Bhaduri, A. Creep and Stress Repture. In *Mechanical Properties and Working of Metals and Alloys*; Springer: Singapore, 2018; pp. 257–314.
70. Mancha, H.; Carranza, E.; Escalante, J.I.; Mendoza, G.; Mendez, M.; Cepeda, F.; Valdes, E. M 23 C 6 Carbide Dissolution Mechanisms during Heat Treatment of ASTM F-75 Implant Alloys. *Metall. Mater. Trans. A* **2001**, *32A*, 979. [CrossRef]
71. Ramírez-Vidaurri, L.E.; Castro-Román, M.; Herrera-Trejo, M.; García-López, C.V.; Almanza-Casas, E. Cooling rate and carbon content effect on the fraction of secondary phases precipitate in as-cast microstructure of ASTM F75 alloy. *J. Mater. Process. Technol.* **2009**, *209*, 1681–1687. [CrossRef]
72. Hassani, F.Z.; Ketabchi, M.; Bruschi, S.; Ghiotti, A. Effects of carbide precipitation on the microstructural and tribological properties of Co-Cr-Mo-C medical implants after thermal treatment. *J. Mater. Sci.* **2016**, *51*, 4495–4508. [CrossRef]
73. Alvarez-Vera, M.; Hernandez-Rodriguez, A.; Hernandez-Rodriguez, M.A.L.; Juárez Hernández, A.; Benavides-Treviño, J.R.; García-Duarte, J. Effect of cooling rate during solidification on the hard phases of M23C6-type of cast Co-Cr-Mo alloy. *Metalurgija* **2016**, *55*, 382–384.
74. Guoqing, Z.; Junxin, L.; Xiaoyu, Z.; Jin, L.; Anmin, W. Effect of Heat Treatment on the Properties of Co-Cr-Mo Alloy Manufactured by Selective Laser Melting. *J. Mater. Eng. Perform.* **2018**, *27*, 2281–2287. [CrossRef]

75. Lu, Y.; Wu, S.; Gan, Y.; Zhang, S.; Guo, S.; Lin, J.; Lin, J. Microstructure, mechanical property and metal release of As-SLM Co-Cr-W alloy under different solution treatment conditions. *J. Mech. Behav. Biomed. Mater.* **2016**, *55*, 179–190. [CrossRef] [PubMed]
76. Yung, K.C.; Wang, W.J.; Xiao, T.Y.; Choy, H.S.; Mo, X.Y.; Cai, Z.X.; Wang, W.J.; Xiao, T.Y.; Choy, H.S.; Mo, X.Y.; et al. Laser polishing of additive manufactured Co-Cr components for controlling their wettability characteristics. *Surf. Coat. Technol.* **2018**, *351*, 89–98. [CrossRef]
77. Yung, K.C.; Xiao, T.Y.; Choy, H.S.; Wang, W.J.; Cai, Z.X. Laser polishing of additive manufactured Co-Cr alloy components with complex surface geometry. *J. Mater. Process. Technol.* **2018**, *262*, 53–64. [CrossRef]
78. Wang, W.J.; Yung, K.C.; Choy, H.S.; Xiao, T.Y.; Cai, Z.X. Effects of laser polishing on surface microstructure and corrosion resistance of additive manufactured Co-Cr alloys. *Appl. Surf. Sci.* **2018**, *443*, 167–175. [CrossRef]
79. Manea, A.; Bran, S.; Baciut, M.; Armencea, G.; Pop, D.; Berce, P.; Vodnar, D.-C.; Hedesiu, M.; Dinu, C.; Petrutiu, A.; et al. Sterilization protocol for porous dental implants made by Selective Laser Melting. *Dent. Med.* **2018**, *91*, 452–457. [CrossRef] [PubMed]

MDPI AG
Grosspeteranlage 5
4052 Basel
Switzerland
Tel.: +41 61 683 77 34

Materials Editorial Office
E-mail: materials@mdpi.com
www.mdpi.com/journal/materials

www.ingramcontent.com/pod-product-compliance
Lightning Source LLC
Chambersburg PA
CBHW061600210926
51850CB00009B/2161
* 9 7 8 3 7 2 5 8 7 8 4 3 7 *